DIRECTIONS IN COMMUNITY HEALTH NURSING

DIRECTIONS IN COMMUNITY HEALTH NURSING

Edited by
Judith Ann Sullivan, R.N., Ed.D. F.A.A.N.

Professor and Head,
Department of Public Health Nursing,
Professor of Public Health,
University of Illinois at Chicago

BLACKWELL SCIENTIFIC PUBLICATIONS, INC.
Boston Oxford London Edinburgh Melbourne

Library of Congress Cataloging in Publications Data
Main entry under title:

Directions in community health nursing.

  Includes index.
  1. Community health nursing.   I. Sullivan, Judith
Ann, 1938–   . [DNLM: 1. Community health nursing.
2. Community health nursing—Trends. WY 106 D598]
RT98.D56   1984   610.73'43   83-21445
ISBN 0-86542-004-1

1 2 3 4 5 6 7 8 9

Blackwell Scientific Publications
Editorial offices at:
52 Beacon Street, Boston, MA, 02108 USA
Osney Mead, Oxford OX2 0EL, England
8 John Street, London WC1N 2 ES, England
9 Forrest Road, Edinburgh EH1 2QH, Scotland
99 Barry Street, Carlton, Victoria 3053, Australia

Distributors

USA
      Blackwell Mosby Book Distributors
      11830 Westline Industrial Drive
      St. Louis, Missouri 63146

Canada
      Blackwell Mosby Book Distributors
      120 Melford Drive
      Scarborough, Ontario, M1B 2X4

Australia
      Blackwell Scientific Book Distributors, Pty., Ltd.
      31 Advantage Road
      Highett, Victoria 3190

Outside North America and Australia
      Blackwell Scientific Publications Ltd.
      Osney Mead
      Oxford OX2 0EL
      England

This book is dedicated to each of its authors.

Each one has taken a highly complex area within their expertise and painstakingly formulated conceptual and operational approaches necessary for effective practice in the community. These approaches then become the basis for determining the direction of community health nursing practice and research.

Despite their many personal achievements and stresses throughout the five years of drafting (and redrafting) these chapters, they each have succeeded in producing a well-spring of ideas that will serve well in the coming years.

JAS

CONTENTS

CONTRIBUTORS

Cheryl Lorane Cox, R.N., Ph.D.
Assistant Professor of Nursing
Department of Public Health Nursing
University of Illinois at Chicago

Christy Z. Dachelet, M.S.
Coordinator of Corporate Planning
Methodist Hospital
Minneapolis, Minnesota

Christine DeGregorio, M.S.P.
Political Science Department
College of Arts and Sciences
University of Rochester
Rochester, New York

Maureen M. Friedman, R.N., M.S.
Instructor of Community Health Nursing
School of Nursing
University of Rochester
Rochester, New York

Barbara E. Hanley, R.N., Ph.D.
Assistant Professor of Nursing
Coordinator for Legislative Affairs
Career Development, Nursing-Health Policy Program
University of Maryland School of Nursing
Baltimore, Maryland

Ruth A. O'Brien, R.N., Ph.D.
Chairperson and Clinical Chief of Community Health Nursing
School of Nursing
University of Rochester
Rochester, New York

Ann Gustafson Robinson, R.N., M.S.
Director of Patient Services
Genesee Region Home Care Association
Rochester, New York

Diane J. Walgren, R.N., M.S.
Assistant Administrator
Boone County Health Department
Madison, West Virginia

Judith S. Warner, M.S.
Adjunct Assistant Professor in Economics
Department of Economics
St. John Fisher College
Rochester, New York

Nancy M. Watson, R.N., M.S.
Senior Associate in Nursing and
Research Associate
School of Nursing
University of Rochester
Rochester, New York

Thomas R. Zastowny, Ph.D.
Department of Psychiatry
University of Rochester
Rochester, New York

PREFACE

This book is one of the most challenging to write. It defines practice via its conceptual roots and then describes these concepts as they have evolved in current practice. The ideas presented by the authors are intended as a guide, not a recipe, for the continual improvement of community health nursing. Toward this end, the topics are covered in sufficient depth to provide the needed direction for the development of a practice that can be very hectic at times.

This book is directed primarily to those with responsibility for leadership in community health nursing: faculty, administrators, practicing clinicians and specialists, and graduate students preparing for these roles. While many professional and lay health care workers and workers in other sectors such as business, agriculture, and politics will be involved in health care planning and delivery, community health nurses are in a key position to provide a direct link between the planners and the patients. Community health nurses have been prepared to identify those persons at high risk of losing health and to initiate and deliver on-site measures of primary, secondary, and tertiary prevention to reduce risk, maintain health, treat minor illness, and care for the chronically ill. This book presents basic information upon which applications in the sub-specialty areas of community health nursing are built.

Part I presents a conceptual approach to the definition of key components that describe the nature and direct the future of this field of practice within the context of its history. It also presents clinical approaches to the three levels of clients for which the community health nurse has responsibility: the individual, the family, and the community.

Part II provides a pointer toward clinical research in this area and recommendations for methods that should be used in investigations, whether from an academic or clinical base. Part III describes basic material on the strategies of power, politics, and economics to use in advancing this field of practice.

Leaders in every area of community health nursing — home health care, primary care, preventive services, and occupational and school health — will find the material in this book applicable to their settings. In addition, this book will prove helpful to deans in nursing and allied health areas where nursing is included, non-nurse administrators, and other policy makers who must set the conditions in which community health nursing can flourish.

Many new applications for the role of the community health nurse have evolved, keeping pace with national priorities. At a time when resources must be distributed more carefully than ever, community health nursing stands out as a versatile, prevention-oriented, and service delivery profession that is well worth the public trust and financial investment.

As editor, I would like to acknowledge the support of specific individuals who assisted in the completion of this book. They include: Judith A. Warner, who gave major assistance in organizing the early phases and continuing help in establishing the integrity of Section III; the faculty and students in community health nursing at the University of Rochester who believed in the purpose and need for this project; my colleagues in clinical agencies who have tested out many of the ideas as they were under development; those colleagues who have provided me with personal experiences and artifacts from the early periods of public health nursing that validate the historical accounts in tangible terms; and the publishers who have given their guidance and patience during the long gestation period of this book.

Producing this book has been for me like planning a symphony and then conducting the orchestra that performs it. While each author speaks for him- or herself, I take the responsibility for the content emphases, level of complexity, and the follow-through of logic from chapter to chapter.

COMMUNITY HEALTH NURSING PRACTICE

Scholars of nursing practice will especially appreciate this section. Chapters 1 and 2 address the development over time of concepts generic to community health nursing and the construction of conceptual frameworks reflecting current-day practice experience.

Chapters 3, 4, and 5 were written by clinician-scholars in active practice. These three chapters include conceptual frameworks that directed the selection of relevant theory, processes, and content explicated at the community, family, and individual levels. Each chapter serves an important role in pointing the direction for further development needed in each of these three basic clinical levels. Moreover, these chapters present the key concepts for implementation in current-day expert clinical practice.

The terms visiting nurse, public health nurse, and community health nurse have all been used at some time to refer to the practice described in this book. Unless a specific point is made of distinctions in the title used, the terms are intended to be used interchangeably.

HISTORY OF NURSING IN THE COMMUNITY: FROM THE BEGINNING

1

Judith A. Sullivan and Maureen Friedman

Community health nursing as a formalized profession in America is only one hundred years old. Its youth as a profession, however, belies the age of its roots, which can be traced back to the ancient Greeks and Romans and to indications of community health nursing practice that have appeared regularly throughout recorded Western history. Before organized community health nursing began in England in 1859, assisting individuals, families, and groups to maintain and improve health and to care for their own ill members was a role at various times assumed by Roman Catholic brothers, both Catholic and Protestant sisters, and wealthy men and women who volunteered their services as charity. Other religious groups as well provided for the visiting of the ill to render care, although their work is not as well documented. The earliest forms of community health nursing practice are attributed to these philanthropic groups and individuals.

Among the earliest legendary ancestors of this profession is Hygeia, the Greek guardian of health. According to Rene Dubos (1971) in his commentary on health and health care over the centuries, the concept of Hygeia originated before the sixth century B.C. Her position was not as a nurse of the sick, but rather as a reminder of the importance of discovering and teaching the natural laws that would ensure a healthy mind and body. She symbolized the belief that living by reason and the natural laws is the basis of health. Health, in turn, was believed to be a positive attribute to which people were entitled if they governed their lives wisely.

Two sisters of Hygeia, Meditrina, the preserver of health, and Iaso, the personification of recovery from illness, represented other aspects of the role later assumed by the community health nurse. Other members of Hygeia's family had related functions: Asclepius, her father, was responsible for mastering the use of the knife and the curative uses of plants — talents later developed further by her two brothers, Machaon and Podalirius. Panacea, Hygeia's sister, provided the knowledge of drugs, either from the earth or from plants, and Epione, Hygeia's mother, symbolized a soothing force (Dubos 1971).

3

Around the fifth or sixth century B.C., Hygeia was relegated to the status of a member of Asclepius's retinue, to be summoned after he had performed his acts of healing. This clear-cut change in role definition between the two gods parallels the Greeks' recognition that maximal receptivity to the teaching of Hygeia often occurred after some threat to health. Later, this same phenomenon was to be manifested in the initiation of health services: first an epidemic occurred, necessitating healing efforts and illness care; this phase was often followed by teaching patients and families about hygienic principles and rules of health.

Specific programs for applying these natural laws to improve health were not described in Western literature except as they were combined with care of the sick in their homes by early religious men and women. Among those who functioned in community settings were the first deaconesses, Tabatha and Phoebe (around A.D. 58), and the Parabolani brotherhood (third century) (Dolan 1978). The early deaconesses perceived the importance of providing for the needy. They visited those in prison, the poor, the sick, and the homeless and brought food, medicines, dressing materials, and compassion. The Parabolani brotherhood was organized during the great plague in Alexandria in the last half of the third century. These men were described as district visitors who cared for and comforted the sick and dying and cleaned infected houses.

Paula, a learned Roman matron of noble birth in the fourth century, converted to Christianity and taught other Christian women to develop their minds through reading and study while increasing their skills in the care of the sick at home. In the thirteenth century, St. Francis of Assisi introduced a new level of intervention. By presenting the plight of the leper population to the community, he took the first steps toward organizing community action in addressing the major health problems of the time (Dolan 1978).

The combination of teaching and care of the sick at home and the mobilization of community groups facing the health concerns of the society were functions clearly established before the seventeenth century as areas of service needed in a community. These functions had been parts of roles of a number of different persons, however. Their combination in one role serves as the conceptual link between the practice of community health nursing by the "pre-professionalized" workers and those later credentialed and employed to provide these services on an ongoing basis.

In early America, recorded evidence shows that concern for general public health measures was part of the Colonial philosophy, and care of the sick at home was one of the voluntary activities undertaken among the earliest settlers. William Bradford, later to be the first governor of Massachusetts, recorded in 1643 his observations on the conditions harmful to the health of the colonists in his account of the Plymouth Plantation, ". . . for it is found in experience that chaing of aeir, famine, or unwholsome foode, much drinking of water, sorrows & troubles &c., all of them are enemies to health, causes of many diseaces, consumers of naturall vigoure and the bodys of men, and shortners of life" (Wish 1962). He concluded that given these hardships it was amazing how many settlers still lived to an old age.

Bradford also described the response of the English settlers to caring for the sick among the Indian tribes, which were nearly decimated by smallpox. He said the settlers ". . . daily fetched them wood and water, and made them fires, got them victualls whilst they lived, and buried them when they dyed" (Wish 1962). Although unaware that they themselves had undoubtedly brought infection to the Indians, the colonists essentially mobilized a community home health aid and hospice service for their stricken neighbors. Community-initiated mutual aid including the delivery of nursing services to the sick at home, continued as the style of implementing public health measures throughout the Colonial period.

Within 35 years after the U.S. Constitution was signed, however, a formalized voluntary service of visiting nurses was begun by the Ladies' Benevolent Society of Charleston, South Carolina. They provided limited nursing care and food for the sick poor during acute phases of illness, especially during epidemics such as yellow fever. During the seventeenth and eighteenth centuries in Europe, the same forces — social reform and the presence of an epidemic (this time, cholera) — brought forth the need for a community-based nursing service for the home bound sick. The service was still offered, however, on a voluntary basis, by both Catholic and Protestant religious orders, organized specifically to provide nursing care for the sick and deprived in the neighborhood (Fitzpatrick 1975).

Summary

The conditions that sparked and sustained community nursing practice in the early Western world are notable. In Greek mythology, each member of Epione and Asclepius's family — and Hygeia in particular — had a role to play in the maintenance of health and the resolution of health problems through the primary, secondary, and tertiary stages. Undoubtedly, actual practice saw servants and slaves pressed into service for care of the ill during normal times. Household leaders (lords and ladies or workingmen and wives) made the decisions about the extent to which health practices were part of the daily routine, while broader programs were needed when epidemics hit.

Subsequently, organized activities by church-related groups were mobilized periodically to provide home health services during these crisis periods. After the epidemics had passed, many of these organizations followed through by providing teaching on hygienic principles and, in at least one case, raising community awareness of (and perhaps action in response to) the problems of a specific vulnerable group.

From the times of the earliest providers, then, education beyond the care of the ill has proved necessary for effective work in community health. Not entirely coincidentally, preventive concepts and social reform were brought forward by the more educated health workers. The epidemics proved to be vehicles for focusing attention on health; few survivors could deny the value of preventing another outbreak if the means were available. This unique combination of events, repeated many times over the early centuries, called for the provision of services that later became institutionalized as community health nursing. Since that time, many applications of the "family care/health education/community action" sequence have been developed. These applications, as they were introduced over the last century, are discussed in the next section.

1880–1900

In the United States institutionalized community health nursing began in the early 1880s. Although only one century had elapsed since the Constitution was ratified, the Industrial Revolution had taken place, bringing with it a surge toward employment in the cities. Between the late 1880s and the early 1900s a period of massive immigration and rapid industrialization brought with it overcrowding in the cities, poor working conditions and inadequate food supplies, and a growing concern for the health of the public. Epidemics of various kinds and in rapid succession led reformers such as C. E. A. Winslow, a physicist and public health worker, Lillian D. Wald, a nurse and social reformer, and others to develop voluntary organizations to improve the health and social conditions of the workers; they were especially concerned with those toiling in sweatshops, child workers, and families with ill members in their homes (Fitzpatrick 1975).

In greater proportions than ever before, these crowded and oppressive environmental conditions existed simultaneously with increasingly frequent epidemics. The effects of these regular outbreaks were presumably countered by voluntary mutual assistance within the community itself: Charleston, South Carolina, and Philadelphia, Pennsylvania, for example, have records of voluntary societies organized for the care and assistance of the sick poor beginning in the early 1880s (Stewart and Austin 1962). Not until the simultaneous occurrence of *seven* major epidemics in the 1880s, however, were visiting nursing organizations established (Maxcy 1956). These associations were formed with the dual purpose of providing care for the sick at home and teaching health principles and sanitary practices to families and community groups.

Leading up to the institutionalization of the first two nursing agencies in 1886 (Boston and Buffalo), a variety of plans for sending nurses into the homes of the sick poor was sponsored by well-educated and public-spirited women's organizations. The Women's Branch of the New York City Mission in 1877 and the Ethical Cultural Society of New York City in 1879 employed graduates of the first classes in schools of nursing to carry out this work. The first formal efforts toward organization of visiting nurse associations were also led by progressive men and women who saw the combination of healing and teaching as the unique and appropriate blend needed for the reforms in health they sponsored. The importance of the second of those functions to the nursing association established in Boston in 1886 is indicated by its name: The Boston Instructive District Visiting Nurse Association (Fulmer 1902).

Three of the pervasive characteristics of pre-professional community health nursing were thus institutionalized into modern practice: (a) the public support for "extra-family" health services inspired by massive threats, such as epidemics, to the health of the community; (b) the provision of curative nursing services, followed by instruction for future prevention, given impetus by the presence of threats to individual and family health; and (c) the preparation of health workers with an education that provides the knowledge and understanding to translate and interpret scientific findings into useful principles of caring for both the ill and the healthy on a community-wide basis.

These three characteristics were present between 1885 and 1900. Also during this period, the first 53 nursing agencies were incorporated in the United States. A list of agencies and a description of the general thrust of the work of this period can be found in a history written by Harriet Fulmer, superintendent of the Visiting Nurse Association of Chicago (1902). She begins by establishing the purposes of the visiting nurse as giving skilled nursing to the sick in their own homes and teaching people "to care for their own sick and carry out the right observance of sanitary laws."

The earliest programs employed few nurses, and their services were largely taken up with care for the sick at home. The epidemics occurring in the late 1800s kept large numbers of victims in bed, cared for by family members. Instruction to families at first consisted of teaching them how to care for the ill person, but before the 1900s, Lillian Wald had added nutrition, sanitation, and housing and work conditions to the material commonly discussed (Stewart and Austin 1962).

By this time, hospital training programs had been established (the first in 1872), and from the beginning these programs recognized that nurses working in community settings needed more education than the hospital alone could provide. Study of family problems and how they interact with social conditions was essential (Wensley 1950). The board membership of the early visiting nurse associations included upper and upper-middle class women who were instrumental in setting the educational standards for this work. Having insight into the relationships between social conditions and health was undoubtedly of great help to the nurses in directing their interventions toward reducing the causes of sickness as well as caring for those already ill. By expecting a broad educational base in the nurses, the agencies were in a position to provide broader services and programs that could be tailored more flexibly to changing community needs. This feature has proven to be one of the most farseeing contributions of the early founders and is as strongly supported today among the community nursing agency boards as it was then.

If community health nursing had been institutionalized in the seventeenth century, it might have been men's work, modeled on the activities of the religious brothers. On the Plymouth Plantation it would have likely attracted both men and women, since both worked full-time at survival tasks, including care of the sick. In Victorian England and America, however, community health nursing was the domain of women of the leisure classes who had the time, interest, and resources to apply to health and "social work." In this context, organized nursing developed primarily as a women's profession, and it took on many of the characteristics associated with women of that period. Fee structures were highly influenced by the charitable visiting that had been done gratis by the benevolent societies.

As early as 1854, Florence Nightingale had insisted that the physicians in the Crimean War theater write their directions for patient care in notebooks. From these directions, she reasoned that she could improve communications between physicians and ward sisters (Freidson 1972). In time, the directions became the physicians' "orders" that were carried into American nursing, and later into community health nursing. In America relationships with physicians, all but one of whom were men at that time, were colored by ascribed sexual roles. After the early stages of their preventive programs, when community health nurses had already established highly successful teaching and counseling programs, the practice of receiving orders (permission) from physicians to see any person, even if not ill, was introduced. Although the majority of the physicians gave this "permission" readily, this procedure represented a limit to nursing practice. Even today, vestiges of this institutionalized permission-seeking persist. Had more of the physicians been women and more of the nurses men, the relationships between nurse and patient may not have been so dependent on the physician's sanction.

Organized medicine had begun in America during Colonial days as European-trained physicians immigrated to the New World. Predating nurses' training by about seventy-five years, medical schools were opened in America to provide local training for physicians. The few schools of quality followed the European (university) model, but many more consisted of little or no training, a laxity stemming from medicine's status as an unregulated trade. By 1890 a medical association was in place that met on a regular basis to discuss pertinent issues. In 1894, at a convention of the American Medical Association (AMA) in New York City, a vote was taken on whether to "approve" nursing (Proceedings, Conference for Professional Nurses and Physicians, 1964). The vote was affirmative; but of more note as an indication of the times was the placing of the issue on the agenda in the first place. Thus, an interprofessional scenario was adopted that would pervade the relationships between physicians and nurses until the present.

In 1892, Lillian Wald and Mary Brewster, who had just completed their education and training in nursing, became appalled with the conditions among the immigrants in New York City. They enlisted the support of a wealthy journalist to underwrite their work in opening what was to become the first settlement house, providing community nursing and social work. It was in this first major demonstration of the role of the community health nurse that the potential of the profession was fully explored. Becoming known as the Henry Street Settlement, its span of responsibility included: representing clients' interests in improving health conditions in housing, work conditions, and neighborhood; visiting and caring for the sick at home; establishing and recruiting needed community services according to the assessment of client needs; and providing health services in schools (Wald 1915). To this day, community health nurses note with pride the accomplishments of their predecessors at Henry Street.

Summary

The conditions produced by the Industrial Revolution (overcrowding, gross inequities in resources and food) provided a fertile breeding ground for epidemics of typhoid, smallpox, and influenza to flourish. No less than seven major epidemics were recorded in the early 1880s. To deal with these conditions, 53 formal associations of visiting nurses were formed across the country between 1885 and 1900. Social reformers who had initiated the role also insisted upon more education for nurses doing work in the community. In so doing, the reformers linked the role of the visiting nurses to that of earlier workers who had conducted family care/health teaching/community action work in the community and in clients' homes.

Before the first major demonstration of community nursing began at the Henry Street Settlement in 1892, the concepts underlying practice had been established after the centuries of response to basic societal community health needs. These concepts were (a) the unit of service (client) is the individual, the family, and/or the community; (b) instruction and counseling for prevention are as important to practice as care and cure; (c) cultural differences must be taken into account in the provision of services; and (d) developing the role behavior and skills for practice requires more education than basic hospital training.

Within the social context of the late nineteenth century, the practice of visiting nursing, as it was then called, was organized on a charitable basis, was provided primarily by well-educated women, and had received the unsolicited sanction of the medical society. This early phase established the premises upon which the further developments in this field were built. The expansionary period that followed the turn of the century is described next.

1900–1910

Contextual Factors Affecting Public Health Nursing

By the turn of the twentieth century, more visiting nurse associations were being initiated across the United States, primarily in urban areas where the needs of the poor in deplorable living conditions were most acute. By 1901, the number of associations had expanded to 58, employing 130 nurses, and grew by 1905 to 200 associations, employing 400 nurses (Goldmark et al. 1923). By 1912 a total of 1000 associations existed across the country (Fitzpatrick 1975). Some of the new associations consulted older, established visiting nurse services to aid in the initiation of their service. In spite of such consultation, however, each new association developed a distinct mode of operation and a character all its own. The uniqueness of each association is most likely related to the variation in the individuals founding them. In some areas, charitable ladies and concerned citizens identified the need for visiting nursing, while in other areas, nurses who came in contact with the poor during their hospital training provided the driving force for creating the service. Some of the associations thus followed the settlement model created by Wald in New York, while others used a strict nursing system providing care to the sick on an hourly or per-visit basis. Among all the associations, care of the sick poor was the initial practice priority. Each new association utilized lay persons in some capacity, most frequently as board members and financial contributors.

Unlike other businesses and professions at the time, visiting nurse agencies had been organized under charitable auspices and as nonprofit institutions. As instruments of social change that "Americanized" the health habits of immigrants and taught them about public health measures, sanitation, and immunizations, the visiting nurse agencies were also supported by government funds to the extent that these functions were part of their work. The first large-scale effort to "sell" services to nongovernmental groups was a contract in 1909 with a national company, the Metropolitan Life Insurance Company (Brainard 1922). Community health nurses visited the company's clients on the supposition that better education and cleanliness in the home would lower mortality and thus preserve company profits. Because this nursing function was congruent with the work they had been doing all along, it was not inconsistent for the profession to expand its funding base beyond charitable and governmental sources. This precedent was to play an important role in multiple funding and reimbursement patterns for community health nursing practice for many years to come.

The Metropolitan Life Insurance Company began its program of visiting nursing service for the company's policyholders. In areas where a visiting nursing organization already existed, the company contracted with the organization to provide service; and where none was yet founded, the company hired its own nurses. The service was generalized, that is, care was given to a variety of age groups for any disease entity. While similar to traditional nursing care, many of the visits were also educational, directing the patient and family to undertake habits that would allow the regaining and maintenance of health.

Three major benefits were offshoots of the Metropolitan program. The first benefit resulted from the company's insistence on very careful reports with data organized systematically to assist in data retrieval. The company wanted to document changes in its policyholders as a result of the service, and it especially wanted to tabulate mortality rates. Brainard (1922) credits the company with "contributing more than any other one factor to the standardizing of reports by visiting nursing throughout the country."

The second benefit of the Metropolitan program was advertisement for visiting nursing. Insurance agents began telling policyholders of the nursing service. Nurses soon dealt with families who had lacked any prior service and were not of society's most indigent class. Thus the visiting nurses' clientele was expanded to include the employed and above-poverty-level persons of their neighborhoods.

The third benefit was the financial backing thus provided to the visiting nursing associations. The income from the insurance program helped to give the associations a sounder financial footing than had previously existed. Private contributions continued to be the largest source of income for all the agencies, but insurance payments grew during each successive year in the early 1900s.

Scope of Practice

Early in the 1900s the client system expanded from a focus on the sick person at home to a focus on the whole family. Although the nurses' first family involvement was to teach family members how to care for the sick person with the emphasis being hygiene and comfort measures, they soon discovered that they were often called back to the same residences when others in the family became ill. Nurses then began to examine the health status of all the family members in addition to giving care and direction to the identified patient. Along with assessing family members for signs of illness and teaching about care of the sick, nurses discovered that they could give the most aid to families if they taught people how to keep themselves healthy. As a result, teaching became focused on how to keep the tenement dwellings sanitary and how to maintain personal hygiene in spite of inadequate facilities. Long before the nation as a whole supported the need for public health standards, visiting nurses were using revolutionary prevention principles in their interactions with families through their teaching subjects such as nutrition and the need for rest and relaxation.

Again it became evident that the scope of this new practice surpassed the training the nurses were receiving in the wards of hospitals during the early 1900s. Visiting families at home necessitated an understanding of social, cultural, and economic factors that often outweighed or compounded medical conditions. Wald and Brewster found themselves pioneering in unknown territory, prescribing family by family for ailments that no physician could cure (Duffus 1938). It is no wonder that Wald saw nursing practice under medical direction as inappropriate. At the Henry Street Settlement, she insisted that nurses should be at the call of the people who needed them, without the intervention of a medical man (Christy 1970). At Henry Street, physicians collaborated with nurses just as the sanitarian workers did. Wald and other visiting nursing pioneers recognized the need for a broader preparation than the hospital-based training program to prepare nurses for this new practice. As a result of their belief that nurses should be highly educated and possess the "right constitution," Wald sought out nurses with some college or additional training to join the practice.

By the early 1900s the demand grew for the care of persons and families in other social classes beside the indigent. Visiting nursing associations expanded their practice to include any family or person requesting service regardless of financial situation. Many of the associations developed a philosophy that a family should be encouraged to pay whatever amount it could afford to maintain its pride. For the first time, a fee policy was suggested to the public to indicate that nursing service was worthy of reimbursement.

The decade 1900–1910 is called the era of specialization of visiting nursing. As the visiting nursing was gaining in popularity and prestige, new settings and more specified disease categories were being emphasized in its practice. The first of these practice "specialties" was originated by Lillian Wald in schools. Wald was especially concerned about the children in her east-side New York neighborhood whom she saw playing in the streets because they were excluded from school for a variety of minor ailments and communicable diseases. Many of the conditions, Wald knew, could easily be treated by a trained nurse.

Wald was aware of the movement in London during the last decade of the nineteenth century to use nurses in schools to conduct inspections of children and to follow up on those children who needed further diagnosis and treatment. The nurses assigned to schools in England were making visits to the homes of children excluded from school to instruct parents on the children's ailments and necessary treatments. Wald saw the efforts in English schools as a natural extension of the work that her nurses were doing in the neighborhood. In 1902 Wald negotiated for one of the Henry Street Settlement nurses to work in selected schools to combat the high expulsion rate caused by illness. The nurse began treating many conditions in her office and visiting homes to teach parents how to continue the treatment. After a one-month trial period for the nurse, the New York Board of Health appointed twelve other nurses to carry on the work. The nurses' intervention enabled many children to remain in school or to return after a brief stay at home (Duffus 1938). This school nursing specialty practiced early diagnosis and treatment and demonstrated the benefits of preventive measures.

Another practice specialty developed during the period was tuberculosis nursing. The mortality rate of tuberculosis at the turn of the century was staggering. As the leading cause of death, tuberculosis was the concern of citizens, scientists, and numerous health professionals. Although Robert Koch identified the nature of tubercle baccilli in 1882, Dr. Osler of Johns Hopkins did not link the home conditions of tuberculosis patients with the rampant spread of the organism until the end of the nineteenth century. He believed that most tuberculosis patients had a poor prognosis because housing, social, and educational interventions were lacking (Brainard 1922).

In 1899 Dr. Osler asked a Johns Hopkins medical student to investigate the status of tuberculosis patients previously diagnosed at the medical center dispensary. The student discovered that the medical plan previously instituted had essentially no impact on the patients because there was no one to follow up and see that recommendations were attended to and that the patients' living conditions improved.

Next, Dr. Osler appointed a nurse to continue where the medical student left off. The nurse followed dispensary patients to teach them the importance of fresh air and nutrition. In addition, the nurse employed relief agencies to aid more individuals and families in need. After six months, the Visiting Nurse Service of Baltimore recognized the value of those nursing interventions and appointed another nurse to augment the tuberculosis work. These two nurses divided the city of Baltimore in half to visit all reported patients. The association soon found that the work far surpassed the capabilities of two nurses, and more nurses were appointed. In 1910 the Baltimore Board of Health recognized the scope of the problem and decided to appoint nurses to continue the practice out of public funds (Brainard 1922). This movement against tuberculosis was the first opportunity for nurses to consider the education of clients and families as their *primary* purpose (Tinkham and Voorhies 1977).

Another specialty that visiting nursing developed during the same decade was the maternal-child nursing specialty known initially as "baby welfare" nursing. This specialty developed in a method similar to that of tuberculosis nursing in that the impetus was the high mortality rate of infants at the end of the nineteenth century. Because the major cause of illness and death among infants was gastrointestinal disease, initial efforts centered around organizing milk stations to distribute properly prepared milk; however, this distribution did not have a profound effect. Dr. Josephine Baker was one of the concerned health care professionals who believed instruction of mothers was needed in addition to milk to achieve a lasting effect. In 1902 in New York City, Dr. Baker sent nurses to visit sick babies and to instruct mothers in baby care (Brainard 1922).

The next revolutionary idea was the establishment of clinics to examine well children at prescribed intervals during the first fifteen months of life. Visiting nurses conducted the clinics and began visiting at home the newborns and infants who came to the clinic. Their purpose was to teach mothers before the children became ill. The nurse was responsible for reinforcing information and advice given to mothers at the clinic sessions (See Fig. 1.1).

Independent of the clinic efforts, visiting nurses began visiting all newborns and some older infants whose births were registered in the jurisdiction. The primary purpose of these nursing visits was to instruct mothers about feeding and hygiene. At the same time, the nurses informed mothers of the clinic services and explained the purpose of examining the children.

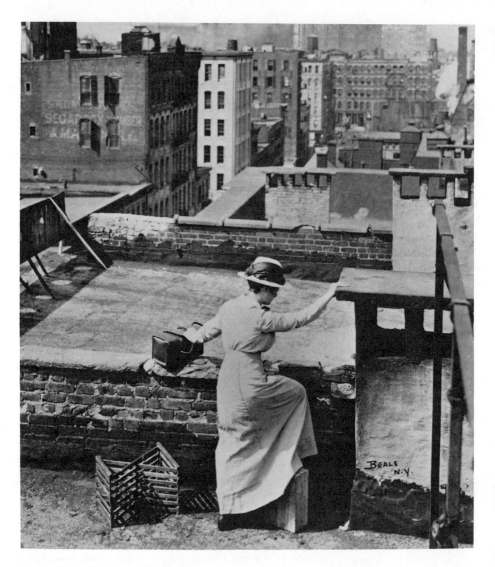

Figure 1.1. Daring and innovative means of travel increased the efficiency of the early home health care programs of the Visiting Nurse Service of New York.

In 1908 the New York Department of Health formed the Division of Child Hygiene, which professed care of the child as a public concern. The nation was awakening to the need for protection of its most valuable resource — children. The division recognized the efforts of visiting nurses with children and hired a staff of nurses to visit all newborns for the primary purpose of educating mothers. These baby welfare nurses gradually expanded the scope of their practice to include the mother during her prenatal and postpartum period. Health care providers were beginning to recognize the impact of the mother's pregnancy on the newborn's health. Birth anomalies and a host of other conditions were suddenly identified as preventable if the mother could be monitored and instructed during pregnancy. The visiting nurses were likely candidates to initiate interventions with pregnant women during home visits and at clinic sessions. As with the tuberculosis nursing, the major intervention was instruction with the aim of preventing illness and disability.

The maternal-child specialty expanded in scope a third time to include the preschool child — care for preschool children was practically nonexistent in the medical system. During prenatal and newborn visits, nurses had observed and interacted with hundreds of preschoolers. The extension of service to a focusing on the preschooler was a natural inclusion in the family approach.

A fourth specialty began to blossom during the first decade of the twentieth century: occupational health nursing, initially called industrial nursing. Before 1900, some individual industries had employed nurses to visit sick employees at home, but not until after 1900 did many industries consider hiring nurses (Fitzpatrick 1975). At first, many small industries contracted with the local visiting nurse service for home visits to their sick employees. Those industries that developed an in-plant health office used the nurse most often for first aid and instruction of employees. Each industry and industrial nurse developed such distinct ways of functioning that categorization of these early services is difficult. Setting of standards and collaboration among industrial nurses followed many years later. The hiring of nurses by industries themselves without linkage to the local visiting nurse service is probably the factor most responsible for the separate development of this specialty and the eventual secession of occupational nurses from the community health nursing association.

Another specialty linked visiting nursing more closely with the hospital. In 1904 the Presbyterian Hospital in New York developed a department of hospital social service. This department used nurses to visit patients discharged from the hospital. In Boston the following year, Dr. Richard Cabot, of Massachusetts General, convinced that the domestic and social conditions of the patient were significant factors influencing that person's diagnosis and treatment (Dock 1912), started to use nurses to visit discharged patients to identify and help rectify unmet needs. Bellevue followed this trend by initiating a social service department in 1906. Lillian Wald suggested a nurse to help the department initiate the follow-up plan. By 1911 forty-three hospitals had developed social service departments according to the pioneer hospitals' plans (Dock 1912).

Specialties continued to rise and change focus as health conditions changed and new needs arose. The development and expansion of a variety of specialties indicated the wide demands for service and an awareness of visiting nursing as an evolving, dynamic entity of nursing. The soon-to-be-coined term *public health nurse* was used for nurses who helped people regardless of their disease, social situation, age, or setting. Such a nurse had a grasp of teaching, social awareness, and resourcefulness that could be employed to meet a multitude of situations.

Summary

The decade from 1900 to 1910 was characterized by expansion of nursing: new associations formed in many new urban areas across the country. The expansion also included new activities and settings for visiting nurses in schools, clinics, and industry working with mothers, children, and the working population. The disease of major concern during this era was tuberculosis, and visiting nurses became instrumental in visiting the afflicted individuals at home to provide direct care and to teach the patient and other family members about the disease and its treatment.

During this decade third-party reimbursement became a factor in visiting nursing. The Metropolitan Life Insurance Company offered visiting nursing service to policyholders who needed care at home. The company documented decreased mortality rates in policyholders who received nursing service while recuperating from illness. It also expanded the visiting nursing clientele to include individuals and families other than the indigent of the community. Visiting nursing associations developed standardized record-keeping mechanisms as a result of the insurance company's emphasis on documentation of results.

Visiting nursing was developing as a valuable service in the period from 1900 to 1910. Families served by visiting nurses recognized that the care and teaching they received made beneficial contributions to their health. In the next decade, public sentiment awakened to the health needs of the population and contribution of visiting nursing.

1910–1920

Contextual Factors Affecting Public Health Nursing

The second decade of the twentieth century was marked by a rise in social consciousness. As the disparity between the rich and the poor of the nation widened, more people became concerned about social injustices and began attempting to narrow this gap. A broad scope of reform programs developed in the areas of housing, labor, education, and health. Voluntary health agencies proliferated as different groups developed programs and agencies for particular diseases and age groups. Tinkham (1977) explains the voluntary health movement by linking the continuing threat of communicable diseases in all communities and the apparent ineffectiveness of health departments because of their lack of power over conditions in the community with the rising social consciousness of a large number of citizens. More voluntary visiting nurse associations developed across the country bringing service to new cities, towns, and neighboring communities. The associations that formed at the end of the 1800s and during the first decade of the 1900s had already passed their infancy and were well established by the second decade.

Within the public sector, citizen concern prompted legislative action. The public health movement was aided by legislation in 1910 that gave authority to the states for the protection of the individual and made the health of the individual a community responsibility (Tinkham and Voorhies 1977). Preventive education measures were beginning to be recognized as the means of keeping the citizens of every community healthy. States and local governments looked to the resources of the local community to put such prevention into full operation. C. E. A. Winslow, a leader in the public health movement, recognized the visiting nurses' service as the effort that most closely approximated the ideals of prevention and brought the preventive philosophy to an individual level. Winslow's 1911 paper, which stated "the nurse [is] the most effective trained person to intervene with individuals," would be quoted many times as the authoritative recognition of visiting nursing's contribution to prevention. He advocated education of the public as the main intervention strategy of prevention. Since nurses were already involved with teaching individuals and families in most communities, the credit was due.

Around the same time that Winslow was praising nurses for their efforts in communities, Lillian Wald coined the title *public health nurse*. Florence Nightingale had used the title *health nurse* to fit her conception of nurses working to improve the health of people by ministering to the sick and teaching the healthy. Wald believed in the same dual purpose of nursing for sick care and for teaching. In addition, she wanted to emphasize the nurse's concern for public welfare. The nurse, according to Wald, was interested in all the conditions that affect people's daily living and overall health. Wald envisioned nursing service as being part of the government's program to aid in the protection and preservation of the health of the nation's citizens. Her choice of titles became popular during the teens and twenties; and public agencies did, indeed, as Wald had hoped, hire more nurses to strengthen programs of prevention in communities.

Then a major controversy about the title *public health nurse* arose. Was this title applicable only to nurses hired by government agencies in their prevention programs? Or was the visiting nurse who continued to teach and to supply direct care to sick individuals also deserving of the title? A variety of health professionals debated these two questions during the period from 1910 to 1920 (Brainard 1919; Fox 1919; Hill 1919; Durkee 1920). At that time, public health nurse, used narrowly, referred to a nurse (usually with visiting nurse background) who worked under governmental auspices for the sole purpose of teaching preventive measures to the public and conducting public health investigations (Fitzpatrick 1975). The broadest use of the term included all visiting nursing activities and the visiting nursing specialties, regardless of employment under governmental or voluntary domain as long as the nurse taught to prevent illness in healthy individuals or to prevent further illness in those already ill. The entire debate could have been alleviated if the idea of levels of prevention had been conceived. That is, the central issue was recognition of primary (before symptoms developed), secondary (early symptomatic), and tertiary (rehabilitative) prevention measures as all being valuable strategies in an overall prevention program. Since prevention was the key to public health nursing in both the voluntary visiting nursing and governmental nursing agencies, then both groups had legitimate claims to the title *public health nurse*.

The debate over this title exemplified the confusion between governmental and voluntarily sponsored nursing functions. The result of the confusion was some dysfunctional practice patterns in this decade that continued through the next two decades in many communities. The governmental public health nurses would visit families to teach preventive health measures and to investigate communicable disease reports. If the nurse discovered that a family needed physical care given to any member, then she would request a nurse from the voluntary agency to also visit the family. The proliferation of specialty nurses only compounded the problem of public and voluntary nurses visiting the same home. A nurse whose specialty was tuberculosis could visit at the same time as another nurse, the "baby welfare" nurse, was visiting the children in the home. During this same decade neonatum ophthalmalia became a concern and special nurses began visiting families with newborns to instill nitroglycerin. As a result, a family could have multiple nurses visiting at home. It is no wonder that Ella Crandall (1915) identified confusion of the purpose of the service, lack of insight (by nurses) into the overall goal, and duplication of territory by the generalized and specialized worker as organizational problems affecting many associations in 1915. Both Crandall's and Wald's recommendations for generalized public health nursing with one nurse per family regardless of the problem or problems were ignored by most agencies until twenty years later when the disadvantage of multiple workers in the same home became even more obvious.

National Organization for Public Health Nursing

The decade of 1910 to 1920 introduced an important organizational factor: the formation in 1912 of the National Organization for Public Health Nursing (NOPHN). The purposes of the organization were to assist in forming standards for the quickly expanding practice and to provide a means for exchanging ideas among public health nurses and their agencies. Many nurses were concerned about the rate at which new agencies were forming without any established standards as criteria for needs or performance evaluation. Since no official network of communication between the agencies and nurses existed, many nursing leaders feared inefficient and ineffective trial and error methods on the part of each new agency.

The new organization prescribed the training that a public health nurse should have for practice. It also examined the postgraduate courses offered for public health nursing and endorsed those programs that incorporated both theory and practice. A major part of the NOPHN's work was consultation to agencies across the country. At the time the organization was formed, more than 1000 agencies employed one or more visiting nurses (Brainard 1922). The executive secretary of the organization traveled across the country to consult with any agency, nurse, or community group employing a visiting nurse. The secretary offered advice on establishing the nursing service, selection criteria for the nurses, and educational programs for nurses. Although by that time nurses were employed by both voluntary and public agencies, the NOPHN's membership consisted primarily of nurses and agencies from the voluntary sector.

A unique feature of the NOPHN was that membership was open to lay persons, that is, non-nurse citizens. The initial rationale for including lay persons was because most voluntary agencies had been founded by lay persons, who continued to serve as board members and policymakers. The early leaders of the NOPHN agreed that lay persons were valuable contributors to the visiting nursing service because of their broad concern for the needs and health of citizens. Lay persons were integral to the organization's setting standards and offering consultation; but their membership made the NOPHN very different from the other two organizations of nursing: the American Nurses Association (ANA) and the National League for Nursing Education (NLNE), which focused primarily on issues internal to the profession.

The NOPHN continued its consultation and standard setting for the next three decades. It became the voice of public health nursing in the country, although its membership never included all the agencies and nurses in public health nursing. This organization finally merged with the American Nurses Association in 1952, when the NOPHN leaders agreed that a unified organization for nursing practice was needed (Fitzpatrick 1975)

Rural Public Health Nursing

The same year that the NOPHN formed, the American Red Cross officially inaugurated rural public health nursing. A few individual nurses had practiced rural public health nursing in the preceding decades, but large-scale efforts to make public health nursing available to all the citizens in nonurban areas were not attempted. Lillian Wald and her colleague Ella Crandall spoke of the great needs in the rural communities and urged the Red Cross to develop this nursing service. The Red Cross recognized that not only were rural areas underserved but many towns also lacked public health nursing services. This Red Cross service developed into the Town and Country Nursing Service.

Rural public health nursing was not a specialty type of public health nursing. The service was generalized; that is, it was a broad-scope practice emphasizing

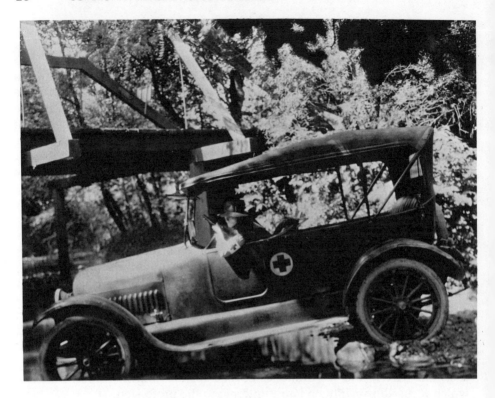

Figure 1.2.   Reaching rural populations challenged the skill and resourcefulness of the public health nurses employed by the American Red Cross.

the whole family, regardless of age, and teaching how to respond to the needs of both ill and healthy family members. The practice included all the specialties developed by that time. The rural nurse was involved in schools, tuberculosis care, maternal-child supervision, and chronic illness management at home (See Fig. 1.2).

Despite the vast needs across the country, rural public health nursing grew very slowly. Some communities failed to call upon the Red Cross to develop the service in their area. Others lacked financing to make the service feasible. By 1915 only 40 or 50 Red Cross public health nurses were employed throughout the entire country (Brainard 1922); and by 1918, the number had increased only to 97. These numbers, however, do not reflect the total rural effort. In the late teens, many states enacted laws that made public health nursing a mandatory service of state health departments. As a result, some of the states and local authorities hired nurses for rural public health nursing.

The biggest surge for rural public health nursing came after World War I when the Red Cross Town and Country Nursing Service reorganized into the Bureau of Public Health Nursing. The bureau consolidated countrywide public health nursing, drawing upon the interest and enthusiasm of citizens and veterans after the war. Many more communities developed public health nursing, resulting in 1300 public health nurses under the Red Cross auspices by 1921 (Brainard 1922).

Maternal-Child Health Practice

The maternal-child nursing specialty expanded in scope during the decade of 1910 to 1920. In 1912, after effective lobbying by Lillian Wald, the federal government created the U.S. Children's Bureau, which was responsible for gathering data about children's health, education, and use in the labor force. The bureau became the reservoir of information related to children and the national center for direction on child-related issues. In 1918, the Children's Bureau together with the Council of National Defense launched a campaign for increased maternal and child health care by declaring 1918 the Children's Year. Public health nursing was used to make the goals of the campaign operational. Nurses became involved in registering births of all newborns, conducting well-child clinics in areas not previously served, and teaching parents and community groups about health problems such as poliomyelitis and lead poisoning. Although some nurses had visited mothers antepartally in the previous decade, the campaign programs made antepartum service available to a greater number of women starting with the first month of pregnancy. Public health nurses essentially managed women's prenatal care by visiting regularly at home during the pregnancy, teaching expectant women critical information, screening for abnormalities, and reporting unexpected signs and symptoms to a physician. They then visited during deliveries at home and provided care to both the mother and baby through the first month postpartum (Fitzpatrick 1975).

Community Focus

At the same time, between 1910 and 1920, public health nursing practice broadened to cover new territories beyond the urban centers, with a new focus on the community. Some of the early leaders like Wald and Crandall had practiced with a broad assessment of an entire neighborhood or community, but not until this period did public health nursing literature clearly articulate the need for the public health nurse to look at the overall community. Stringer (1914) identified factors that every public health nurse should include in a community survey, emphasizing the need to survey the community to identify needs of the population and gaps in services. If the public health nurse was to be a general practitioner, according to Stringer, she needed to have a broad overview of the community to keep her practice relevant.

This community assessment strategy was a shift from the earlier methods that developed nursing service in response to the current epidemic or highest mortality disease. The community assessment approach emphasized nursing as one of many services available in a community. For nursing to continue to focus on "public health," the nurse needed to examine all the services offered, assess the characteristics of the community, and identify discrepancies. Although Stringer's article was specific enough to urge every nurse to put the community approach into practice, how widespread the community assessment strategy became during the teens and twenties is not clear.

Boundaries of Practice

With public health nursing broadening in scope, its boundaries became more diffuse. The nurse-physician boundary was often unclear, especially to the physician. Edna Foley (1913) described the variance in physician understanding of public health nursing and proposed methods such as standing orders to clarify these boundaries. Some physicians welcomed public health nurses into the community to care for families with a sick member. Others were suspicious, possibly threatened by nurses whom they mistakenly understood to be practicing medicine. Mary S. Gardner (1926), in her classic text on public health nursing, prescribed a set of ethics for the public health nurse to follow in an effort to minimize the friction between medicine and public health nursing. The practicing public health nurse, however, had difficulty living with such ethics as "never criticize the physician; never suggest the patient change doctors." Just as Foley had hoped that standing orders would clarify public health nursing practice, Gardner hoped that a set of published ethics would help the nurse-physician relationship. Unfortunately, such strategies may actually have hampered the independence of public health nursing and inadvertently given medicine a control that was not appropriate.

Preparation for Practice

The broadened public health nursing practice made further education for nurses entering this field an obvious need. Before 1910, some visiting nurse associations had developed their own programs to educate new nurses for practice; all of them recognized that the practice required skills that the training from the basic hospital program did not foster. In 1910, Teachers College at Columbia University was the first institute of higher education to assume any responsibility for the education of public health nurses (Tinkham and Voorhies, 1977). Teachers College initiated an eight-month public health nursing course for nurses who had completed a hospital-based program and were to be employed by a public health nursing agency. This course covered hygiene and sanitation, health problems (tuberculosis, infant mortality), sociology, and social psychology; at the same time students gained practical experience through affiliation with a public health nursing agency (Brainard 1922). By their supervised experience at a health department, visiting nurse service, or public health clinic, the trainees gained insight into the application of their new knowledge in the broader community.

Following the lead of Teachers College, other agencies and universities soon began to form collaborative relationships offering theory and field experience. By 1921, 15 colleges and universities offered courses in public health nursing that were coupled with work in a public health nursing agency for field experience (Tinkham and Voorhies 1977). By 1923, some 13 colleges and universities had combined programs that offered 2 years of nurse's training at a hospital, 2 years of college liberal arts, and an additional year in the specialty of public health nursing. The students earned a nursing diploma plus a baccalaureate degree (Goldmark et al. 1923).

In addition to a broad preparation that included study of social factors, public health nurses needed teaching skills with a health emphasis. Kalisch (1978) cites a high degree of communicative ability as one of the most valuable of such skills for this practice. The interpersonal nature of public health nursing also called for tact and sensitivity in dealing with a variety of social and hygienic problems. Student nurses were able to learn how to interact with families in a constructive manner through field experience under a senior public health nurse. Realizing that more than the "right constitution" or personality was required to practice public health nursing, young nurses turned to their role models for examples of how to teach and conduct home visits.

At the end of the 1910–1920 decade, the postwar period marked an increased — but largely unsatisfied — demand for public health nursing service. Nurses were commonly expected to return from war duty and enter public health nursing. Instead, many registered nurses on their return sought employment with hospitals, which meant that those institutions were no longer depending on student nurses to supply their staff. Public health nursing agencies were forced to compete for the experienced nurses, and the shortage, especially of those with a postgraduate public health nursing course, continued into the early twenties.

The end of the decade also marked the initiation of a major study on nursing education conducted by a committee composed of public health nurses, public health leaders, and nurse educators with Josephine Goldmark, a social scientist, as secretary. In 1918 Adelaide Nutting of the NOPHN approached the Rockefeller Foundation to launch a study on public health nursing and educational preparation. The issue of a postgraduate course or integration of a public health nursing course into the basic program for all nurses had been debated by the NOPHN for many years. The study, which became known as the Goldmark Report, was expanded to examine the broader issue of nursing education in general, with the final report issued the next decade, in 1923 (Goldmark et al. 1923)

Summary

The decade from 1910 to 1920 was the period of awakening of communities' responsibility for the health of their citizens. A surge occurred in efforts to educate citizens about health and illness, primarily through public health nurses educating families at home.

The birth of the National Organization for Public Health Nursing (NOPHN) indicated a desire by public health nurses to develop standards for their rapidly expanding practice. The organization launched efforts to consult with associations across the country and to develop criteria for entry into practice.

The public health nursing practice boundaries expanded further in this decade. Rural public health nursing developed in many communities under the auspices of the Red Cross. Rural practice was generalized and dealt with both sickness care and health promotion.

Public health nurses increased their involvement with both pregnant women and healthy children as a result of the Children's Bureau campaign to improve the health of these groups. Both clinic services and home visiting by nurses for health promotion with mothers and children were expanded during the decade.

A new strategy for practice, community assessment, was also developed during the teens. Rather than being a reactive approach, the community assessment method emphasized analyzing the population and services offered so that public health nurses could plan the best programs to meet community needs before disaster struck. The strategy was introduced during the teens, but its implementation was not widespread until many decades later.

During the 1910–1920 period, two major dilemmas arose in nursing practice. One concerned the proper boundary between public health nursing and medicine. The literature indicates some dysfunctional norms and ethics were developed to minimize the confusion between the two practices. The end result appeared to be a willingness by some nursing leaders to give control of public health nursing practice to physicians.

Second, no best method of educating nurses for public health nursing practice had been accepted. There was general agreement that education and training beyond the hospital training program was needed. A trend began of offering a postgraduate training program for nurses entering public health nursing. Eventually in some colleges and universities, the programs were incorporated into college degree granting programs for nurses. The subsequent variety of courses and programs for public health nursing led the NOPHN to approach the Rockefeller Foundation to study the issue of education for public health nursing practice. The study (called the Goldmark Report) that ensued was published in 1923 after being expanded to examine nursing education in general.

1920–1930

During the 1920s, public health nursing had reached a peak in expansion of services for both urban and rural areas. The number of nurses in this field had grown from 130 in 1901 to 11,000 in 1921 (Goldmark et al. 1923). In addition, political and organizational efforts alike strengthened public health nursing practice.

Fitzpatrick (1975) calls the decade 1920 to 1930 the period of consolidation and cooperation with other groups for joint effort at improving community health. All the states had health departments by 1920 and these employed a variety of workers, nurses making up the largest group (Tinkham and Voorhies 1977). Public health nurses were no longer the sole professionals delivering health education to citizens, but they continued to have a monopoly on individual and family health education in the home. Other workers within public health departments used primarily mass media methods to develop programs of health education.

The voluntary sector of nursing practice formed the National Health Council in 1920, with the purpose of helping voluntary groups to plan and share resources to improve public health. To further that goal the National Organization for Public Health Nursing joined the council. The council was the first organized effort by voluntary groups to address the duplication of services.

As health departments expanded their programs and hired more nurses, the voluntary nursing associations needed to specify further their role in communities (Brainard 1922). The private agencies used their freedom from the public mandate and flexibility in programming to be the testing ground for new services and programs. In many communities, a private agency supplemented the public nursing program and rounded out the overall nursing service available.

Amid the effort to consolidate, three important events occurred that were to shape the direction of public health nursing as a discipline for the next 50 years. These three events were:

- the passage of the Shepard-Towner Act in 1921
- the publication of the Goldmark Report in 1923
- the initiation of research on public health nursing by the NOPHN in 1924.

These events set important directions in practice, education, and research, respectively, and are discussed in more detail below.

Public Health Nursing Practice

The twenties marked expansion in practice in maternal-child services as a result of the Shepard-Towner Act of 1921. The act gave money to the states on a matching basis to enable each state to establish a program for the promotion of the welfare and hygiene of mothers and infants in both rural and urban areas that were previously underserved (Rothman 1978). Public health nursing used the funds to expand services to women during their pregnancies and then to assist with deliveries and to provide postpartum care at home. Clinic services were also expanded to offer more well-child conferences for infants and preschoolers. Public health nurses were conducting many more maternal-child home visits during the twenties to offer health promotional instruction with an emphasis on teaching mothers about the nutritional and developmental needs of children.

Aside from the fact that the Shepard-Towner Act provided far more services for mothers and children, it represented a new pattern of allocation of funds by Congress, whereby money was given to states on a matching basis for a predetermined health program. The sponsors of the Shepard-Towner Act assumed that no rival in the private sector had yet staked out the field of preventive health care. In assigning this task to each state, they assumed that physicians who were engaged in private practice primarily focused on treating ill children. Women reformers, educated in the community-oriented approach to the improvement of health and welfare conditions, led campaigns in their local communities to establish municipal bureaus of child hygiene and baby health stations to educate parents about the rules of hygiene, sanitation, growth and development, and illness prevention. The Shepard-Towner Act provided for the costs of this program, to be carried out largely by public health nurses (Rothman 1978). By taking a greater role in the definition of health services to be provided to the public, the federal government also provided the financial underpinnings for services by public health nurses employed by official agencies. As the first such legislation of its kind, the Shepard-Towner Act also officially legitimized the role of nurses in the promotion of health and welfare of mothers and infants. The effect of public policy on nursing practice thus cannot be underestimated, though the ultimate importance of this particular act was undercut by a change in medical practice.

Gradually during the 1920s, physicians began to expand their domain to include not only control over treatment of disease but control over prevention as well. In the early 1920s, Drs. John Dodson, Haven Emerson, L. Emmett Hall, and Frank Billings gave presentations at the AMA to convince their colleagues that (a) preventive care was vital to their patients' health and, therefore, they should be offering it; (b) skills in counseling on nutrition and well-child care could be developed and incorporated into office practice, in a method similar to current practice; and (c) since the AMA was behind this movement, physicians could not be accused of recommending periodic health examinations for their own benefit (Rothman 1978) — instead they were offering the public a preventive model for medical services.

In 1927 the Shepard-Towner Act was dropped as the federal government responded to pressure to shift the responsibility of preventive health care from public agencies employing public health nurses to private doctors. By 1930 physicians had shifted their practice from the sickroom and emergency calls to office visits by appointment and examinations of the healthy. Thus, the 1930s mark a period when public health nurses continued to offer preventive care but without financial backing or authority to deliver it. Nevertheless, the demonstrated success of health services delivered by public health nurses and partially funded by the government created a pattern that would recur in a number of health programs in the future.

Public Health Nursing Education

Improvements in the education of public health nurses were becoming increasingly necessary as the gap between the expansion of services and availability of educational opportunities became greater. When Adelaide Nutting approached the Rockefeller Foundation in 1918 for funds, she was applying for support for a program at Johns Hopkins for public health nursing education. What ensued was the appointment of the Commission for the Study of Nursing Education. At first the charge to the committee was to study "the proper training of the public health nurse," but later it was expanded to include all of nursing.

The Goldmark Report in 1923 influenced both nursing practice and education. The report recommended that public health nursing principles should be included in all basic nursing programs instead of just postgraduate programs. All nurses could thereby have a broader perspective of practice with a family-centered approach. The report criticized the common practice within many public health agencies of giving instruction but no physical care. The major criticism was based on findings of duplication of services in many communities, where nurses from public agencies visited families to give instruction but then referred these families to the voluntary agencies if any physical care were needed. The report encouraged generalization of public health nursing service, with one nurse giving care and instruction to the whole family. It suggested that the specialist nurses give consultations to the generalized staff nurses. Sixty years later this suggestion is still being realized.

The major recommendations of the Goldmark Report were gradually adopted within the next two decades. Postgraduate public health nursing courses were incorporated into basic curricula primarily of baccalaureate programs. The generalist public health nurse became the norm in most agencies, both public and private. The conflict over the public health nurse's involvement in prevention and teaching versus that of the visiting nurse was finally laid to rest. Both publicly funded and privately funded public health nurses were expected to teach, to prevent disease and promote health, and to give direct care when necessary.

By 1925, more than 1800 hospital training schools existed, and 25 colleges offered two years of liberal arts followed by three years of hospital training. Although from the beginning, higher education had been recommended at least for public health nurses, only 368 students were enrolled in the 25 colleges. Viewed in this context, the recommendations of the report were probably revolutionary. It supported not only a complete reversal of the prevailing educational model, but also the integration of public health studies and public health nursing within the basic curriculum in nursing.

Public Health Nursing Research

The first two formal studies of public health nursing were published in 1924, in the *American Journal of Public Health* and *Public Health Reports,* and were abstracted later by Hilbert (1959) in her comprehensive review of research in community health nursing. It seems strange that a practice field that had been in existence for forty years and had grown so rapidly had not been subject to evaluation research earlier in its history. The need for service apparently had appeared so obvious that the emphasis in the early years had been put entirely on the expansion of practice, and not on education or research.

The first study was a survey of the qualifications of superintendents and supervisors in public and private agencies in 83 cities. The findings indicated that, in the private agencies, the qualifications were higher and the ratio of supervisors to staff was lower. The American Public Health Association (APHA) Committee responsible for the study recommended that the nursing services be coordinated under a single director, and the nurse director be given more freedom in the selection of the nurses. This measure was believed to be necessary to upgrade the nursing staff to the level of the private organizations.

The other study published in 1924 was a survey of the standards for duties, qualifications, experience, and salaries of nursing staff in public health nursing in state health programs. Ways to coordinate the nursing work of the health departments with that of voluntary agencies to avoid duplication and waste were also investigated.

In 1926 a comparative study of generalized and specialized nursing elaborated upon the best pattern for organizing public health nursing services. The findings of the study were amazingly definitive. In the census tracts where generalized service was provided, the public health nurses saw 27 percent more families, gave sickness care and health supervision to 46 percent more individuals, and made 40 percent more home visits than nurses in specialized programs. Such data supported the conclusion that the provision of generalized nursing services in the community maintained the lowest cost per visit and minimized duplication of effort. Coming only three years after the Goldmark Report, this study provided the supporting documentation for the recommendations for nursing education in this report. Although no other studies of the organization and administration or of personnel policies were done during the 1920s, these topics have continued to be a periodic source of study until the present.

In 1925, the first study of a clinical educational setting was reported by Jane Allen of Teachers College of Columbia University. Minimum requirements were set for establishing an educational experience in rural health nursing, and an experimental program was developed. This study was indeed unusual, considering the educational milieu of the time. Another study of public health nursing education was not to be reported until the late 1940s.

Research on practice was reported as early as 1925 in a survey of child health in 86 cities in the United States. In this survey, information was collected not only on the programs provided, but also on the health habits of school children. Infants received the most care, whereas prenatal and preschool children were less frequent recipients. The implications for health departments, and public health nursing in particular were discussed in terms of standards of personnel, types of programs to offer, and coordination of efforts with voluntary agencies.

Another interesting study followed two years later correlating the growth of public health nursing services with a decline in infant mortality. Spurious factors were accounted for, and the author claimed "it is possible to estimate the average saving of life that may be expected from a given amount of effort," at least in retrospect. This study represents the first published effort to estimate quantitatively in terms of lives saved the value of the public health nurses to the health of the community. Until the 1940s, clinically oriented research was conducted almost exclusively in the field of maternal-child health. Only one study of nursing services in the home for those with chronic illnesses was reported in 1929, and two on communicable disease were reported in the 1930s.

Another area of research appeared in a series of three papers in 1927 and 1928 on time and costs of nursing service programs in the community. The investigator, Emma A. Winslow, studied child health demonstrations sponsored by the Commonwealth Fund. From her collection of information, she estimated that about 50 percent of a nurse's time was available for the clinical programs in home visits, conferences, school health services, and education. She projected that "office work, travel, vacation, and sick leave will occupy 40–50% of total working time, no matter what the type of program." She also estimated that an allowance of approximately one nurse per 4000 would safely assure the maintenance of "desired" standards of service, and she later estimated the costs of various units of service based upon salary data.

Although the methods used were the forerunners of later techniques of planning and budgeting, the Winslow studies were the only ones available for at least a decade, and they were used extensively in the consultation to agencies given by the NOPHN. By this time, 3267 organizations nationwide employed 11,152 full-time public health nurses, with twice as many public as private. The rapid proliferation of agencies in conjunction with the existence of other organizations to serve the needs of public health nurses (such as the ANA, APHA, and NLNE) prompted a study by Mary S. Gardner in 1926 of the functions of the NOPHN and its role in national health and nursing work. Although no radical changes were recommended, several statements relating to the budget, amount of work that could be done, and work with other organizations on a variety of projects were proposed.

Summary

The expansion in public health nursing activities peaked during the 1920s and was combined with a struggle to maintain involvements begun during the earlier decades. The major program that expanded in scope and communities served was the maternal-child nursing service, which was supported by the Shepard-Towner Act of 1921 until it was dropped in 1929.

During both the 1920s and 1930s public health nursing began collaborating with other health professionals to improve the health of families and the community. With the efforts to distribute public health nursing throughout the country, the majority of public health nurses were employed by public agencies where nurses learned to collaborate with a variety of public health workers (See Fig. 1.3). Generalized services were recommended by the Goldmark Report and supported by research findings as the best organization of services.

Preparation of nurses for practice in public health nursing had been an issue from the inception of public health nursing. The Goldmark Report, published in 1923, made recommendations about the preparation of public health nurses, the practice of public health nursing, and nursing education in general. The report recommended incorporating the postgraduate public health nursing course into the basic curriculum of nursing education programs. The end result would be a nurse more broadly prepared for institutional or public health nursing practice.

Research on public health nursing was published for the first time during the 1920s. The majority of the studies related to organizational, administrative, and cost surveys, but one study appeared on public health nursing education and three on clinical practice. Each study was an important beginning, laying the groundwork for further investigations.

By the end of the decade, the practice of public health nursing was firmly established in terms of the dimensions important to the development of a professional discipline. The basic concepts of generalized practice were established and a model for financial support had been demonstrated, an important study recommending the educational requirements in institutions of higher learning had been reported, and research on the practice had begun.

THE NEXT HALF-CENTURY: 1930–1980

The 1930s

By 1930, the provisions for establishing nursing as a profession were in place. According to Freidson (1972), the criteria of a profession include (a) prolonged

Figure 1.3.   (next page) Extending health care services to families in the remotest areas was a successful undertaking of the Frontier Nursing Service.

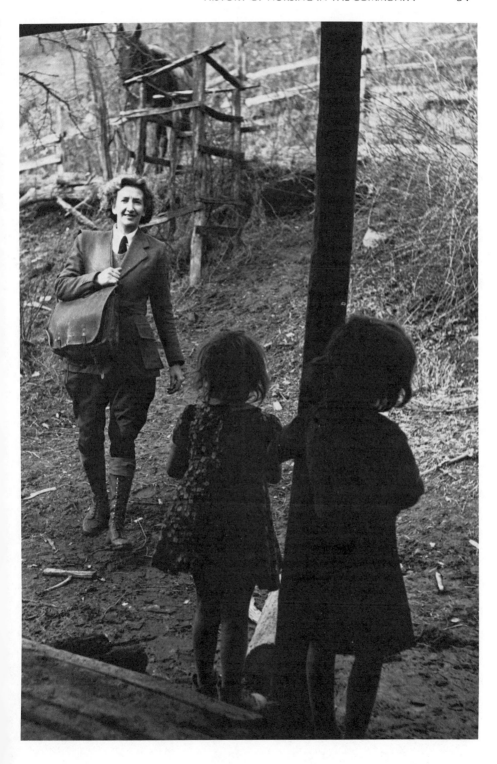

specialized training in a body of abstract knowledge, and (b) collectivity or service orientation. The underlying characteristic of the first criterion is autonomy over education and training, admission and licensure, and influence upon most legislation affecting the profession. The Goldmark Report provided the blueprint for the "prolonged specialized training," and the research appearing on nursing education and practice began to provide validation of, as well as new information about, the body of abstract knowledge on nursing. Data on public health nursing had been a prominent component of the Goldmark Report and, in fact, its collection was the impetus for the report. Public health nursing also qualified as a profession under Freidson's criteria as a highly autonomous specialty that had formally campaigned for and initiated service in many different settings for the past 50 years.

The practice of public health nursing had grown rapidly, and by 1930, a large number of people (both nurses and non-nurses) were committed to this practice and ready to move ahead with the legislative and economic supports necessary to its continuing development. The timing, however, could not have been worse. The nation's economic upheaval during the Great Depression in 1929 and the aftereffects during the thirties created turmoil for public health nursing. Although there was still great need for the services of the public health nurses, little money was available to the agencies, so many qualified public health nurses throughout the country were unemployed. Under the New Deal, the Federal Emergency Relief Act and Civil Works Administration created short-term programs, as stopgap measures that provided work for many citizens, including nurses. Most of the short-term health programs created at this time were for services in communicable disease control, clinic services for pregnant women, and health examinations for children in schools. When the economy began to stabilize, some nursing leaders speculated that the ranks of public health nursing might have become so stripped that few of the pre-Depression programs could be reestablished; and some of this apprehension proved valid.

The most important government program to influence public health nursing during the 1930s was the Social Security Act of 1935. Through this act health and social services were provided under government auspices. Tax support was again available for maternal-child health programs, for crippled children, and for those with rheumatic fever, venereal disease, and mental illness. As a result, programs for mothers and infants and care to the ill at home experienced a growth spurt. At the same time, though, the economic stress encountered by many families during this period had resulted in a multiplication of needy families. To meet this demand, many nurses were employed whose training was limited to a hospital diploma. These nurses brought with them a more limited vision of nursing in the community and nursing's relationship to medicine. To cope with the increasing variety of preparation, procedure books were developed to cover nearly every area of practice, leaving little to the imagination. Service programs were thus kept in place; but educational and clinical research programs, as recommended by the Goldmark Report, were not implemented.

From 1935 onward, government support for the work of public health nurses became a prominent source of financing. Although such support helped public health nursing to survive, the field suffered by losing the philanthropic support and interest of an elite lay public; as a consequence, it also lost its emphasis on higher education, its leadership in social activism, and support for its preventive care focus, which had taken the form of teaching and counseling. On the other hand, support from the Social Security Act provided the first step toward regaining the professional vitality that had marked the earlier periods.

During the 1920s and 1930s, the NOPHN received more requests than ever for consultation, guidance, and materials to help deal with the new programs; and yet its prepared nursing staff had shrunk in agencies throughout the country. The NOPHN maintained the position that public health nurses needed further education beyond the basic hospital training; but in light of the nation's economy, the organization also recommended that agencies offer as much training and supervision as feasible for nurses who were entering the field unprepared.

Besides preparation of staff, the NOPHN was confronted with agency funding dilemmas. Donations from the wealthy, which had been many voluntary associations' major source of funds, were sharply curtailed during the Depression. Other possible sources of funding for services, such as tax revenues and health insurance, were explored. In some communities, the voluntary and public agencies, each having its own public health nurses, combined into a single agency to reduce administrative costs and duplication of effort.

During the 1930s, public health nursing practice broadened to incorporate new specialties in nursing and to reflect changes in prevalent diseases. Orthopedic nursing developed during this period and became incorporated in public health nursing. The orthopedic specialty practiced in the community created a more rigorous rehabilitation approach for stroke victims and a more comprehensive approach for the rehabilitation of children with orthopedic problems. At the same time, acute diseases were being replaced by chronic diseases as the major cause of mortality and morbidity. Public health nursing practice had to undergo a similar shift, with its new emphasis on chronic ailments. The resulting practice found nurses visiting individuals with cardiac problems, especially those who had experienced myocardial infarctions, and individuals with diabetes in need of instruction and assistance.

Early in the century, public health nursing practice had emphasized the influence of social factors on health. In the 1930s, the psychological impact on health became well known, and public health nursing developed a philosophy of individualizing care to incorporate the role of psychological factors into the process of healing.

By the end of the thirties, the focus of nursing on the entire community had been reaffirmed and was generally accepted within public health nursing. In 1922, Brainard wrote that the public health nurses' domain is the entire community, and the NOPHN definition of public health nursing in 1929 proclaimed the service as "an organized community service . . . rendered . . . to the individual, family, and community." The NOPHN was less clear, however, about the means for delivery of service to a community other than through individuals and families in need of instruction and direct care. Because public health nurses were assigned to geographic units rather than according to their specialties, the staff manifested an intuitive sense of the community as client. The agency leadership participated in, and sometimes initiated, efforts to determine community needs and introduce programs to deal with them. More explicit and systematic approaches to "nursing a community" would wait for a few more decades.

A broader perspective on health using a team approach to care for individuals and families was also developed in the 1930s. Collaboration between medicine, nursing, social work, and psychology was finally recognized as important in developing approaches to improve health of individuals. In addition, some agencies put a greater emphasis on discharge planning from hospital to home (Crain 1933). If public health nurses were to be involved in post-myocardial infarction and diabetic teaching, for example, it was critical that hospitals coordinate with the local public health nursing agencies to plan for clients being discharged who were in need of this service. During this period, hospitals and agencies developed mechanisms of communication to facilitate the linking of hospital and home care. Discharge planning programs to this day remain impossible to carry out without interdisciplinary and interagency collaboration.

The thirties also marked a period when nurses and administrators in agencies began program evaluation. With funding scarce, agencies needed to set priorities and evaluate the effects of their current programs. Program evaluation studies were begun in a number of agencies as a means of self analysis. Some of the studies looked at nursing activities and rated the process used in the nurse-family interaction (Hilbert 1959). Others looked at the overall community and described the nature of the service and clientele. The trend of studying the service delivered and the nature of the community receiving it was an important advance in the administration of public health nursing and a step toward improving service.

The 1940s–1960s

One year before the United States became involved in World War II, Senator Robert Wagner introduced a bill to incorporate the National Health Program (Kalisch and Kalisch 1978), which would provide for a system of health care for all citizens. Although nursing groups were highly supportive of this effort, the leadership of the AMA, the American Hospital Association (AHA), and the American Dental Association (ADA) testified against it. Later that summer, the Senate committee stated that it wished to give the bill further study. An amended bill was not reintroduced as expected, and the issue did not appear in President Roosevelt's 1940 campaign. This pattern of national health insurance bills being tabled after AMA opposition was to recur a number of times in the next 40 years despite strong approval of such bills by many groups, with nursing among the most vocal.

After the entry of the United States into World War II, in 1942, many nurses were needed in the military. Hospitals and public health agencies alike were again depleted of their pool of nurses, and alternative measures were taken to replace them, in quantity, if not quality. Programs were set up for licensed practical nurses, and nurses' aides and volunteers were recruited as well.

The years of World War II brought important changes to preparation for nursing as well. Since so many additional nurses were needed for duty, both at home and on the front, government support was needed to prepare the numbers required in as short a time as possible. In 1941 Frances Payne Bolton introduced a bill that included the first large-scale commitment of federal funds for nursing education. This first allocation of money was used to prepare unprecedented numbers of nurses at the basic levels during the war effort.

By the time the war was over, hospitals had moved away from relying heavily on student staffing and were competing with public health agencies for nurses to care for the patients. The competition provided nurses with bachelor's degrees many opportunities to join hospital and public health agencies as staff nurses as well as to fill leadership positions in both settings. A long time would pass, however, before enough well-educated nurses were available to fill the public health nursing positions created to meet the demands for care. In 1948 a report by Esther Lucille Brown (1948), sponsored by the Russell Sage Foundation, again called for collegiate education for public health nurses, with the study of public health nursing and related sciences built into the basic curriculum. According to the report, only four NOPHN-accredited programs offered this preparation, and three of those were part of university offerings. Many more would be needed for the basic preparation of public health nurses, and the public sector was charged with the responsibility for providing this education.

The Brown Report also recognized the need for both academic (at all levels) and professional training, not only to provide leadership in the practice areas but also to carry on "desperately needed research, writing, publication, and consultation related to the improvement and extension of nursing care" (Brown 1948). The second allocation of federal funds for nursing education, which followed in 1956, provided for graduate as well as baccalaureate training. The money was distributed to colleges with graduate and undergraduate nursing programs for their enlargement, and to other colleges for the institution of such programs.

In 1959 the spring issue of *Nursing Research* published 232 abstracts of research in public health nursing conducted between 1924 and 1957 (Hilbert 1959). This number represented all the reports of research in the public domain that could be found through a two-year search conducted by Hortense Hilbert of Teachers College, under a grant from the National Institutes of Health (NIH), U.S. Public Health Service. As a result of the search, Hilbert had determined that 1924 was the earliest year in which a report based on a systematic investigation had been published. Although at least one study in every year since 1924 met her definition, 50 percent of the studies had been conducted during the last six years covered by the report (1953–1959). In the first third of the 33 years reported, an average of 2.3 studies per year was reported; in the second third, an average of 4.5 studies per year; and in the last third, an average of 14.0 studies per year. Most striking in the types of studies conducted was the increase in clinical investigations. Although maternal and child health services had been the only clinical area regularly investigated before 1951, after that time other clinical areas such as school health, care of the chronically ill and handicapped, and mental health began to be more regularly studied. This increase in published research on public health nursing serves as evidence of a serious attempt to heed the advice given in the Brown Report.

In 1963 a report was prepared by the Surgeon General's Consultant Group on Nursing. This report provided specific goals for nursing manpower and services toward which national efforts should be directed (HEW 1963). Although the total number of nurses had grown since 1920, the proportion of those who were in public health nursing and school health nursing had remained at 6 percent. Similarly, although the number of nurses with bachelor's degrees had increased substantially, only 10 percent of all nurses had this preparation at the time of the Surgeon General's report. Projections for this field were to more than triple the number of public health nurses with bachelor's degrees in preventive care and home health services by 1970. The Surgeon General's report also provided a blueprint for achieving these goals through federal support for nursing education at all levels and for increased numbers of research fellowships and research grants.

This federal support, channeled toward the goals set out in the report, at last provided an adequate recruitment pool for public health nursing agencies. Many agencies began to fill their director and supervisory positions with nurses who held master's degrees. Preparing the nurses for the staff and agency leadership positions in public health nursing absorbed most of the time of the public health nursing educators during the remaining years of the fifties and throughout the sixties. But by the end of the sixties, there was an appreciable increase in the proportion of public health nurses who held at least a bachelor's degree. From 10 percent in 1942, 42 percent held bachelor's degrees in 1972 (Kalisch and Kalisch 1978).

Another piece of legislation was passed in 1966 that had an enormous impact on the programs offered by public health nursing agencies. Title XVIII of the Social Security Act, entitled "Health Insurance for the Aged and Disabled," commonly known as Medicare, went into effect on July 1, 1966. The federal government by that act provides health insurance with two components for the elderly and disabled. One component, Part A, provides basic protection against hospital cost and related posthospital services. The other component, Part B, comprises a voluntary insurance plan for outpatient therapy, physicians' services, and some limited home health benefits. Since Medicare specifies what home health services are reimbursable, many home health agencies tailor their public health nursing and related services to provide only those services that meet the criteria. These are primarily short-term skilled services relating to an acute illness or episode; long-term, maintenance, and preventive home health care services are not covered by Medicare and are therefore offered in limited instances by many home health care agencies. Unfortunately, therefore, one result of the Medicare legislation in many communities is the neglect of long-term care needs of elderly clients because of lack of funding.

The Medicare regulations did, however, result in some spinoff benefits for public health nursing practice similar to the benefits to practice that came from the Metropolitan Life Insurance Company 57 years earlier. The Medicare regulations specified case record documentation of the skilled service provided and required professional personnel to advise the certified home health agency on professional matters. As a result, public health nursing administrators and staff began to scrutinize their practice and improve documentation of the service rendered and the resulting client impact. Public health nursing practitioners improved the utilization of appropriate level nursing personnel to provide the level of client care required. The professional nurse in the public health nursing agency, most often with baccalaureate preparation, became a skilled care manager and practitioner who set up the plan for home health services and determined the type of service required.

An important event in education for community health nursing practice also occurred during the sixties. A nurse-physician pair developed the first ongoing training program for nurse practitioners at the University of Colorado in 1965. The initial purpose for the program was to staff a series of neighborhood health centers set up by the city of Denver. The nurses were prepared to care for well children and to diagnose and treat common problems of ill children in situations where physician backup was available (Silver et al. 1966). The subsequent evaluations that were conducted on the results of this practice supported the position that nurses could successfully take a prime role in the delivery of primary care in the community. This growing trend would eventually revolutionize nursing practice and, ultimately, nursing education. By 1975 about 5800 nurses had been prepared in primary care practice, and by 1980, this number had tripled. Most had taken positions in health centers, public health agencies, schools, colleges, occupational settings, and similar places (Sultz et al. 1979). The importance of this role expansion for nursing was in the opening of the gate to a much broader role for nurses (primary care providers to patients) and to a much wider array of community settings than had been customary in the more recent decades. Those who practiced in the traditional agency settings could thus expand their practice.

A second event that provided a resource for graduate nursing education was a series of monographs published by the Western Interstate Council on Higher Education in Nursing (WICHEN) (1967). One of these focused on community health nursing and provided a theoretical basis for practice, that is, a conceptual framework based on the key concepts emerging from theories and from experience in the practice field. By the time this report was published, the term *public health nursing* had been replaced by *community health nursing* in an attempt to describe better the work in this field. The newer term was intended to show a commitment to the concept of high-level wellness for the whole community, and not only for selected segments of the population. The importance of this monograph lies in its lucid presentation of a theory base for practice with the intent that the theory be subsequently tested, and in the identification of key concepts for inclusion in community health nursing graduate programs. These concepts are high-level wellness, stress, socialization and the interstitial role of the nurse, communication, and problem-solving and decision-making. Dialogue was beginning to converge among educators in public health nursing around the nation on the appropriate content for master's programs, and a variety of types were developed. In general, the concepts defined in the WICHEN monograph were found in most programs at that time, and it laid the groundwork for future program development as well.

The 1970s and 1980s

The evolution of practice, education, and research described above had, by the 1970s, served to reaffirm and develop broad support for community/public health nursing as a key community service as well as an academic discipline. The events of the 1970s could have taken place only upon such a base without causing complete breakdown in communication within the profession. In a nutshell, these events were (a) the development of separate programs at the master's level for delivering care to individuals and families using the practitioner model, and to the community using either the epidemiologic model or the group advocate model, (b) the expansion of practice opportunities into new fields such as ambulatory/primary care and health care planning, and (c) the movement of relatively large numbers of public health nurses into doctoral programs and the ensuing demand for an increase in scholarly clinical research in the field. The consequences of these three major events can be seen in documents produced throughout the 1970s.

In a conference held in 1973, leaders in public health and public health nursing presented papers on the nature of public health nursing practice, its function within the health manpower system, and the relationship in this field between education and practice (HEW 1973). The conference report reflected the excitement generated in the discussion as further clarification was reached on the direct care and community focus of practice. For the first time, resolution of public health nursing's multiple and distinct competencies was addressed. Emphasized throughout the conference was the need for public health nursing to be reality oriented, that is, responsive to the lifestyles of people, societal values and structures, differing cultures, and the health needs of families and communities as defined by the population. These values are clearly reminiscent of those expressed throughout the history of public health nursing; but articulated within the context of advanced education and research emphasis, the reaffirmation of these values also served as a guidepost to future program planning. These concepts paved the way for more definitive documents on definition (American Public Health Association 1980), and standards (American Nurses Association 1973).

At the international level, these same values are reflected in a technical report on community health nursing prepared by a World Health Organization (WHO) Expert Committee (1974). This report also expresses great concern for the inappropriate preponderance of nursing education in acute care services, while the majority of health problems can be dealt with by community-focused and primary care services. Within the recommendations for change is included encouragement to form a *system* of nursing care that includes all those who deliver nursing services in addition to nurses, such as family members, lay healers, and often other professional workers. The dual emphasis on delivery of direct care and community-focused services is prominent throughout the report.

The WHO report places the efforts in the United States to develop further programs in both primary care and community-focused nursing services within the mainstream of thinking among world leaders. Two publications (HEW 1976, 1977) in the mid 1970s by the Division of Nursing, USPHS, in fact, underline the intensity of effort to accomplish these goals. One publication reports on a conference held to develop curriculum guidelines for family nurse practitioner (FNP) programs. A series of workshops and meetings followed this conference that produced curriculum guidelines for FNPs and a fledgling organization to encourage the further development and evaluation of FNP practice (National Task Force 1980).

The other publication reported the development of a demonstration curriculum for "community nurse practitioners." Rather than focus their efforts on individuals and families, the students in this program learn to apply the nursing process to aggregates and to work with community groups toward achieving health-related goals. At last the concepts developed so early in American public health nursing practice were receiving serious attention through the articulation of specific curricular components and practice expectations. These curricular directions not only hold importance for schools of nursing but for schools of public health as well (Milbank Memorial Fund Commission 1976). Course content in public health education as applied to nursing, especially the programs emphasizing the aggregate approaches, is most efficiently obtained through existing study of epidemiology, biostatistics, and the delivery of health care services. Where schools of public health and of nursing develop the content together, both master's and doctoral programs in community health nursing can be greatly enriched.

At the close of the decade, differences among educators surfaced over whether "community" health or "public" health was the best designation for nursing practice in this field. Assuming that a population base is used for decisions on program planning, and that outreach constitutes a component of the program to treat those who do not present themselves for care as well as those who do, the difference is semantic. All programs using a public health philosophy must prepare students to offer whatever services they are being educated to provide on the basis of (a) population need (risk), and (b) the development of strategies to reach those in need (outreach). These assumptions imply a core of knowledge integrating both public health and nursing sciences, bolstered by experiences in applying these skills to client (individual, family, group, or community) needs.

By 1980, the graduates of the new programs in public health nursing had brought their skills into a wide variety of settings and roles (Archer 1976). Community planners, outreach program directors at health maintenance organizations (HMOs), primary health care providers, researchers, health care providers in public health programs, and nursing directors in community-based programs, such as home care and hospice programs, all became viable career roles for graduates of these programs.

Many of the early nurses with master's degrees were recruited into careers in teaching because of the desperate need for educators in the new programs. As academicians seeking tenure, however, they recognized the increasing prevalence of doctoral preparation as a career necessity: many graduates of these new master's programs sought out doctoral programs to advance their educations. Over time, doctoral programs have become better suited to the specific career demands presented to the graduates, who must perform in both the research and clinical worlds as well as in education. At present, three options are open to those seeking doctoral preparation to enhance their public health nursing careers: (a) selecting any of about 26 nursing PhD or DNS programs, (b) electing a DPH program within a school of public health, or (c) identifying a related scientific field (e.g., sociology, political science) and applying the concepts of the latter two degree types to solve nursing problems (HEW 1976b). Eventually, specialization in public health nursing at the doctoral level in schools of nursing will undoubtedly become a reality.

The vigorous growth in graduate education for community health nurses is paying off in the emergence of more research with specific relevance to the field, tighter research designs, and greater efforts to develop theory to guide practice. In response to the demand for the dissemination of the experiences — research, clinical, and teaching — of these master and doctorally prepared graduates, two new journals are in preparation for release in 1984.

The major organizations responsible for conveying thought and action for the continued development of community health nursing are the newly reorganized Division of Community Health Nursing within the American Nurses Association, the Public Health Nursing Section of the American Public Health Association, and the Council of Community Health Services within the National League for Nursing. A new organization, the Association of Graduate Faculty in Community Health/Public Health Nursing was established in 1978, and serves as an influential forum for deliberation by all those interested in graduate education in the field. Although divisiveness has characterized the interrelationships among these organizations at times in the past, there is now a distinct sense of collaboration among them. Representatives of each organization have put forth considerable effort to share ideas and cooperate on projects in the interest of the continuing development of the discipline.

SUMMARY

The year 1986 marks the centennial for public health nursing in the United States. Within this century, the entire unfolding of public health nursing as a full profession has taken place. Those who watch from outside, serve in supportive capacities, or read about its development out of interest can observe with fascination the evolution of a profession. For those who have played a role in its development, the profession has offered an exciting career.

The last half century solidified the practice of public health nursing into a profession by specifying and refining the curricular designs, broadening the base of financial support for practice and education, and developing the research that provides empirical evidence on the quality and effectiveness of the practice. This development should serve as the foundation for more definitive intervention programs — organized in collaboration with others in the community, tested using sophisticated evaluation methods, and offered to the public at an unprecedented level of quality in the next century. Public health nursing has had a proud history, which portends a brilliant future.

REFERENCES

American Nurses Association. Standards: community health nursing practice. Kansas City, Missouri, 1973.

American Public Health Association Newsletter. The definition and role of public health nursing in the delivery of health care. 1980 (June), Working Draft III.

Archer, SE. Community nurse practitioners: another assessment. Nurs Outlook 1976; 24:499.

Brainard A. Why the visiting nurse is a public health nurse. Public Health Nurs 1919; 11:488.

Brainard A. The evolution of public health nursing. Philadelphia: Saunders, 1922.

Brown EL. Nursing for the future. New York: Russell Sage Foundation, 1948.

Christy T. Portrait of a leader: Lillian D. Wald. Nurs Outlook 1970; 18:50.

Crain G. The patient goes home. Am J Nurs 1933; 33:233.

Crandall EP. The relation of public health nursing to the public health campaign. Am J Public Health 1915; 5:225.

Dock L. A history of nursing. Vol. 3. New York: Putnam, 1912.

Dolan J. Nursing in society: a historical perspective. Philadelphia: Saunders, 1978.

Dubos RJ. Mirage of health. New York: Harper & Row, 1971.

Duffus RL. Lillian Wald: neighbor and crusader. New York: MacMillan, 1938.

Durkee CJ. Am I a public health nurse? Am J Nurs 1920; 20:319.

Fitzpatrick ML. The National Organization for Public Health Nursing 1912–1952: development of a practice field. New York: National League for Nursing, 1975.

Foley E. Standing orders. Am J Nurs 1913; 13:451.

Fox E. Is a visiting nurse a public health nurse? Public Health Nurs 1919; 11:575.

Freidson E. Profession of medicine, a study of the sociology of applied knowledge. New York: Dodd, Mead, 1972.

Fulmer H. History of visiting nurse work in America. Am J Nurs 1902; 2:411.

Gardner MS. Public health nursing. 2nd ed. New York: MacMillan, 1926.

Goldmark J et al. Nursing and nursing education in the United States. New York: MacMillan, 1923.

Hilbert H. Extending hospital care to the home. Public Health Nurs 1949; 41:378.

Hilbert H. Abstracts of studies in public health nursing (1924–1957). Nurs Res 1959; 8:42.

Hill HW. Is the visiting nurse a public health nurse? Public Health Nurs 1919; 11:486.

Kalisch P, and Kalisch B. The advance of American nursing. Boston: Little, Brown, 1978.

Maxcy KF. Preventive medicine and public health. 8th ed. New York: Appleton-Century-Crofts, 1956.

Milbank Memorial Fund Commission. Sheps C, chairman. Higher education for public health. New York: Prodist, 1976.

The National Task Force on FNP Curriculum and Evaluation. Jelenek DE, Umland BE, eds. Guidelines for family nurse practitioner curriculum planning. March 1980.

Proceedings of the First National Conference for Professional Nurses and Physicians: Medical and nursing practice in a changing world. Sponsored by the American Nurses Association and American Medical Association. Williamsburg, Virginia, 1964.

Rothman S. Women's proper place: a history of changing ideals and practices, 1870 to the present. New York: Basic Books, 1978.

Silver HK, Ford LC, and Day LR. The pediatric nurse practitioner program. Expanding the role of the nurse to provide increased care for children. JAMA 1966; 204:298.

Stewart I, and Austin A. A history of nursing. New York: Putnam, 1962.

Stringer E. What every public health nurse should know. Am J Nurs 1914; 14:976.

Sultz HA, Henry OM, and Sullivan JA. Nurse practitioners: USA. Lexington, MA: Lexington Books, 1979.

Tinkham C, and Voorhies E. Community health nursing: evolution and process. 2nd ed. New York: Appleton-Century-Crofts, 1977.

U.S. Department of Health, Education, and Welfare. Toward quality in nursing: needs and goals. Report of the Surgeon General's consultant group on nursing. Washington, DC: February 1963.

U.S. Department of Health, Education, and Welfare. Redesigning nursing education for public health. Washington, DC: Conference report, May 23 to 25, 1973.

U.S. Department of Health, Education, and Welfare. Current directions in family nurse practitioner curricula. Pickard CG, Watkins JD, eds. Washington, DC: January 1976.

U.S. Department of Health, Education, and Welfare. The doctorally prepared nurse. Report of two conferences on the demand for and education of nurses with doctoral degrees. Washington, DC: March 1976.

U.S. Department of Health, Education, and Welfare. The development and implementation of a curriculum model for community nurse practitioners. Washington, DC: August 1977.

Wald LD. The house on Henry Street. New York: Henry Holt, 1915.

Wensley E. The community and public health nursing. New York: MacMillan, 1950.

Western Interstate Commission on Higher Education. Defining clinical content, graduate nursing programs, community health nursing. Boulder, CO, February 1967.

Winslow CEA. The role of the visiting nurse in the campaign for public health. Am J Nurs 1911; 11:909.

Wish H, ed. Of Plymouth Plantation: the Pilgrims in America. New York: Capricorn Books, 1962.

World Health Organization. Community health nursing. Report of a WHO expert committee. Geneva, 1974.

CONCEPTUAL FRAMEWORK: A BASIS FOR COMMUNITY HEALTH NURSING PRACTICE

2

Diane J. Walgren

Because nursing is a practice profession, nursing knowledge is valued by its usefulness to nurses in making actual nursing care decisions (Crawford et al. 1979). This knowledge yardstick, which is common in the professions, contrasts sharply with the standard of measure in the physical sciences and the arts, where knowledge is valued for its own sake (Diers 1979). The source of the value measurement for professional knowledge is the implied societal obligation that professions exist to improve the state of the world (Diers 1979).

If nursing knowledge must be useful, then it must assist the nurse in evaluating health conditions and in developing sound judgments about changes needed to improve those conditions. With the rapid proliferation of new knowledge, maintaining a current knowledge base is a difficult task. Compounding the problem is the tremendous variety in nursing roles that have evolved over the past decade.

In order to deal with the knowledge explosion, along with the differences in knowledge required by the varying nursing roles, the nurse clinician must work within a method of organizing knowledge. A conceptual framework developed from personal experience in nursing practice can furnish that organization because it provides a structure for analyzing the nursing process. The conceptual framework guides the nurse clinician in determining the need for nursing, in selecting a nursing intervention, and in predicting the outcome relevant to the setting and client situation. In addition, with a conceptual framework, the nurse can evaluate new knowledge for relevance to personal practice and can organize and store knowledge for later retrieval. Thus a conceptual framework for nursing practice provides a guideline for lifelong learning (King 1971), as well as a mechanism for directing and maintaining clinical practice.

In community health nursing, a conceptual framework is especially important because of the generalist nature of the community health nurse role, which has historically encompassed the entire life span and all levels of prevention from health promotion to rehabilitation (Leavell and Clark 1965). The variety of practice settings, services, and clients in community health make the framework essential for determining the usefulness of the mass of data accumulated in clinical practice. A totally different conceptual framework for each community health nurse clinician is not advocated; but within the basic concepts of community health nursing, which have historical roots, each nurse must tailor the practice guidelines to suit the specific practice. This chapter was developed to assist community health nurse clinicians in developing such a conceptual framework for nursing practice. The topics to be addressed are nursing theory development, nursing theory analysis, and conceptual framework development.

NURSING THEORY DEVELOPMENT

Theory is knowledge in development. To understand the kind of knowledge needed for nursing practice and how to develop it, one must understand theory.

Definition of Theory

Explanations of what constitutes a theory vary. Hardy defines a theory as sets of interrelated hypotheses that are subject to reformulation and refinement (Hardy 1974). Ellis defines theory as a coherent set of hypothetical, conceptual, and pragmatic principles forming a general frame of reference for a field of inquiry (Ellis 1968). Either definition is correct, but in order to understand them, one must know that a theory is (a) a group of precisely defined *concepts* (b) organized by specific propositions or hypotheses about their relationships to each other.

Concepts are simply abstractions of real world occurrences (Williams 1979). They are the word symbols by which people categorize all observations, feelings, and experiences for later recall and use (King 1971). Concepts are the elements of a theory. Some sources differentiate between "concepts" and "constructs," with the former referring to observable phenomena such as trees or cars and the latter referring to nonobservable phenomena such as self or love (Williams 1979). For the purposes of this chapter, however, the word *concept* will refer to both types of abstractions since nursing deals with both types of phenomena.

The process of developing categories or concepts to explain real life events is a process that nurses need to bring to the conscious level. Nurses have frequently been known to say, "I don't know why I did that! It was just instinct." That explanation, as the basis of a nursing judgment, is simply not true. The nurse may not have been aware of the process involved in making the nursing decision, but previous knowledge and/or experience were undoubtedly involved. By becoming more aware of these conceptualizations, nurse clinicians can develop a structure for identifying and organizing new information and making it accessible for use in clinical practice.

Propositions are the other major component in a theory. A proposition is a statement describing the relationship between two or more concepts. If the statement is tentative, then it is called a *hypothesis*. In a theory, the propositions must be systematically interrelated and empirically tested (Williams 1979).

Dickoff and James, Ellis, and Hardy all discuss factors to consider in evaluating a theory, though the ones chosen vary from author to author. One helpful set of criteria for a theory is that of the National League for Nursing, which states that a theory should

1. include a set of postulates and definitions of terms used in the postulate.
2. be explicit in its boundaries and its concerns and limitations.
3. be internally consistent, with concepts logically interrelated.
4. be congruent with empirical data.
5. be capable of generating hypotheses.
6. contain generalizations that go beyond the data.
7. be verifiable and stated in such a way that it is possible to collect data to prove or disprove it.
8. explain past events and predict future ones (Faculty-Curriculum Development 1975)

Definition of a Conceptual Framework

What relationship does a theory have to a conceptual framework? Dickoff and James describe a theory as a conceptual system or framework invented for some purpose (Dickoff and James 1968). This statement suggests (and most authorities agree) that all theories contain conceptual frameworks (Dickoff and James 1968; Ellis 1968). The opposite is *not* true, however: not all conceptual frameworks are theories. Williams (1979) addresses the issue of distinguishing conceptual frameworks and theories very well:

The distinction between a theory and a conceptual framework, admittedly somewhat fuzzy, appears then to be a matter of the range of phenomena included and the degree of specificity of the concepts and hypotheses. Conceptual frameworks are broader, more general, and more vague. They are not easily submitted to empirical testing. Theories, by contrast, tend to deal with more limited phenomena, to be more precise (even to the point of including quantifiable relationships), and to have their concepts sufficiently well defined to allow for empirical testing.

For the purposes of this chapter, a *theory* is composed of precisely defined concepts, preferably quantifiable, with specific hypotheses regarding the interrelationship of the concepts. In contrast, a *conceptual framework* refers to a group of concepts and their relationships and is more general in nature and broader in scope. A conceptual framework should serve as the blueprint of a house, with theories as the walls.

Classifications of Nursing Theories

Theories are developed for the purpose of describing, explaining, predicting, and controlling phenomena (Jacox 1974). In fact, the four kinds of nursing theory identified by Dickoff and James (1968) are directly related to these four purposes. These authors recognize:

1. factor-isolating theories.
2. factor-relating theories (situation-depicting theories).
3. situation-relating theories.
4. situation-producing (prescriptive) theories.

Factor-isolating theory is the most basic kind of descriptive theory. It simply isolates factors and labels them. This type of theory also provides descriptive definitions as well as labels. Diers uses the nursing diagnosis project as an example of this type of theory. The project's goal is simply to identify nursing diagnoses that are independent (isolated) and describe the characteristics that are common to each diagnosis (Dickoff and James 1968).

Factor-relating theory relates the factors or describes the linkages between concepts. This type of theory is often called descriptive in other disciplines. In this type of study one merely looks at the relationships among factors or concepts.

Situation-relating theory is predictive or explanatory. Actual predictions about the concept relationships are made and then tested. Examples are learning theory and behavior modification. This type of theory includes both causal theories ("if x, then y") and correlational theories that do not include prediction (x and y vary together, but x does not necessarily cause y or y cause x) (Hardy 1974; Diers 1979).

Situation-producing theory contains prescriptions for activities to bring about the goals defined within the theory. This level of theory subsumes the other three and is the one that is needed in the nursing profession (Dickoff and James 1968). Theory at this level would give the practitioner the prescription for the nursing action that would result in a specific goal.

Diers (1979) has found no examples of prescriptive theory as such in the literature. Jacox (1974), in addressing the issue of theory development in nursing, claims that the behavioral and social sciences are behind the physical sciences in the development and testing of theories. Furthermore, she characterizes the applied fields, such as nursing and social work, as even less developed. Given these limitations in the development of nursing theory, the need for advanced nurse clinicians to study nursing theory becomes clear: one of their goals must be to develop their own conceptual frameworks for practice;

and then, as they test their frameworks in practice; they will help build a scientific foundation for nursing.

THEORY ANALYSIS

Four theories with special relevance to community health nursing practice will be summarized here. Each one contains concepts, constructs, and assumptions that are commonly thought to be related to practice. From this perspective, each of these theories suggests concepts that should be considered for inclusion in the clinician's own conceptual framework.

The Theoretical Basis of Nursing (Martha E. Rodgers)

Rodgers (1970) bases her conceptual model of nursing on the life process of humans, which is "characterized by wholeness, openness, unidirectionality, pattern and organization, sentience and thought." Human life is likened to a Slinky, the child's toy with undulating spirals. These represent the rhythms of nature. People are seen as constantly interacting with their environment in consistent patterns that form an energy field. The energy or electrical field then moves in Slinky-like fashion, expanding and contracting but moving unidirectionally through the age span.

Rodgers (1970) describes the life process as homeodynamic, not in the sense of achieving equilibrium but in the sense of achieving new dimensions. She has identified specific principles — synchrony, helicy, and resonancy — that "postulate the way the life process is and predict the nature of its evolving." Each of these principles, according to this theory, is useful in the practice of community health nursing.

The principle of *synchrony* refers to the state of both the environmental and human fields at any particular point in space and time. Although a nurse may select a specific time to assess a family, he or she does so with the knowledge that the family is not static. The principle of synchrony also implies that the past cannot be repeated; for example, Rodgers (1970) believes that adult behaviors cannot be interpreted as developmental because of the differences in space–time in which they occur.

Helicy refers to the unidirectional yet rhythmical nature of the life process. For example, menstrual cycles recur at certain intervals, yet each one brings a woman closer to the cessation of her childbearing years. In community health nursing the identification of certain patterns of events allows the nurse to predict their occurrences and to prepare clients to manage these life events. Recognizing the phases of loss, for example, would help a nurse give proper care to an individual working through the death of a spouse.

The principle of *resonancy* "postulates that change in pattern and organization of the human field and the environmental field is propagated by waves."

Thus, changes in the life process occur by repatterning of both man and the environment (Rodgers 1970).

All of these principles describe a way of perceiving man and the life process. They are postulates and need to be tested on real life phenomena to verify their scientific value. In order for nursing to continue to assist people to achieve their maximum health potential, nursing must increase its knowledge of the life process and man's response to life changes. This knowledge could then be applied in clinical practice.

The Adaptation Model of Nursing (Sister Callista Roy)

Roy describes nursing as a scientific method of providing care for the ill or potentially ill. Her adaptation model for nursing care is composed of three elements: the recipient of nursing care, the goal of nursing, and the nursing activities. Roy's model (1976) resembles Rodger's theory in that an understanding of man is the major premise. People, the recipients of nursing care, are viewed as biopsychosocial beings who are in constant interaction with a changing environment. They have biological, psychological, and sociological needs that they must satisfy to maintain integrity. To deal with the constantly changing environment while maintaining this integrity, people exercise both innate and acquired coping mechanisms (Roy 1976). An example of an innate mechanism is the increase in heart rate with exercise. An acquired mechanism is the placement of a footboard to prevent foot drop.

Coping mechanisms can be either positive or negative, depending upon whether the action taken preserves or compromises the individual's integrity. Applying sunscreen while spending a day on the beach would be a positive adaptation, while not applying it and becoming sunburned would be a negative adaptation. To determine whether any response is adaptive or maladaptive, a nurse using this model would analyze the focal stimulus or degree of change, contextual stimuli that refer to all other concurrent stimuli, and any additional influences such as attitudes or beliefs (Roy 1976).

Roy has tentatively identified four adaptive modes that people use to respond to both internal and external environmental changes. These are *physiological needs, self-concept, role-function*, and *interdependence*. Each of these modes has been further subdivided into specific need areas with specific adaptive problems identified for each need area. An example would be role conflict and role failure, which are adaptive problems of the role-function mode. Roy views the goal of nursing to be the promotion of human adaption in each of the adaptive modes, in all varying states on the health-illness continuum from death to peak wellness.

In applying the Roy adaptation model to the nursing process, the nurse's first assessment is the client's condition in each of the adaptive modes. From this assessment the nurse identifies maladaptive behaviors or behaviors that need reinforcing. Each of these behaviors is then subjected to a second-level assessment, which refers to identification of the focal, contextual, and residual stimuli. Having clearly identified the behaviors requiring change or reinforcement, the nurse states the goal in behavioral terms and develops approaches to achieve it (Roy 1976).

Historically, community health nursing has had a generalist approach to practice. Roy's model is especially applicable in that it applies to all stages of wellness and illness yet does not limit itself to a particular age or medical condition. Also, the idea of analyzing adaptive behavior objectively prior to developing nursing actions is especially beneficial in the delivery of nursing services to groups of people from various cultures.

Toward a Theory for Nursing (Imogene M. King)

King's discussion of nursing theory focuses initially on the description, development, and utilization of a conceptual framework. This discussion is easily comprehended and thus provides an excellent resource for the beginner in conceptual development. The discussion progresses from concept definition and its relationship to theory development to theory sources and their relationships to nursing. Prior to describing her general framework for nursing, King reviews societal changes that are influencing nursing. She specifically mentions the information explosion, the changes in types of educational programs, and the increasing demand for specialization. These changes are the reason that nursing needs a "unifying focus" (King 1971). King (1971) believes that a conceptual framework can provide the mechanism for this unification. Her frame of reference for nursing is based upon the following belief:

Nurses, in the performance of their roles and responsibilities, assist individuals and groups in society to attain, maintain, and restore health. In the process of functioning in social institutions, nurses assist individuals to meet their basic needs at some point in time in the life cycle when they cannot do this for themselves. An understanding of basic human needs in the physical, social, emotional, and intellectual realm of the life process from conception to old age, within the context of social systems of the culture in which nurses live and work is essential and basic content for learning the practice of nursing.

King (1971) identifies four concepts in her conceptual framework for nursing, which she calls *social system, perception, interpersonal relationships,* and *health.* She views people as interacting with their environment and nursing as having a responsibility to "influence the environment and exert some control over it". This idea definitely relates to community health and the agent, host, and environment relationships that epidemiology has used to study disease causality for years (Leavell and Clark 1965). Other King ideas that relate to community health nursing are: (a) the client defined as an individual or group, (b) the goal of nursing as the attaining, maintaining, or regaining of health, and (c) the concept of health perceived as a continuous adaptation to internal and external stresses.

The Nature of Nursing (Virginia Henderson)

Henderson, one of the earlier theorists, begins her discussion of nursing by documenting the need for the nursing profession, whose services affect human life, to define its services. She then presents the complications nursing faces in accomplishing such a task. Included in that list are the variety of roles and positions nurses fill, educational modes and levels of preparation, and certification and licensing criteria (Henderson 1966).

Henderson believes that the nurse should be as independent a practitioner as possible and sees the goal of nursing as the assistance of the patient in his or her activities of daily living. The nurse should focus on the patient's entire life and assist the patient in improving all aspects of that existence, not just the ones affected by an illness. This goal requires the nurse to do more than simply carry out physician orders. In addition, the nurse identifies potential health problems, develops and monitors improvement programs, or counsels and refers patients and their families to other agencies for assistance. For example, a mother who visits a pediatrician because her child has an ear infection might be counseled by the nurse to contact the La Leche League for assistance with her own concerns about breast feeding. Another example is assisting a healthy client to improve his health status by developing and maintaining an exercise program.

Henderson (1966) views nurses as the authority on *basic nursing care*, which she describes as

. . . helping the patient with the following activities or providing conditions under which he can perform them unaided:

1.   Breathe normally.
2.   Eat and drink adequately.
3.   Eliminate body wastes.
4.   Move and maintain desirable postures.
5.   Sleep and rest.
6.   Select suitable clothes — dress and undress.
7.   Maintain body temperature with the normal range by adjusting clothing and modifying the environment.
8.   Keep the body clean and well groomed and protect the integument.
9.   Avoid dangers in the environment and avoid injuring others.
10.   Communicate with others in expressing emotions, needs, fears, or opinions.
11.   Worship according to one's faith.
12.   Work in such a way that there is a sense of accomplishment.
13.   Play or participate in various forms of recreation.
14.   Learn, discover, or satisfy the curiosity that leads to normal development and health and use the available health facilities.

This view of nursing, as merely a supplement to independent functioning of the patient and family, parallels closely the practice of community health nurses, especially at the individual level. One example is home health care, where nurses enter the home primarily to provide assistance to the family until they are capable of managing the situation themselves. In this type of nursing care delivery, the nurse determines the aspects of daily living with which the family needs assistance, develops with the family a plan to improve those areas, and then gradually decreases assistance as the family becomes more self-sufficient. In addition, using this framework, the nurse would screen all of these areas of self-care to determine if nursing intervention was needed in any other area.

These 14 activities of daily living have been very useful to community health nurses as a guide for identifying the nursing services needed by a family. Number 9, which refers to environmental hazards, encompasses the entire scope of prevention, including immunizations, sewage disposal, pollution education, and traffic laws. The actual nurse role in each of these areas varies widely from counseling individual patients to testifying at Senate committee hearings. Nurses who know the value of environmental controls need to work to effect their enactment and enforcement. Remember however, as Henderson suggests, that the nurse should *assist* the patient, not *do for* the patient. Identifying the need for a safe play area to keep children out of the street is fine, but the nurse should not assume the responsibility of securing one. Instead, the nurse might assist the neighbors in the process of organizing and developing a plan to find a solution to the problem (Henderson 1966).

All four of the preceding nursing theories identify the importance of people's interaction with their environment and the changes that are constantly occurring. This characteristic makes them all very applicable to community health nursing, which strives to provide health services to clients (whether family, group, or community) in their own environment.

All of the theories refer to health as a continuum, but only Roy identifies one end of the continuum as illness. Henderson does recognize functions with which a client may need help, but does not call this situation illness. Henderson's concept of health expressed here is broad, encompasses all aspects of life, and corresponds to the general nature of community health nursing practice.

From these theories, the significant concepts are identified that are thought to influence the health of clients. These concepts, then, become the analyses of variables, which can be specified at the operational level. These operational level variables are then ready for empirical testing in practice settings.

Both Roy and Henderson discuss the concepts they view relevant to the assessment of the *individual,* such as self-concept, sleep, and rest. Rogers and King, on the other hand, cite factors such as synchrony, and social system, which are applicable to either the individual, family, or the community. The theory selected as a potential guide to practice should include concepts reflecting the nature of the practice in which the nurse is engaged.

COMPONENTS OF A CONCEPTUAL FRAMEWORK

Analyzing a developed nursing theory acquaints the nurse clinician with concepts that have been identified and described by others, as well as with the process of constructing a conceptual framework.

An additional benefit of the process is the opportunity to examine new concepts and new perspectives of thinking. This section discusses some of the major considerations for developing a conceptual framework for community health nursing. First, several assumptions and philosophical statements will be examined for their potential contribution to, or extension of, a conceptual framework. Second, definitions of community health nursing practice are presented for the reader to identify additional major ideas that could be expressed as concepts for inclusion in a framework. Third, the Standards of Community Health Nursing Practice developed in 1973 are given to provide the structure within which the framework must function. Last, recognition is made of the fact that observation of practice is the best and most direct means of deriving practice-relevant concepts. Elements of conceptual frameworks developed for specific practice purposes are likely to draw from both theory and practice statements (deductive approach); and empirical observations of clinicians as presented in this section (inductive approach).

Philosophy and Basic Assumptions

Philosophical beliefs are the foundation for the manner in which one relates to the world and, consequently, the way one practices nursing. These underlying beliefs must be delineated prior to the development of a conceptual framework for practice because they will undoubtedly determine which theories and concepts will be relevant to a personal practice framework.

Philosophical statements frequently describe beliefs about people, nature, rights, health, and life. Below are some philosophical statements about community health nursing.

1.   The consumer is viewed as a client rather than a patient in an effort to emphasize his or her active participation in the securing of health care (Tinkham and Voorhies 1977; Fromer 1979).
2.   Health is a basic human right and quality health care should be equally available to all people (Freeman 1970; Hall and Weaver 1977).
3.   Consumer needs dictate the setting and mode of health care delivery (Freeman 1970; Hall and Weaver 1977).
4.   The emphasis of community health nursing care is the promotion of health (Archer and Fleshman 1979; Benson and McDevitt 1980).

One can see how such beliefs influence the manner in which nursing care is delivered. When developing a conceptual framework for practice, one must first describe one's personal philosophy of life as it relates to health and its maintenance. From this statement are derived the basic assumptions about the provision of nursing care. These assumptions may be stated with or without justification, but together they form the "givens" of the practice. Some examples of basic assumptions selected from student conceptual framework papers follow:

1. Man is ever dynamic and capable of change (Grover 1978).
2. Families are more than the sum total of the individual members (Duncan 1978).
3. Health cannot be perceived as a need if other, more basic needs have not been met (Robinson ME 1978).

Basic assumptions, then, reflect the nurse's perception of the world and how it functions. These perceptions obviously also affect the nature of practice.

Thus the initial step in developing a conceptual framework for community health nursing practice requires that the nurse identify and describe the beliefs held about people, society, and health. An additional possibility is the enumeration of premises that the nurse considers to be true and on which all further statements and discussions will be based. These statements then constitute the philosophical basis for a personal conceptual framework for practice.

Definition of Community Health Nursing Practice

Building a conceptual framework for practice permits the development of a working definition of community health nursing practice. This section presents some of the facets of a community health nursing definition.

Defining a clinical practice involves describing its client focus, practice activities, and goals. Although never simple, this task in community health nursing is especially difficult due to the traditionally generalist perspective of the community health nurse. The following are varied sample definitions of community health nursing:

1. Community Health Nursing is a synthesis of nursing practice and public health practice applied to promoting and preserving the health of populations. The nature of this practice is general and comprehensive. It is not limited to a particular age or diagnostic group. It is continuing, not episodic. The dominant responsibility is to the population as a whole. Therefore, nursing directed to individuals, families or groups contributes to the health of the total population. Health promotion, health maintenance, health education, coordination and continuity of care are utilized in a holistic approach to the family, group and community. The nurse's actions acknowledge the need for comprehensive health planning, recognize the influences of social and ecological issues, give attention to populations at risk and utilize the dynamic forces which influence change (Standards of Community Health Nursing Practice 1973).

2. Community nursing is a learned practice with the ultimate goal of contributing, as individuals and in collaboration with others, to the promotion of the client's optimum level of functioning through teaching and the delivery of care (Archer and Fleshman 1979).
3. Public health nursing is a field of specialization within both professional nursing and the broad area of organized public health practice. It utilizes the philosophy, content, and methods of public health and the knowledge and skills of professional nursing. It is responsible for the provision of nursing services on a family centered basis for individuals and groups at home, at work, at school, and in public health centers. Public health nursing interweaves its services with those of other health and allied workers and participates in the planning and implementation of community health programs (Hanlon 1979).
4. Community health nursing is seen as a population-based obligation, realized through a multidisciplinary ecologically oriented effort and utilizing concepts and skills that derive both from generic nursing and from public health practices. It focuses on nursing the *community* in contradistinction to nursing *in* the community. Family nursing care is seen as an essential aspect of health care of the population, and the community health nurse's responsibility is seen as encompassing but not being limited to this aspect of the program (Robischon 1975).
5. Public health nursing synthesizes the body of knowledge from the public health sciences and professional nursing theories. The implied overriding goal is to improve the health of the community by identifying sub-groups (aggregates) within the community population which are at high risk of illness, disability, or premature death and directing resources toward these groups. This lies at the heart of primary prevention and health promotion. Public health nursing accomplishes its goal by working with groups, families, and individuals as well as by functioning in multidisciplinary teams and programs. Success in the reduction of risks and in improving the health of the community is dependent upon a full range of consumer involvement, especially from those groups at risk as well as the community and its members, in health planning, in self help, and in individual responsibility for personal health habits which promote health and a safe environment (Public Health Nursing Section 1980).

All of these definitions specify the client and the goals of community health nursing. The client to whom community health nursing is directed may be an individual, family, group, or community. In developing a framework of practice it is important to include a clear definition of which level of *client* is being addressed: this will influence the method of intervention selected.

All the sample definitions agree that a central goal of community health nursing is health promotion. The term *health promotion* here refers to the three levels of prevention: primary (health promotion and specific protection), secondary (early diagnosis, prompt treatment, and disability limitation), and tertiary (rehabilitation) (Leavell and Clark 1965). Both client and goal are aspects of community health nursing that should be addressed in a personal practice definition.

Another important aspect of a personal definition of community health nursing is the activities of the practice, which include practice setting and nursing activities. See Tables 2.1 and 2.2 for an idea of the variety of practice settings

Table 2.1. Practice Setting

Health Oriented	Non-Health Oriented
Health department — local, state	Schools
Visiting nurse services	Colleges
Hospitals — discharge planners	Industries
Outpatient departments	Community planning
Health maintenance organizations	Research foundations
Physician offices	Consulting firms
Comprehensive health centers	Professional organizations

and the diversity of nursing activities. Table 2.1 presents examples of practice settings in both health oriented and non-health oriented agencies. Table 2.2 classifies nursing activities into direct, semi-direct, and indirect.

With so many possible practice sites and nursing activities, guidelines must be found for use in controlling the quality of practice. The American Nurses Association's *Standards of Community Health Nursing Practice* provides a general structure. Although specific criteria for measuring quality of care are also needed, these standards at least identify evaluation areas. They are as follows:

Standard I — The collection of data about the health status of the consumer is systematic and continuous. The data are accessible, communicated, and recorded.
Standard II — Nursing diagnoses are derived from health status data.
Standard III — Plans for nursing service include goals derived from nursing diagnoses.
Standard IV — Plans for nursing service include priorities and nursing approaches or measures to achieve the goals derived from nursing diagnoses.

Table 2.2. Classification of Nursing Activities

Direct	Semi-direct	Indirect
Case finding	Teaching	Planning program
Triage	Supervising	Evaluating
Assessments	Consulting	program
Treatment	Evaluating staff	effectiveness
Referral	Providing direct	Controlling service
Teaching	client services	delivery
Follow-up		Policy department
Evaluating client care		
Collaboration		

Reprinted with permission from Archer and Fleshman 1979.

Standard V — Nursing actions provide for consumer participation in health promotion, maintenance, and restoration.

Standard VI — Nursing actions assist consumers to maximize health potential.

Standard VII — The consumer's progress toward goal achievement is determined by the consumer and the nurse.

Standard VIII — Nursing actions involve ongoing reassessment, reordering of priorities, new goal setting and revisions of the nursing plan (Standards of Community Health Nursing Practice 1973).

Therefore, in the development of a personal practice definition of community health nursing, the nurse's own current practice should be compared to the legal definition of nursing and the established national standards.

In summary, a definition of community health practice should concisely describe the client focus, nursing activities, and goals of the clinical practice. The process presented here for formulating a personal practice definition included critical study of various definitions of community health nursing, a description of the client, consideration of practice sites, nursing activities, standards, and goals. From this diversity of information the nurse selects the pieces with which to forge a personal framework for community health nursing suitable to the specific practice situation. The framework can be as broad or as narrow as the nurse desires, depending upon the purpose for its use. The dimensions, when nurse specific, assist in setting priorities for services at all levels, from individual client care to group programs and even agency goals.

In identifying concepts from observation of practice, a nurse must be certain that the concepts are reflective of personal philosophy and definition of community health nursing practice. (See Fig. 2.1.) Otherwise the concepts will not be useful when implemented in practice. If the concepts identified in a practice seem to be in conflict with personal philosophy or practice definition, then either the concept definition or the practice philosophy must be adjusted. It is possible that changes in practice have occurred without any analysis of the significance of these changes in relation to practice definitions and personal beliefs about nursing care. However, any conflict between concepts of current practice and personal beliefs or practice definitions must be resolved in order for the conceptual framework to be really useful to the clinician in making practice decisions.

Having identified concepts from observations of clinical practice, the nurse must then select a concise definition for each one. The definitions may be original, quoted, or a combination of both. A very useful reference for this phase of concept derivation is King's *Toward A Theory of Nursing* (King 1971). The concept definitions in a conceptual framework should be abstract and flexible enough to allow for alteration over time. King (1971) suggests that one of the purposes of a conceptual frame of reference for nursing is to assist practitioners in accommodating new knowledge throughout the lifelong process of learning. As a result, nurse clinicians should anticipate evolutionary

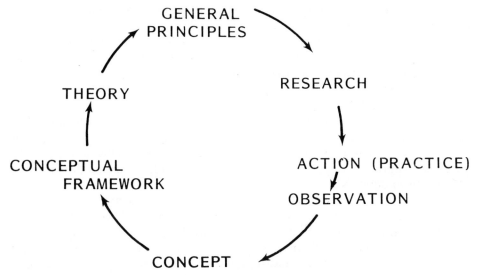

Figure 2.1.   Process of concept development for practice

changes in their personal conceptual frameworks from the acquisition of new knowledge. This process is to be expected and not avoided.

Selection of the concepts or ideas that have particular significance for a personal practice is followed by their being labeled and defined. For the novice in conceptual development, a one-word label for each concept provides a simplicity that is often helpful. *Health* is an example of a one-word label for a complex concept. However, in defining a concept, the meaning for a particular framework must be explained. Health could be defined in either of the following ways depending on the nurse's purpose.

Health refers to high-level wellness, to an integrated method of functioning that is oriented toward maximizing the potential to which the individual is capable. It requires that the individual maintain a continuum of balance and purposeful direction within the environment where he is functioning. (Dunn 1961)

Health is a state of complete physical, mental, and social well-being and not merely the absence of disease or infirmity. (World Health Organization 1980)

If the nurse desires to apply these concepts in clinical practice, they would have to be operationally defined. Two such examples follow:

Client states he is not sick.
Client is at low risk for a specific illness compared to general population.

An operational definition should be as concrete and objective as possible. The more explicit the definition the easier it will be to operationalize in practice.

Such clarity will also facilitate subsequent application and investigation of the conceptual framework.

It is at this point in conceptual framework development that the spotlight turns to clinical practice. Having identified and defined the concepts, a clinician must delineate and describe their relationship to one another to formulate a useful nursing process guide. Again, the clinician should investigate any theory or portion thereof that has personal appeal, especially from an experientially derived belief system. Many great discoveries have been made unexpectedly, and this process of testing the relevance of concepts and theories from new perspectives is another means of promoting creative nursing interventions. The only criterion that must be met is that the concept be explained sufficiently to be well understood.

In review, concepts should be derived from and reflective of the nurse's clinical practice. The process of constructing a conceptual framework includes identification of concepts that are relevant to the practice situation and that may be accomplished by theory analysis or practice observation. The concepts are then labeled and defined. Lastly, the manner in which the concepts relate to one another is described. This last step is important because it delineates the application of the framework to the nursing process.

PRACTICAL APPLICATIONS: DEVELOPMENT OF CONCEPTUAL FRAMEWORK MODELS

One method of presenting a conceptual framework is in a visual model that may assist the readers' understanding. This includes the use of a graphic model or a visual picture of the relationships of the major concepts. Included here are several samples, drawn from student papers, of visual conceptual framework models plus brief explanations of their relationship to nursing practice. The conceptual framework model in Figure 2.2 depicts health as a concept of self that includes having self-worth and control over the environment. The goal of nursing is to increase these aspects of the client's self-concept. The model uses concepts from systems theory and Becker's "Health Belief Model" to describe the interaction between the client and his or her environment (Becker and Maimon 1975). The client can be an individual, family, group, or community. However, changing the client definition also changes the scope of the primary and secondary suprasystems (Robinson A 1978).

In applying the nursing process to this model, the nurse assesses the client's concept of a health need by examining all the inputs from the suprasystems and by identifying the *modifying factors* and *cues to action* that are contributing to the client's state of health (Public Health Nursing Section 1980). The nurse then devises a plan to assist the client in clarifying his or her perceptions and interpretations of the inputs. Nursing care goals and strategies for achieving them are formulated with the client. In addition, criteria are identified for evaluating the success or failure of the nursing actions. In this model, nursing

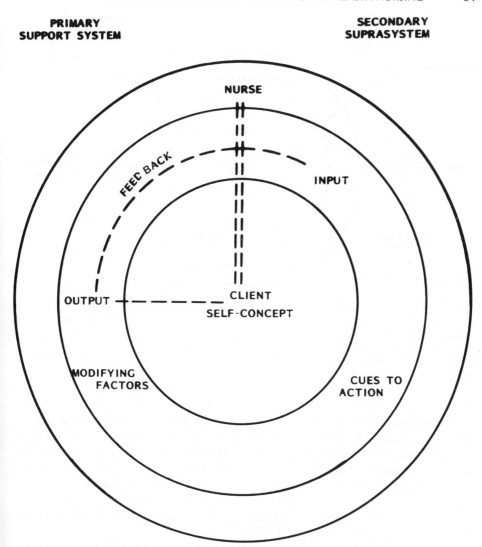

Figure 2.2. Client receptiveness to change model

interventions foster self-worth of the client by improving self-regulation, which results in an enhanced self-concept.

The model in Figure 2.3 emphasizes the relationship between the nurse and the individual client (Casaw 1978). Health is viewed on a continuum from illness to high wellness. The four major influences on a client's health status are categorized as biological, environmental, health care systems, and lifestyle (Lalonde 1974). The goal of nursing is to assist the client in managing each of these influences in order to improve his or her health.

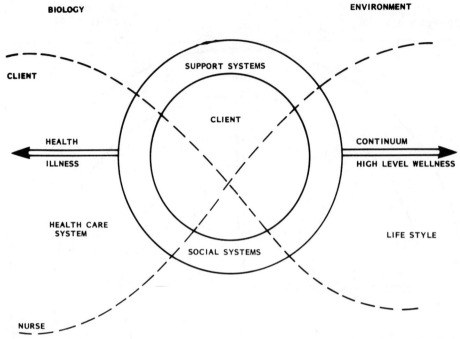

Figure 2.3.   Reciprocal interaction between client health continuum and nurse's role in wellness care: A model

The dashed lines in Figure 2.3 represent the client's relationship to the nurse. This relationship varies from dependency in severe illness to near, but not absolute, independence. It is assumed that the nurse could always offer the client some suggestions for improving his or her level of health, especially since high-level wellness is defined as " . . . an integrated method of functioning which is oriented toward maximizing the potential to which the individual is capable" (Dunn 1961). In this model the client could also be defined as a family, group, or community.

In applying this model to the nursing process, the nurse assesses the inputs and outputs of the environmental, biological, lifestyle, and health system influences on the client. Then a plan for nursing care is developed, which considers the client's support systems, with the goal of moving the client along the health continuum toward better health (Casaw 1978).

The model presented in Figure 2.4 views the client as a system that interacts with other systems. While defining the client as an individual, the model depicts a unidirectional progression of life from birth to death (Rodgers 1970). The double axes for the life process and health status indicate that a person could be healthy at death. Health is defined as an optimum level of mental, physical, and social functioning (World Health Organization 1980).

The nurse using this model in nursing practice assesses the client's developmental stage, health status, and support systems. A plan of care is then

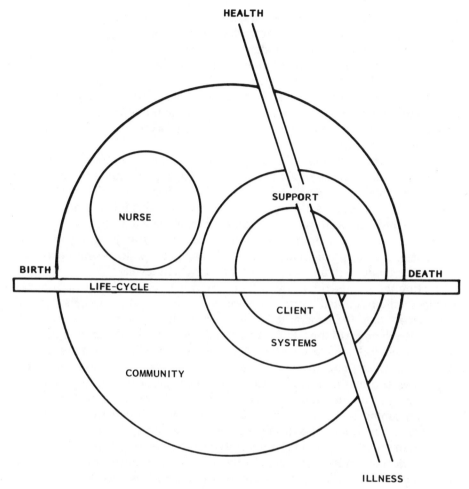

Figure 2.4.   Client systems assessment model

developed to improve the client's health. This plan of care could be implemented at any system level, i.e., individual, family, or community (Robinson, ME 1978).

These models, although simplistic in nature, are presented as examples of how other nurses combine concepts and theories to develop their own personal framework for practice. In addition, Figures 2.2–2.4 demonstrate how a visual model can clarify the written explanation of a conceptual framework.

Clinical Application to Community Health Nursing

The "pilot study" phase of developing a conceptual framework for practice gives the clinician an opportunity to experiment with practicing community health nursing using the framework. Two issues must be considered in applying a specific conceptual framework to nursing practice: (a) the translation of aspects of the conceptual model to all phases of the nursing process (assessment, planning, implementation, and evaluation), and (b) the use of the model in the delivery of direct nursing service. Having thoroughly analyzed the research on the theories and concepts incorporated into the conceptual framework, the nurse clinician will be aware of the framework's strengths and weaknesses. The nurse can then adapt for the weaknesses in the application of the framework to the nursing process.

Following such careful, detailed preparation, the clinician must then test the framework in a current clinicial setting by using it to guide the delivery of nursing services in a real life situation to real life clients. (Results from research testing various elements of practice are discussed in detail in another section.) Since the nurse clinician will be functioning on at least one, and perhaps more than one, client level (individual, family, or community) during the development of a conceptual framework, it is anticipated that the situations used to test the model will include more than one client level.

Testing the framework in the actual provision of community health nursing services will undoubtedly uncover some of its values and limitations. Since the clinician adapted for some of the previously known disadvantages, evaluation of the effectiveness of the adaptations should be possible. Evaluating the assets of the framework should include a description of specific characteristics of the conceptual model and their influence on the aspects of the nursing process, i.e., types and methods of data to collect, client participation in plan of care, strategies for nursing interventions and criteria and mode of evaluation.

In explaining the evaluation of the framework subsequent to testing, the nurse clinician should specifically address the advantages and disadvantages of the framework for guiding community health nursing practice. It is through such work that nurses will more clearly articulate the concepts of clinical practice. These concepts then can serve as a guide for research and curriculum planning.

Implications for Education and Research

A conceptual framework for nursing practice is a method of organizing knowledge so that it is useful to the nurse in making judgments about the provision of nursing care. Conceptual frameworks when used as a basis for educational or research programs serve the same purpose: the provision of a structure for decision making.

After constructing a conceptual framework for community health nursing and applying it to the nursing process in an actual practice setting, the nurse can describe the implications of this practice perspective for community health nursing education and research. Identifying these implications is not difficult, because the framework developer has already thoughtfully considered the concepts and theories that compose the framework and has actually experimented with the framework in clinical practice.

In speculating about the educational implications of a particular framework for community health nursing practice, a clinician would probably identify concepts and/or content areas that would need to be learned in order to deliver nursing care within the framework. There might even be some courses identified as prerequisites. Sources providing more information for the learner, such as books and periodical references, would be of assistance. In addition, having actually practiced nursing from the framework, the author could describe a clinicial experience that would facilitate applying this framework to practice. Some characteristics perhaps to mention are agency structure, practice site, nursing activities, and client response or outcome. Any clarification of helpful or detrimental aspects regarding the learning of clinical practice from the particular framework would be informative. For example, if the conceptual framework defined a family as an open system, then an understanding of systems theory would be essential for anyone attempting to use this framework in clinical practice.

In commenting on the implications for research of a specific practice perspective, a nurse should first identify any concepts, theories, or portions thereof that have already been investigated. On the other hand, if the concept differs in some way or if it is entirely new, this information, too, should be conveyed. The discussion should also include clues or suggestions that would be of assistance to anyone attempting to conduct research utilizing the framework for community health nursing practice.

Requiring nurses to consider the research possibilities of a practice framework, especially the nurse involved in advanced study or expanded practice, has a hidden agenda. Ideally the nurses will identify some aspect of the framework that could be thoroughly developed into a research question for a thesis, dissertation, or other research project. One advantage in this sequence is the considerable amount of literature review that will have been already completed. Another advantage lies in the drawing of practice and research closer together. Since nursing is a practice profession, the value of research is measured by its usefulness in making clinical practice decisions. Nurse clinicians in active practice would logically be most likely to identify phenomena whose study would provide useful information about that particular practice. Then, since they were interested in the research study from its inception, the translation of the findings into practice would be facilitated.

Another possibility is that the suggested research ideas may appeal to someone else because the framework is clearly developed or because the examples are real, thus making the "task" of doing "research" much more appealing.

Creation of a Framework

The final step in the development of a conceptual framework for practice is the written product. The development, in writing, of a conceptual model for practice is a difficult task. One nurse likened the experience to that of childbirth, requiring strenuous and exhausting work but resulting in exhilaration with the finished product (Casaw 1978). The synthesis that occurs in the writing of the conceptual framework is essential to its utility and thus to the birth of new ideas.

The actual task of explaining the model that is the design for personal practice requires the reconceptualization of all theories and concepts studied into unique combinations and innovative applications. In addition, the nurse must then demonstrate how the conceptual model could be used in applying the nursing process. This demonstration should clarify the influence of the model on each aspect of the nursing process: assessment, planning, intervention, and evaluation. The framework must be consistent with the nurse's beliefs about practice and contain original ideas or combinations that reflect those beliefs.

Several problems may arise in the production of a paper that describes a conceptual framework for practice. One is concept selection, definition, and labeling. A review of the literature will quickly show that there is no one definition of even what a concept is. However, there are commonalities. The nurse must either compile a definition or use one from the authorities, with the purpose of defining the concept for that paper, not for the entire profession. Basic concepts should be chosen cautiously as well in order to limit the difficulty of determining their relationships to one another. The use of an authority's definition for any concept must be accompanied by a critical analysis to determine whether it is suitable to the nurse's personal beliefs about nursing practice. Of great importance is the ability to enumerate why the chosen definition is significant to a particular nursing practice model.

Labeling is another potential problem area. Nurses must be comfortable in defining "their" concepts and using them as such. An important point to remember for the novice is that one-word labels provide a useful simplicity.

Another possible problem area is that of attempting to cover all aspects of community health nursing practice without sufficient background or experience. For example, in community health nursing the client may be an individual, family, group, or community. If a nurse has never really practiced community level nursing intervention or has not had additional theory on nursing a community, it would be best to limit the framework focus to the individual or family. Undoubtedly, the practice framework will undergo evolutionary changes with additional education and experience, but for the first attempt a nurse should limit the focus to the most familiar client. Otherwise, in attempting to relate the framework to an unfamiliar client, the nurse will have difficulty explaining how the framework is applied in practice.

SUMMARY

Although the production of a conceptual framework for community health nursing is difficult, the effort required to create the model ensures that the nurse can easily explain to others — be they peers, non-nursing colleagues, or clients — the perspective utilized in making clinical judgments. This is perhaps the most significant benefit of a conceptual framework for practice. By clarifying the parameters of clinical judgment, the nurse supplies the health care consumers and providers with the data needed to predict service expectations. This predictability will decrease the confusion regarding the community health nurse clinician role.

In addition to providing direction for practice, a conceptual framework can form the basis of a visual model. Models can show relationships among concepts, and serve as guides for planning programs of research and education. The guidelines for model building given in this chapter will provide the community health nurse leader with the basic tools for designing the central elements and relationships to be addressed in any health program.

REFERENCES

Archer SE, and Fleshman RP. Community health nursing patterns and practice. 2nd ed. North Scituate, MA.: Duxbury Press, 1979.

Becker MH, and Maimon LA. Sociobehavioral determinants of compliance with health and medical care recommendations. Med Care 1975; 13:10.

Benson ER, and McDevitt JQ. Community health and nursing practice. Englewood Cliffs, N.J.: Prentice-Hall, 1980.

Casaw PO. Conceptional framework for community health nursing. Unpublished manuscript. Rochester, NY: University of Rochester, 1978.

Crawford G, Dufault K, and Rudy E. Evolving issues in theory development. Nurs Outlook 1979; 27:346.

Dickoff J, and James P. Theory of theories: a position paper. Nurs Res 1968; 17:197.

Diers D. Research in nursing practice. Philadelphia: Lippincott, 1979.

Duncan KM. Conceptual framework for community health nursing with families. Unpublished manuscript. Rochester, New York: University of Rochester, 1978.

Dunn HL. High level wellness. Arlington, VA: Beatty, Ltd., 1961.

Ellis R. Characteristics of significant theories. Nurs Res 1968; 17:217.

Faculty-curriculum development: part III   conceptual framework — its meaning and function. New York: National League for Nursing, 1975.

Freeman RB. Community health nursing practice. Philadelphia: Saunders, 1970.

Fromer MJ. Community health care and the nursing process. St. Louis: Mosby, 1979.

Grover S. Conceptual framework of nursing. Unpublished manuscript. Rochester, NY: University of Rochester, 1978.

Hall JE, and Weaver BR, eds. Distributive nursing practice: a systems approach to community. Philadelphia: Lippincott, 1977.

Hanlon JJ. Public health administration and practice. St. Louis: Mosby 1979.

Hardy M. Theories: components, development, evaluation. Nurs Res 1974; 23:100.

Henderson V. The nature of nursing. New York: Macmillan, 1966.

Jacox A. Theory construction in nursing: an overview. Nurs Res 1974; 23:4.

King IM. Toward a theory for nursing. New York: Wiley 1971.

Lalonde M. A new perspective on the health of Canadians. Ottawa, Ontario; Dept. of National Health and Welfare, 1974.

Leavell HR, and Clark EG. Preventive medicine for the doctor in his community — an epidemiologic approach. 3rd ed. New York: McGraw-Hill, 1965.

Public Health Nursing Section. The definition and role of public health nursing in the delivery of health care (working draft III). Newsletter. American Public Health Association, June 1980.

Robischon P. Community nursing in a changing climate. In: Spradley BW, ed. Contemporary community nursing. Boston: Little, Brown, 1975.

Robinson A. The process of nursing the client self-concept: a conceptual framework for community health nursing. Unpublished manuscript, Rochester, NY: University of Rochester, 1978.

Robinson ME. A health potential model for community health nursing. Unpublished manuscript, Rochester, NY: University of Rochester, 1978.

Rodgers ME. An introduction to the theoretical basis of nursing. Philadelphia: F.A. Davis, 1970.

Roy SC. Introduction to nursing: an adaptation model. Englewood Cliffs, N.J.: Prentice-Hall, 1976.

Standards of community health nursing practice. Kansas City, Missouri: American Nurses Association, 1973.

Tinkham CW, and Voorhies EF. Community health nursing evolution and process. New York: Appleton-Century-Crofts, 1977.

Williams CA. The nature and development of conceptual frameworks. In: Downs FS, Fleming JW, eds. Issues in nursing research. New York: Appleton-Century-Crofts, 1979.

World Health Organization Constitution. In: Benson ER, McDevitt JQ. Community health and nursing practice. Englewood Cliffs, N.J.: Prentice-Hall, 1980.

COMMUNITY AS CLIENT   3

Nancy M. Watson

Community health nursing has had a long history of supporting practice with a community viewpoint. However, it has only been recently that community health nursing has endorsed a systematic process of community diagnosis as being an essential characteristic of community health nursing practice (American Public Health Association 1982). Accounts of early community health nurses suggest that needs of communities were determined inductively through living and working in them, rather than systematically through community diagnosis. Now many community health nursing leaders regard community diagnosis as the keystone to responsible community health nursing practice (Williams 1977; Freeman 1981). Numerous other health professions also support practice that considers the health of populations, rather than individuals. The interdisciplinary group of professionals in public health have historically viewed community diagnosis as the basis for action to control disease and improve health (McGavran 1971; Sheps 1976).

Community diagnosis is *the identification of health problems in communities or populations for the purpose of preventing them at the community or population level.* Actual practice of community diagnosis by community health nurses is probably rare. Williams has suggested several barriers to "the planning, delivery and evaluation of nursing services that are in touch with community needs" (Williams 1977). One barrier, and perhaps the most fundamental, is the failure of community health nurses to recognize or value the distinction between clinical practice, which focuses on the health of individuals and families and public health practice, which focuses on the health of populations. Failure to make this distinction is not unique to community health nurses. Few health professionals grasp this crucial difference.

THE RATIONALE FOR COMMUNITY DIAGNOSIS AND TREATMENT

Support for community diagnosis and treatment stems from the realization that people's ability to control disease is limited by their ability to identify the sources of risk to disease and change them. As McGavran (1971) pointed out, the most expert and successful treatment of sick individuals will not reduce the incidence of health problems. The prevention of health problems is not possible through early diagnosis and treatment of individuals. It is only possible through systematic reduction of risk in communities (a) by reducing individuals' exposure to risk or (b) by changing individuals' reactions to exposure.

Advocates of a community approach to health recognize that treatment, no matter how excellent and early, cannot prevent health problems from occurring. Treatment can speed recovery, reduce mortality, and prevent complications and disability — but it cannot protect others from the health problem. Preventive health efforts should emphasize reducing individuals' exposure to such risks as smoking, hypertension, obesity, lack of exercise, and social isolation or changing individuals' reactions to unavoidable exposure — through such traditional public health approaches as immmunizations as well as through other approaches such as the use of seat belts, development of social support groups, sheltered living situations, crisis intervention, and support services for the infirm. By reducing risks in these ways, health problems can actually be avoided.

The Need for Community Diagnosis

In order to focus efforts on existing community health problems, systematic community diagnosis is required. This belief is based on certain assumptions derived from epidemiology, which is "the study of the distribution and determinants of diseases and injuries in human populations" (Mausner & Bahn 1974). These assumptions are

- that the distribution of health problems is not static, but changes over time, even within the same community.
- that the distribution of health problems varies between communities, even at the same point in time.
- that the distribution of health problems in communities is not necessarily reflected in the health problems for which care is sought or provided.

Because health problems that exist in specific populations are not predictable or necessarily known to care providers, it is necessary to diagnose them. Existing health problems change from population to population as well as over time. What once was a health problem may no longer be so today, while new, more significant problems could present health issues that were insignificant earlier. Similarly, a large number of individuals seeking treatment for certain problems does not automatically justify characterizing them as the population's most common health concerns. Other problems for which treatment is not sought could be more widespread or significant, such as hypertension, alcoholism, depression, child or spouse abuse, or venereal diseases. Therefore, before introducing a health program into a community, the existing health problems must be recognized by prevalence. By not making this determination, community health services can fail to deal with the most significant health problems in the community that need attention. Instead they deal with health problems that have been traditionally addressed or for which attention is demanded or money available.

The Basis for Being Able to Treat Communities

In addition to these reasons for assessing or diagnosing communities, there are additional assumptions that are the basis for a community-wide treatment approach. First, health problems are not distributed randomly or evenly in communities, but it is possible to identify patterns in the way health problems occur in communities through epidemiology. This identification of patterns is essential to being able to treat communities. Otherwise, it would not be possible to determine what groups in communities were at increased risk. Second, through epidemiology it is also possible to identify the circumstances that increase risk of specific health problems, such as family history, genetic makeup, other diagnoses, environmental exposure, and behaviors. Some of these risk factors are potentially changeable — for example, certain behaviors and environmental exposures that increase risk may be changed. Exposure to unsafe housing, lack of supportive care, inability to feed oneself, and social isolation are changeable risk factors, just as toxic substances and air pollution are in theory. Being able through epidemiology to identify changeable risk factors is essential to being able to treat communities by reducing these risks.

Limitations of Community Diagnosis and Treatment

There are limitations to what community diagnosis and treatment can address. First, this process cannot solve all health problems. It is not a panacea and it will not eliminate the need for treatment of health problems. It does open up, however, the possibility of preventing those health problems that have known risk factors which theoretically can be changed and for which we have the skills to effectively bring about change. Fortunately, some theoretically changeable risks have been identified for our current leading causes of death (heart disease, cancer, stroke and accidents) — risks such as smoking, hypertension, carcinogens in the work place, and driving while intoxicated or at fast rates of speed (See Table 3.1). The methods to bring about change in these risks are less well known and agreed upon.

THE PROCESS OF COMMUNITY DIAGNOSIS AND TREATMENT

Any nurse responsible for program decisions in an organization or organizational unit that serves a defined population has the potential of practicing community diagnosis and treatment. Nurses in leadership positions — in official and unofficial health agencies, voluntary agencies like the Red Cross or the Heart Association, industries, schools, home care agencies, HMOs, neighborhood health centers, nutrition centers, senior citizen housing projects, and day care centers for the elderly — may have responsibility for making program decisions for the population served. These nurses, along with others, help

Table 3.1.   Major Causes of Death in 1981 and Associated Risk Factors

Cause	Percent of All Deaths	Risk Factor
Heart disease	38.2	Smoking,* hypertension,* elevated serum cholesterol* (diet), lack of exercise, diabetes, stress, family history
Malignant neoplasms	21.3	Smoking,* worksite carcinogens, environmental carcinogens, alcohol, diet
Cerebrovascular diseases	8.3	Hypertension,* smoking,* elevated serum cholesterol,* stress
Chronic obstructive pulmonary diseases	3.0	Risk factors not included
Pneumonia and influenza	2.7	Smoking, vaccination status*
Motor vehicle accidents	2.6	Alcohol,* no seat belts,* speed,* roadway design, vehicle engineering
All other accidents	2.5	Alcohol,* drug abuse, smoking (fires), product design, handgun availability
Diabetes mellitus	1.7	Obesity*
Chronic liver disease and cirrhosis	1.5	Alcohol abuse*
Atherosclerosis	1.4	Elevated serum cholesterol*
Suicide	1.4	Stress,* alcohol and drug abuse, and gun availability

* Major risk factors (Office of Disease Prevention & Health Promotion).

From: HHS. Health United States-1980. 81-1232, p. 274; and NCHS. Monthly Vital Statistics Report 31:13, December 1982, Table E.

determine what services are offered, to whom, by whom, where, when, and for what purpose. Their decisions are crucial in deciding what health problems these programs address and how they address them. They are, therefore, in positions to determine whether or not programs address health problems that are significant and reduce risk. They have the option of using or not using a community approach.

The use of a community approach requires knowledge and skills beyond clinical and administrative competence alone (Sheps 1976). Graduate preparation in the public health sciences of epidemiology, biostatistics and community assessment, planning, and evaluation is needed in graduate nursing education if nurses are to be able to participate effectively in " . . . policy analysis and development and the use of epidemiology in making practice decisions" (Williams 1977). The purpose of this chapter is to outline some of the basic skills required to diagnose and treat communities or populations based on an epidemiologic perspective.

The Basic Steps of Community Diagnosis and Treatment

Although the process of diagnosing and treating communities has been previously described by epidemiologists (Cassel 1974) as well as by community health nursing authors (Leahy et al. 1977; Tinkham and Voorhies 1977; Freeman 1981) the basic steps of community diagnosis and treatment have not always been clear. These are the same as those for treating an individual patient. To diagnose and treat a community, it is necessary to (a) assess or diagnose health problems, (b) develop a plan of treatment, (c) implement that plan, and (d) evaluate the results. However, for a community the methods used to do this diagnosis are quite different, as are the means for intervening, which will be shown later in the chapter.

Prediagnosis Steps
Identification of the community or population.   Before beginning a community diagnosis, it is necessary to be clear about the community or population that is being diagnosed. Most often the community is defined by a professional's responsibility for direction of a program(s) for a given population. Regardless of whether or not this population is chosen or assigned, for the purposes of diagnosis, it (a) *must be clearly identifiable.* A specific set of boundaries in time and space makes it possible to determine who is and who is not involved.

Second, the community or population (b) *must have demographic and health status data that is either already available or obtainable.* Since few organizations have the resources to collect their own data, population groups that already have demographic and health status data are most often selected. The majority of these populations are defined in terms of place of residence according to political and geographic units of towns, cities, counties, and states. Schools and places of work also often have demographic and health status data available. It is impractical to select smaller groups by place of residence, such as a neighborhood, without existing data or without the ability to get it. It is, however, possible to select small populations when data is obtainable through surveys or special studies.

Finally, the focus of a community diagnosis (c) *should not be arbitrarily limited to specific demographic or diagnostic groups.* A community diagnosis that arbitrarily focuses on the elderly of an area unnecessarily excludes other age groups from consideration. Only the health problems of that one age group would be diagnosed, which presumes the precedence of their health problems over those of other age groups. Similarly, a community diagnosis that focuses on arthritics only identifies the health problems of arthritics without considering whether or not arthritis is a significant health problem in the community to begin with.

Administrative responsibility for programs sometimes requires that the focus of a community diagnosis be limited. An organization may have a focus limited to a specific demographic or diagnostic group, such as the elderly or adolescents or people with arthritis or heart disease. From the organization's perspective, it is not possible to ask what the needs of the broader population are — because the organization is only aimed at addressing the needs of its one chosen group. This limitation is basic to all categorically defined health organizations: they lack the flexibility of focusing on different health problems and different demographic groups according to the changing problems in the community. This lack of flexibility (a) limits the health problems identified to those of that specific group and (b) does not determine their relationship to health problems of other groups. Within these limitations, however, it is possible to apply the principles of community diagnosis and treatment to specific demographic and diagnostic populations.

Analysis of demographic characteristics.   The next step is to determine the demographic makeup of the community. Just as in a clinical diagnosis it is necessary to know the age, sex, and race of a patient in order to understand what is normal or abnormal, similar data are necessary when diagnosing a population. Basic questions about the demographic characteristics of the community are

1.   What are the characteristics of people in the community? (Demographic composition — age, sex, race.)
2.   What changes are occurring in the characteristics of people in the community? (Dynamics — births, deaths, migration.)

Communities vary in demographic composition and can change over time. Table 3.2 shows changes in the age composition of the United States over time (National Center for Health Statistics 1978). Demographic composition can affect mortality within the community. Communities with a high proportion of elderly are more likely to experience a high mortality than communities with a low proportion. Sex and racial composition can similarly affect mortality. For example, blacks in the United States have higher age-adjusted mortality rates than whites in all of the ten leading causes of death except suicide. Men have higher age-adjusted death rates than women. (See Table 3.3.) By knowing the demographic composition of a community or population it is possible to determine if differences in the distribution of these mortality-prone demographic groups (a) are present and/or (b) have changed over time. Without knowledge of the communities' demographic composition and changes, these differences in communities' health status data could not be accurately interpreted.

It is also necessary to know how the demographic composition is being changed — its dynamics. How and at what rate are people coming into or leaving the community or population — through births, deaths, and migration in and out of the community or population? These dynamics account for all movement into and out of a community. Taken together they provide a picture of the stability of the people in the community. Even considering a community that has changed very little in size, the dynamics present in that community could result in a great deal of change in individuals over time.

Table 3.2.   United States' Demographic Composition by Age of Residents in 1940, 1960, 1970, and 1976

Age Group (yrs)	Percent of Total Population in Age Group*			
	1976	1970	1960	1940
All ages	100.0	100.0	100.0	100.0
Under 5	7.1	8.4	11.3	8.0
5–9	8.1	9.8	10.4	8.1
10–14	9.2	10.2	9.4	8.9
15–19	9.9	9.4	7.4	9.4
20–24	9.1	8.1	6.0	8.8
25–29	8.3	6.6	6.1	8.4
30–34	6.6	5.6	6.7	7.8
35–39	5.5	5.5	7.0	7.2
40–44	5.2	5.9	6.5	6.7
45–49	5.4	6.0	6.1	6.3
50–54	5.6	5.5	5.4	5.5
55–59	5.0	4.9	4.7	4.5
60–64	4.3	4.2	4.0	3.6
65–69	3.9	3.4	3.5	2.9
70–74	2.8	2.7	2.6	2.0
75 and over	4.1	3.8	3.1	2.0

* Enumerated as of April 1 for 1940, 1960, and 1970 and estimated as of July 1 for 1976.
From: NCHS. Facts of Life and Death. 1978, p. 2.

Interpreting death rates of a community over time requires consideration of differences in the community's composition. If significant differences in the proportion of mortality-prone persons by age, sex, or race are present over time in the community, crude rates should not be used for comparison over time. Instead, age-specific, sex-specific, or race-specific death rates should be used. These rates would more validly compare like-groups over time. By adjusting rates for age, sex, or race according to where the differences in distribution have occurred, a single adjusted rate can be calculated for valid comparisons of death rates over time. United States' death rates in crude form and age-adjusted form are shown in Tables 3.3 and 3.4 (National Center for Health Statistics 1977, 1982).

Interpreting birth rates of a community over time can present similar problems. A community's composition in terms of the proportion of females of childbearing age can affect the birth rate. When significant differences in this respect are found in a community's composition over time, this difference must be taken into consideration when comparing the resulting birth rates. This end can be accomplished by comparing age- and sex-specific birth rates for the community at two or more points in time. In other words, the real population at risk of giving birth (females 15–45 years old) is used to produce a rate specific

Table 3.3   United States' Age-Adjusted Death Rates for 1940–1979 by Race and Sex

| | Age-Adjusted Death Rate per 1,000 Population§ | | | | |
| | White | | All Other | | |
Year	Male	Female	Male	Female	Total
1979*	7.5	4.1	10.0	5.9	5.9
1978*	7.7	4.3	10.3	6.1	6.1
1977*	7.8	4.3	10.5	6.2	6.1
1976*	8.0	4.4	10.7	6.4	6.3
1975*	8.1	4.5	11.0	6.5	6.4
1974*	8.4	4.7	11.5	6.9	6.7
1973*	8.7	4.8	12.1	7.4	6.9
1972†,‡	8.8	4.9	12.3	7.5	7.0
1971*	8.8	4.9	12.1	7.5	7.0
1970*	8.9	5.0	12.3	7.7	7.1
1969‡	9.1	5.1	12.7	8.0	7.3
1968‡	9.2	5.2	12.9	8.3	7.4
1967‡	9.0	5.1	12.1	8.0	7.3
1966‡	9.2	5.3	12.4	8.3	7.4
1965‡	9.1	5.3	12.2	8.3	7.4
1960	9.2	5.6	12.1	8.9	7.6
1955	9.1	5.7	11.9	9.1	7.6
1950	9.6	6.5	13.6	11.0	8.4
1945	10.7	7.5	14.5	11.9	9.5
1940	11.6	8.8	17.6	15.0	10.8

* Excludes deaths of nonresidents of the United States.

† Based on a 50 percent sample.

‡ Rates revised.

§ Adjusted to age distribution of U.S. population as enumerated in 1940.

From: NCHS Facts of Life and Death. 1978, p. 29; and NCHS. Monthly Vital Statistics Report. 31:6, Supplement, September, 1982, Table 2.

to them. This age- and sex-specific birth rate is called a fertility rate. United States' birth and fertility rates are shown in Table 3.5 (National Center for Health Statistics 1982).

Step I: Assessment/Diagnosis of a Community
The first step in diagnosing a community is to determine what the health problems are. A variety of health status data are needed to answer the following questions:

1.   What health problems are occurring in the community? (New cases or incidence rates.)

Table 3.4. United States' Crude Death Rates for 1940–1981 by Race and
Sex

| | Crude Death Rate per 1,000 Population | | | | |
| | White | | All Other | | |
Year	Male	Female	Male	Female	Total
1981 (est.)	9.7	8.0	8.9	6.3	8.7
1980 (est.)	9.8	8.0	9.4	6.5	8.7
1979*	9.6	7.7	9.2	6.4	8.5
1978*	9.8	7.8	9.4	6.5	8.7
1977*	9.8	7.7	9.5	6.6	8.6
1976*	10.0	7.8	9.7	6.7	8.8
1975*	10.0	7.8	9.9	6.7	8.8
1974*	10.3	8.0	10.3	7.1	9.1
1973*	10.6	8.2	10.8	7.5	9.3
1972*,†	10.7	8.2	11.0	7.5	9.4
1971*	10.7	8.1	10.9	7.6	9.3
1970*	10.9	8.1	11.2	7.8	9.5
1969‡	11.0	8.2	11.5	8.0	9.5
1968‡	11.1	8.2	11.7	8.2	9.7
1967‡	10.8	8.0	11.0	7.9	9.4
1966‡	11.0	8.1	11.4	8.2	9.5
1965‡	10.9	8.0	11.2	8.2	9.4
1960	11.0	8.0	11.5	8.7	9.5
1955	10.7	7.8	11.3	8.8	9.3
1950	10.9	8.0	12.5	9.9	9.6
1945	12.5	8.6	13.5	10.5	10.6
1940	11.6	9.2	15.1	12.6	10.8

* Excludes deaths of nonresidents of the United States.

† Based on a 50 percent sample.

‡ Rates revised.

From: NCHS. Facts of Life and Death. 1978, p. 29; and Monthly Vital Statistics Report. 30:13, December 1982, Table 5.

2. What health problems are present in the community? (Existing cases or prevalence rates.)
3. What health problems are causing deaths in the community? (Deaths or mortality rates.)
4. Are these health problems increasing in the community or greater than in other areas? (And could this be due to differences or changes in composition?

Epidemiologists are mainly concerned about three aspects of health in communities or populations — incidence, prevalence, and mortality. Incidence is

Table 3.5. United States Birth and Fertility Rates for 1940–1980*

Year	Birth Rate per 1000 Population	Fertility Rate per 1000 Women Aged 15–44 Years
1980	15.9	68.4
1979	15.6	67.2
1978	15.0	65.5
1977	15.1	66.8
1976	14.6	65.0
1975	14.6	66.0
1974	14.8	67.8
1973	14.8	68.8
1972	15.6	73.1
1971	17.2	81.6
1970	18.4	87.9
1969	17.9	86.1
1968	17.6	85.2
1967	17.8	87.2
1966	18.4	90.8
1965	19.4	96.3
1960	23.7	118.0
1955	25.0	118.3
1950	24.1	106.2
1945	20.4	85.9
1940	19.4	79.9

* Beginning in 1970, excludes births to nonresidents of the United States.
  Births in 1940 up to and including 1955 have been adjusted for underregistration.

From: NCSH. Monthly Vital Statistics Report. 31:8 Supplement, November 1982, Table 1.

the occurrence of health problems or new cases. The term signifies the extent to which health problems are *developing* in a community. Prevalence, on the other hand, indicates the extent to which health problems *exist* in a community. Prevalence is defined as existing cases, not just new cases. Prevalence is what would be used to estimate service demands for a treatment program. Mortality is, of course, the extent of deaths caused by a health problem.

The availability or obtainability of these types of data for populations is problematic. Ideally, all three types of data should be considered. In reality, only one — mortality data — is usually readily available on the health problems of geographic areas such as cities and counties and, sometimes, census tracts. Incidence and prevalence data on specific diseases or conditions are very limited. The rate of occurrence of health problems in communities is available systematically on reportable diseases only, most of which are not reliably reported. Incidence of reported cases by state and region is published weekly by the Center for Disease Control. Table 3.6 is an example of the type of data available on reportable diseases.

Incidence of nonreportable diseases is not systematically available. However, incidence and prevalence data is available (Smith 1981) for a variety of selected diseases and conditions, based on national probability samples, through the Health Interview and Health Examination Statistics published by the National Center for Health Statistics. These data can be used to estimate incidence or prevalence of health problems for populations with known demographic compositions. Using such an estimate assumes that the rate of incidence or prevalence in the national data for various age–sex–racial groups is similar to that of those groups in the community. Because the demographic composition in a community is unique, national sample rates produce a specific estimated number of cases for each demographic group, which taken together result in a characteristic estimated rate for that community.

Estimates of incidence and prevalence are especially useful and necessary when considering health problems that do not result in death. These health problems do not show up in mortality rates and would otherwise be undocumentable. Chronic conditions such as diabetes, hypertension, asthma, or senility may not result in death but may be significant health problems. Other problems include conditions like venereal disease, measles, upper respiratory infections, as well as events such as food poisoning or injuries.

Other data on incidence and prevalence of health problems are available in communities from services not officially concerned with health. The frequent police calls for "family disturbances," cases of juvenile delinquency, vandalism, child abuse, battered spouses, and rapes all represent events that may be indicative of problem behaviors in the community. Although these available data are not perfect, they are a beginning measure of problems that are not likely to be reflected in a community's mortality data.

Disease-specific mortality data are generally systematically reported and available on individual communities through official health agencies. Mortality data represent only one outcome of a health problem — death, which is not always significant for health problems — and therefore, is limited in its usefulness. Table 3.7 shows the United States' crude mortality rates for 1981 and 1900 by cause of death (National Center for Health Statistics 1978, 1982).

Why is it so important to get data on health problems in communities? Unless the existence of a health problem can be documented, there is no basis for a community health program. A health problem cannot be assumed to exist in a community just because other communities are affected, or because a community has more older or younger people or has more Hispanics or Puerto Ricans. Having a large elderly population in a community does not necessarily mean that a community needs services for the elderly. They may already have services that meet their needs. Before a case can be made for services in a

Table 3.6.   United States' Cases of Specified Notifiable Diseases, 1975–1979 and 1980

	Number of Cases Reported	
Reportable Disease	1980*	1975–1979†
Venereal diseases (civilian)		
gonorrhea	1,000,188	1,001,673
syphilis, primary and secondary	27,237	23,724
Chicken pox	184,308	182,250
Hepatitis, viral		
type A	28,155	30,874
type B	18,292	15,091
type unspecified	11,828	8,795
Tuberculosis	27,425	30,329
Measles	13,406	26,915
Mumps	8,438	20,964
Asceptic meningitis	7,341	4,691
Rabies in animals	6,218	2,971
Rubella (german measles)	3,803	16,210
Meningococcal infections (civilian and military)	2,662	1,819
Malaria	1,916	531
Pertussis	1,612	1,570
Typhys fever, tick-borne (Rocky Mountain spotted)	1,132	1,050
Encephalitis, primary	1,107	1,185
Typhoid fever	492	405
Tularemia	223	144
Leprosy	222	NA‡
Brucellosis	176	222
Trichinosis	124	NA
Psittacosis	103	NA
Tetanus	74	84
Leptospirosis	74	NA
Typhus fever, flea-borne (endemic, murine)	73	NA
Botulism	69	NA
Congenital rubella syndrome	47	NA
Plague	18	NA
Cholera	9	NA
Polio		
total	8	NA
paralytic	6	NA
Diphtheria	5	86
Anthrax	1	NA
Rabies in man	0	NA

* Cumulative first 52 weeks.

† Median.

‡ NA = Not available.

From: CDC. Mortality and Morbidity Weekly Report. 30:1, January 2, 1981.

Table 3.7.   United States' Crude Mortality by Cause of Death for 1900 and 1981

Rank in 1981	Cause of Death	Crude Mortality Rate per 100,000 Population	
		1900	1981
	All causes	1719.1	866.4
1	Diseases of the heart	137.4	330.6
2	Malignant neoplasms	64.0	84.3
3	Cerebrovascular diseases	106.9	71.7
4	Accidents and adverse effects	72.3	44.5
5	Chronic obstructive pulmonary diseases	*	26.1
6	Pneumonia and influenza	202.2	23.7
7	Diabetes mellitus	11.0	15.2
8	Chronic liver disease and cirrhosis	12.5	12.9
9	Atherosclerosis	*	12.5
10	Suicide	10.2	12.3

* A comparable category of cause of death was not classified in 1900.

From: NCHS. Monthly Vital Statistics Report. 30:13, December 1982, Table E; and Facts of Life and Death, 1978, Table 26.

community, the existence of a problem — to be addressed by those services — must be established.

Once the existence of health problems has been established in whatever way possible, the next step is to determine if these health problems are greater in one community than others. In order to answer this question most fairly, it is necessary to consider the demographic composition of the community and the communities to which it is being compared. Differences in the magnitude of health problems in communities could be due to differences in composition of the communities alone or due to real differences in risk between communities — not related to demographic composition. By comparing health data adjusted or standardized for demographic composition, differences between communities are given a possible cause.

Unlike a clinical diagnosis, a community diagnosis requires more than establishing the presence of a health problem. More than one health problem is always present in a community, and therefore community diagnosis requires additional prioritizing of health problems for community action. Establishing the significance of an existing health problem involves comparing the rate of the problem to that of others. The incidence, prevalence, and/or mortality of an existing health problem may be identified as significant by virtue of the size of the (a) rate alone, (b) rate relative to other health problems, (c) rate relative

Table 3.8.   Criteria for Selecting a Health Problem for
Community Treatment (i.e., Systematic Reduction of Risk)

1. Significance of the problem
2. Level of community awareness and priority
3. Ability to reduce risk
4. Cost of reducing risk (economic, social, ethical)
5. Ability to identify the target population (i.e., those at highest risk)
6. Availability of resources to intervene (i.e., to reduce risk)

Adapted from WHO. Criteria to be considered in selecting a preventive
health action. In Report of the First Interdisciplinary Workshop on Psychosocial Factors and Health. Stockholm, October 11–15, 1976.

to that of other communities of similarly composed populations, and/or (d) increase in rate over time within the community.

In addition to the objectively measurable dimensions of an existing health problem, however, the level of felt need or concern in the community for a health problem may determine its actual chances of catalyzing community health action. Significance of health problems to a community is based on the perceptions of its members. This measuring rod may be quantified by considering various health problems in terms of their impact on the community, such as (a) lives lost, (b) years of life lost, or (c) earnings forgone due to the health problem.

Whether or not a significant health problem warrants community treatment is, however, a much different question. In order to make this determination, a number of judgments must be made. In 1976 an interdisciplinary World Health Organization (WHO) work group (1976) attempted to answer this question. They developed criteria for deciding whether or not a health problem in a community was appropriate for preventive community action (see Table 3.8). First and foremost, they insisted that a health problem must be significant in some objective sense — in terms of the number of people affected or the consequences resulting from it, such as disability or death. Second, the health problem must be recognized by the community and given high priority. Third, the health problem must have known risk factors that are, at least in theory, changeable. Fourth, the cost of reducing risk of the health problem must be acceptable to the community. In other words, the community must be willing to pay the price for whatever action is proposed. Fifth, the resources necessary to reduce risk of the health problem must be available. These requirements must be met by all proposals to reduce risk in communities.

Step 2: Development of a Community Treatment Plan
Once a health problem has been identified as warranting community treatment, the next step is to develop a plan of treatment. In order to develop a community treatment plan, the following basic questions must be answered:

Table 3.9.   Natural History of Disease Levels of Prevention*

Stage of Susceptibility	Presymptomatic Disease	Clinical Disease	Outcomes
			Cure
	Biological	Clinical onset	Disability
	onset (signs)	(symptoms)	Death
Primary prevention	Secondary prevention		Tertiary prevention
(reduction of risk)	(early diagnosis		(reduction of disabilitty
	and treatment)		and/or prevention of
			complications)

* Adapted from Mausner JS, Bahn AK. Epidemiology: An introductory text. Philadelphia: W.B. Saunders, 1974; 6–10.

1. Who is at greatest risk of the health problem? (Demographically — age, sex, race, etc.)
2. What factors that are changeable increase risk of the health problem? (Inherited/biological, environmental, behavioral.)
3. What can most effectively reduce risk among those at greatest risk? (To select the most effective approach.)
4. What can be done in the community to reduce risk among those at greatest risk? (A program plan.)
5. How much change in the health problem is desired over what period of time in the community? (Operational objective.)

Determining who is at risk of contracting a health problem means establishing the natural history of the problem (Mausner and Bahn 1974). How is the biological or actual onset of the condition defined? How is the clinical onset of the condition defined? What are the outcomes of the condition? Knowledge of these points provides a guide for reducing risk by planning intervention before biological onset (See Table 3.9).

Community treatment is based on the risk factors associated with a health problem. To determine the nature of risk factors associated with a given health problem, differences in incidence (i.e., occurrence of new cases) rather than prevalence (i.e., distribution of existing cases) or mortality (i.e., deaths) are required. Prevalence is affected by differences in length of illness and of rate of recovery and/or survival. Incidence alone reflects the rate of occurrence of a disease. Only by determining differences in incidence can risk be established. Interpretation of these epidemiologic findings demands a sound understanding of epidemiologic principles; otherwise, the correct target group and risk factors cannot be identified. Usually, high standards for evidence of risk factors are required — such as well-designed cohort or case control studies, preferably done in a number of settings.

Risk factors associated with health problems can be viewed as those that are readily changeable and those that are not. One way of categorizing risk factors is according to

1. Demographic characteristics — specifically sex, age, race, marital status, socioeconomic status, etc. (Not readily changeable.)
2. Inherited/biological characteristics — such as genetic traits, physical conditions such as obesity, high blood pressure, other disease processes, etc. (May or may not be changeable.)
3. Environmental exposures — physical aspects of the environment such as climate, pollution, housing, noise, toxic substances, etc., as well as psychosocial aspects of the environment such as social isolation, highly competitive work setting, loss of a significant other, other forms of psychological stresses (Most are changeable.)
4. Behavioral characteristics — such as certain patterns of food consumption, use of cigarettes, alcohol or other drugs, exercise, rest or work habits, etc. (Most are changeable.)

Demographic and some inherited/biological risk factors are used to identify high-risk groups in a community or population that most warrant attention. Behavioral and environmental risk factors provide a basis for designing ways to reduce those risks. In this way, identification of risk factors can focus intervention on reducing risk among those in the community where risk is greatest. Table 3.1 shows some of the risks known to be associated with the leading causes of death in the United States in 1981 (HHS 1981; National Center for Health Statistics 1982).

Before decisions are made about a plan for community treatment, alternative approaches should be systematically considered. Selection of an approach to reduce identified risk factors requires analytic skills to interpret the results of evaluation studies in order to select the most effective approach — not just the approach most popular or "in." All alternative approaches should be evaluated — from legislation to mass media to health education to service provision — to determine which one or two approaches have the most evidence of effectiveness.

A wide range of approaches are relevant to a community's health. Any approach that positively affects the course of a health problem or disease in a community is health relevant and therefore is a potential community health intervention. Health professionals most often consider intervention only in terms of those activities they perform. This viewpoint greatly limits the range of interventions considered. The impact of traditional diagnostic and treatment approaches on health is small in relation to that of environmental and behavior factors (Dever 1980). Therefore, it is important for health professionals to broaden their perspective on interventions that they consider as appropriate to treat communities.

Once this groundwork has been laid, a plan of community treatment can be formulated that focuses on reducing risk among those at greatest risk, using the most effective method or methods possible. As a part of this plan, a program objective should be developed that clearly specifies the extent to which the plan is expected to change the health problem, among what group of people, where, and over what period of time. Such a statement should contain the five components suggested by Deniston et al. (1968) as being necessary to adequately evaluate a program. Specifically, Deniston suggested that a program objective should outline "(a) what — the nature of the situation or condition to be attained (or changed), (b) extent — the quantity or amount of the situation or condition to be attained (or changed), (c) who — the particular group of people or portion of the environment in which attainment is desired, (d) where — the geographic area of the program, and (e) when — the time at or by which the desired situation or condition is intended to exist." Program objectives should *not* include how these conditions are to be obtained, as that involves program activities. A clearly stated program objective commits those responsible for implementing it to a clear goal, not to a predetermined set of activities. It focuses attention on the achievement for which program activities are implemented, not on the activities themselves.

In 1979, National Health Goals were formulated by the Surgeon General for each of five age groups in the United States' population (HEW 1979). These goals focus attention on specific desired changes in the health status of each age group in the United States by 1990. They specify what, the extent, who, where, and when desired changes are to be achieved. They are actually operational objectives for health programs in the United States during the 1980s. They include the following:

1. By 1990, to reduce infant mortality by at least 35%, to fewer than 9 deaths per 1,000 live births (in the U.S. population).
2. By 1990, to reduce deaths among children ages 1–14 years by at least 20% to fewer than 34 deaths per 100,000 (in the U.S. population).
3. By 1990 to reduce deaths among people ages 15 to 24 by at least 20% to fewer than 93 deaths per 100,000 (in the U.S. population).
4. By 1990 to reduce deaths among people ages 25–64 by at least 25%, to fewer than 400 deaths per 100,000 (in the U.S. population).
5. By 1990 to reduce the average annual number of days of restricted activity due to acute and chronic conditions by 20%, to fewer than 30 days per year for people aged 65 and older (in the U.S. population).

These goals have been further operationalized in a Health and Human Services (HHS) publication (1980) titled *Promoting Health and Preventing Disease: Objectives for the Nation*. In this publication, additional operational objectives are identified more specifically, as well as possible intervention strategies, their relative strength, the principal assumptions underlying these strategies, and national and local data sources to monitor their achievement. This information should be a useful resource to those planning health programs throughout the 1980s.

Step 3: Implementation of Community Treatment
Once a program plan for reducing risk has been developed, implementation follows. Implementing a program is the aspect of community treatment with which health professionals are probably most familiar. Unfortunately, all too often, implementation of community programs occurs without professionals' having first assessed and diagnosed the community or having considered whether or not reduction of risk is possible. Equally deficient is the extent to which health professionals actually select intervention methods based on their effectiveness. From a community diagnosis and treatment point of view, any method of implementation of community programs that is not based on assessment and diagnosis of community needs, consideration of the possibility of reducing risk (i.e., primary prevention), or an analysis of a possible intervention's effectiveness should be questioned as to its value.

Step 4: Evaluation of Community Treatment
In order to complete the process of community diagnosis and treatment, community treatment (i.e., programs) must be evaluated by answering the following basic questions:

1. Was the program carried out? (Document program activities.)
2. Was the program acceptable to the community? (Document community exposure to the program.)
3. Was the health problem changed as desired? (Document the outcome of the program.)
4. Was the program effective overall and why or why not? (Interpret the overall evaluation findings.)

Evaluation of community treatment documents whether the program was carried out, the target group received the treatment, and the desired change in the health problem was achieved. These are simple questions, but they are difficult to answer. They require good preparation in program evaluation, preferably from an epidemiologic point of view because community treatment is aimed at changing the distribution of health problems in population groups. Evaluation of community treatment is complex and demands skill and the willingness to invest the time, effort, and money. Failing to evaluate community programs, however, risks continuing ineffective programs that in the end could be more costly. Table. 3.10 summarizes these basic steps in diagnosing and treating a community.

COMMUNITY HEALTH NURSING PRACTICE BASED ON COMMUNITY DIAGNOSIS AND TREATMENT

It is not known to what extent a community diagnosis and treatment approach is actually applied in community health nursing practice. Some speculate that

Table 3.10.   Basic Steps to Diagnose and Treat a Community

Assessment/Diagnosis of a Community
  1. Identify the community
  2. What are the characteristics of people in the community? (demographic composition—age, sex, race)
  3. What changes are occurring in the characteristics of people in the community? (dynamics—births, deaths, migration)

Development of a Community Treatment Plan
  1. What health problems are occurring in the community? (new cases or incidence rates)
  2. What health problems are present in the community? (existing cases or prevalence rates)
  3. What health problems are causing deaths in the community? (deaths or mortality rates)
  4. Are these health problems increasing in the community or greater than in other areas? (Could this be due to differences or changes in composition?)

Implementation of Community Treatment
  1. Who is at greatest risk of the health problem? (demographically—age, sex, race, etc.)
  2. What factors increase risk of the health problem that are changeable?
      (inherited biological—genetic traits, physical conditions)
      (environmental—physical & psychosocial conditions)
      (behavioral—smoking, eating habits, exercise)
  3. What can most effectively reduce risk among those at greatest risk? (to select the most effective approach)
  4. What can be done in the community to reduce risk among those at greatest risk? (a program plan)
  5. How much change in the health problem is desired over what period of time in the community? (operational objective)

Evaluation of Community Treatment
  1. Was the plan carried out? (document activities)
  2. Was it acceptable to the community (document exposure)
  3. Was the health problem changed as desired? (document outcome)
  4. Was the program effective? (interpret findings)

it is quite rare (Tinkham and Voorhies 1977). The majority of community health nurses' practice probably involves the provision of a wide variety of direct care services to individuals and families, as described by Archer (1976). Provision of these services occurs in either homes or clinics or other noninstitutional settings. Whether or not these services are based on a community diagnosis and treatment approach is determined by the community health nurses responsible for planning, administering, and evaluating those services. The nature of their decisions regarding the what, where, why, and how of community health nursing practice determines whether or not services are based on a community diagnosis and treatment approach.

Although it is not known to what extent community health nursing services are based on a community approach, it is possible to speculate on what these services would look like if they were. Community health nursing services based on a community diagnosis and treatment approach would

1. Be directed toward significant health problems that exist in the community or population, not just health problems brought to public attention or for which service is usual or demanded or reimbursed.
2. Be focused on groups in the community or population known to be at greatest risk of developing identified health problems, not just those individuals who seek service.
3. Be aimed at reducing risk of developing identified health problems (primary prevention), not just at early diagnosis and treatment (secondary prevention) or prevention of complications and reduction of disability and discomfort (tertiary prevention).
4. Utilize acceptable methods of intervention known to be most effective in achieving the desired health outcome, rather than traditional methods of unknown effectiveness.
5. Have operational objectives that specify the nature and amount of change(s) in the identified health problems to be achieved over a specified period of time in the community or population.
6. Determine their effect on achievement of desired changes in identified health problems over a specified period of time in the community or population.
7. Be continuously evaluated as to need and effectiveness in light of new and changing community health problems, knowledge of risks, diagnostic/ treatment and management modalities, existing community resources; and effectiveness of intervention methods.

Although most of community health nursing practice does not currently meet these expectations, an increasing number of community health nurses are being prepared at the graduate level to practice and value community diagnosis and treatment. As a result, it appears likely that major changes in community health nursing practice may gradually begin to occur in the near future. More and more community health nursing services will begin to "grasp and deal effectively with the opportunity to identify and promote improved health levels in significant risk groups under their care." Community diagnosis and treatment will really be practiced. Community health nursing's rich heritage of concern for communities will have been put into action with a sound scientific base.

REFERENCES

American Public Health Association. The definition and role of public health nursing practice in the delivery of health care. Am J Public Health 1982; 72(2):210–212.

Archer SE. Community health nurse practitioners: another assessment. Nurs Outlook 1976; 24.

Cassel JC. Community diagnosis. In: Omran AR, ed. Community medicine in developing countries. New York: Springer, 1974.

Centers for Disease Control. Morbidity and Mortality Weekly Report, Atlanta, Georgia.

Deniston OL, Rosenstock IM, and Getting VA. Evaluation of program effectiveness. Public Health Rep. 1968; 83(4):323–334.

Dever GEA. Holistic health — an epidemiological model for policy analysis. In: Dever GEA, ed. Community health analysis: a holistic approach. Germantown, MD: Aspen Systems Corporation, 1980.

Freeman RB. Community diagnosis: keystone of public health practice. In: Freeman RB, Henrich J. Community health nursing practice. 2nd ed. Philadelphia: Saunders, 1981.

Health and Human Services. Health United States 1980. Washington, DC: U.S. Government Printing Office, 1981.

Health and Human Services. Promoting health and preventing disease: objectives for the nation. Washington, DC: U.S. Government Printing Office, 1980.

Leahy KM, Cobb MM, and Jones MC. Focusing on communities. In: Leahy KM et al. Community health nursing, 3rd ed. New York: McGraw-Hill, 1977.

Mausner JS, and Bahn AK. Epidemiology: an introductory text. Philadelphia: Saunders, 1974.

McGavran. EG. What is public health? Printed monograph. Chapel Hill, NC: School of Public Health, University of North Carolina, 1971.

National Center for Health Statistics. Monthly vital statistics report.

National Center for Health Statistics. Vital and health statistics. Series 10 — data from the health interview survey.   .

National Center for Health Statistics. Vital and health statistics. Series 11 — data from the health examination survey and health and nutrition examination survey.

National Center for Health Statistics. Facts of Life. 1978.

Sheps C. Public health defined. In: Sheps CB, ed. Higher education for public health: a report of the Milbank Memorial Fund Commission. New York: Prodist, 1976.

Smith SS. Major data systems of the National Center for Health Statistics. Public Health Rep 1981; 96(3):200–201.

Tinkham CW, and Voorhies EF. Gathering pertinent data about the community; Analysis of data and identification of community nursing needs; Developing a nursing plan of action for the community; and Implementing and evaluating a nursing plan of action for a community. In: Tinkham CW, Voorhies EF, eds. Community health nursing: evolution and process, 2nd ed. New York: Appleton-Century-Crofts, 1977.

U.S. Department of Health, Education and Welfare. Healthy people: the Surgeon General's report on health promotion and disease prevention. Washington, DC: U.S. Government Printing Office, 1979.

Williams CA. Community health nursing — what is it? Nurs Outlook 1977; 25(4):250–254.

World Health Organization. Criteria to be considered in selecting a preventive health action. In: Report of the First Interdisciplinary Workshop on Psychosocial Factors and Health. Stockholm, October 11–15, 1976.

FAMILY AS CLIENT 4

Ruth A. O'Brien and Ann G. Robinson

The emergence of the 1980s heralded a growing consensus among organized nursing bodies and professional leaders as to the nature and direction of community health nursing practice. Both the Division of Community Health Nursing of the American Nurses Association (1980) and the Public Health Nursing Section of the American Public Health Association (1982) articulated position papers supporting identification of the first and foremost concern of community health nursing as the promotion and preservation of the health of communities. Attaining this goal means directing program planning and implementation toward identified high-risk aggregates. Individual, family, or group intervention modalities are utilized to effect the desired change in health behavior of the at-risk population.

Evidence linking family functioning to individual well-being and effective health behavior continues to accumulate. Community health nursing traditionally has advocated a family orientation in the delivery of its services. In reality, much of its efforts have been aimed at solving the health problems of referred individuals, with other family members being considered a support system for helping the individual cope with his or her concern. The complexity of health issues, stresses, and strains confronting contemporary families may, at times, necessitate a more sophisticated family-focused approach. With a family-focused approach, as contrasted to a family-oriented approach, no single family member serves as the referent point for service. Rather, the family is viewed as having specific health responsibilities and the extent to which family processes support these functions is the focus for service. Assessments of the family as a group are made and interventions are directed toward helping the family grow in its abilities to meet its health responsibilities.

Although the ideas represented by a family-focused approach are not entirely new, community health nurses have been impeded in moving in this direction by the lack of a coherent conceptual framework for working with the family as the primary unit of service. The purpose of this chapter is to present a conceptual model for family-focused intervention, derived from the analysis and synthesis of selected theories of family functioning and pertinent research studies. Specifically, the family as a system with distinctive developmental phases is examined and its health functions are delineated. Family structure and processes that affect the fulfillment of its designated health functions are identified and definitions of family competence are explored. Finally, applications of the model to goal-directed interventions with families are illustrated.

THE FAMILY AS A SYSTEM

Family interaction and behavior can be viewed from a systems perspective, using general systems theory as a conceptual foundation. The family, as a living system, is a collective of individuals who manifest some degree of interdependence in their interactions with each other and the environment. Every system has both subsystems and suprasystems. The subsystems are smaller subcomponents of the focal system, whereas the suprasystems are larger environmental systems of which the focal system is a part (Friedman 1981). For example, when the family is the focal system, the suprasystem would be its sociocultural group or community and the subsystems would be sets of family relationships (husband-wife dyad, parent-child dyad, sibling-sibling dyad) or the individual members themselves.

Each system possesses certain characteristics such as wholeness, structure, and function. Watzlawick, Beavin, and Jackson (1967) note that while components within a system may be described by their attributes, it is the relationship between the components and their attributes that tie the system together. Because of these relationships, a system behaves not as a simple composite of independent elements, but as a coherent and inseparable whole. Thus, an assessment of the family's competence in meeting its health responsibilities cannot be obtained by summing the attributes of each family member. Rather, an appraisal of family competence necessitates an assessment of how family processes either impede or foster health.

In systems terminology, the processes utilized by the system to accomplish its aims describe the functioning of the system. The structure of a system refers to the arrangement of its parts at any given time, notably its composition and organization. Structure and function are interrelated in that the structure of a family influences how well it is able to fulfill its aims and responsibilities (von Bertalanffy 1968; Lazlo 1972). The subsystems of a family must be integrated much as the meshing of the gears in a finely tuned engine to facilitate attainment of common goals. Thus, the extent of family integration is a critical parameter for the nurse to assess when trying to understand the difficulties a given family is experiencing in meeting its health responsibilities.

The term *equifinality* further denotes the progressive complexity of interaction patterns found both within the family and between the family and its environment (Lazlo 1972). That is, the traditional cause–effect relationship is inconsistent with a systems perspective. Relations among parts are reciprocal, not unilateral. The behavior of one family member affects and influences the behavior of other family members; the environment both shapes and is modified by family behavior. Hence, systems that appear to have the same initial conditions may generate quite different products. Families having similar attributes may function quite differently in fulfilling their health commitments.

Furthermore, in examining family processes, the how of interactions is often more relevant than the what — the content (Janosik and Miller 1979). The how of interactions defines the relationships that exist among family members, while the reciprocity denotes the contribution of each member to the existing relationships. An example of the importance of this principle may be found in a spousal argument over the wife's allowing the couple's 10-year-old son to attend a movie with a group of friends. After much heated discussion, the husband acknowledges he did not object to his son having gone to the movies with his friends, but he felt his wife should have consulted him before giving the son permission. Hence, the essence of the argument is a relationship issue rather than a substantive one. In assessing family competence, the nurse needs to guard against focusing on the content of expressed concerns to the exclusion of family processes related to those concerns. Bandler, Grindler, and Satir (1976) note that when families understand how they arrived at where they are, they can influence and change the process to get what they want.

The family, like all living systems, is open, in that it exchanges materials, energies, and information with its environment (Lazlo 1972). Through such transactions, the family has the potential to replenish its energy and to change and grow. Families, however, vary in the extent of openness to environmental interchange and change. All families develop patterned and organized ways of functioning that provide self-regulation of the system. The pattern and organization of family functioning, while never totally stable, are manifested in the repetition or redundancy of certain events and in the nonoccurrence of others (Watzlawick et al. 1967). One value to the nurse of this characteristic is that an assessment of family interaction patterns may be initiated at a variety of points (Janosik and Miller 1979). The patterns of interaction remain similar regardless of the vantage point from which they are approached, thus enabling the nurse to predict a family's possible responses to anticipated events.

When circumstances within the family or environment stimulate a change in the family's customary mode of functioning, processes within the family act to either foster or impede the change. Negative feedback is directed toward maintaining constancy, whereas positive feedback produces system mutations that accommodate change (Lazlo 1972). Families that have developed more rigidly patterned and organized ways of functioning tend to evidence more resistance to change (Beavers 1977). In assessing family functioning, the nurse seeks to identify those patterns that are detrimental to health. Awareness that one family member's behavior affects that of others and vice versa should help the nurse to focus on the family as the client rather than on the individual member who may manifest the actual concern.

To summarize, a systems perspective of the family suggests that in the assessment of family competence, the nurse needs to consider (a) the unified wholeness of the family, (b) the complexity of family interaction and the reciprocal nature of the relationships among members and between the family and its environment, (c) the how of family process as opposed to the content, and (d) the repetitive pattern and organization in family behavior.

HEALTH RESPONSIBILITIES OF THE FAMILY

The assessment of the family's competence to foster the health and well-being of its members presupposes a clear understanding of its health care responsibilities. Remarkably few articles have addressed the subject in any systematic manner. One notable author attributes the cursory treatment of the subject to the pervasive assumption that, in highly industrialized and technological societies, many functions formerly performed by families have been absorbed by specialized agencies. Yet, as she so aptly documents, the professional care system serves as the locus of health activity only during episodic intervals in an individual's life (Pratt 1976).

That the family has the principal responsibility for assisting its members to develop a personal identity compatible with the surrounding culture and for acting as a buffer against life strains and stresses is the consensus of a number of theorists (Ackerman 1958; d'Abate 1976; Beavers 1977). In speaking to this issue, Ryder (1974) asserts that the individual in a technologically advanced society has an even greater need for emotional support from his or her family. He notes that the competitive and impersonal environment of an occupational structure for an adult or of an educational structure for the child is stressful: it asks much of the individual in discipline and conformity and provides little in emotional warmth. According to Ryder, the family serves as an oasis for the replenishment of the person coping with the achievement-oriented struggles of the outside world. Parsons (1971) further comments that while it has long been accepted that the family is the primary agent in the emotional and social development of the child, the family as the primary basis of security for the adult has been recognized only more recently. Similar conceptualizations of family effectiveness in supporting mental health are presented by Sedgwick (1981) and Lewis et al. (1976).

From a socialization and educational perspective, the family serves as the basic societal unit within which members acquire values about health and health care, knowledge about how and when to use professional care services, and personal health practices relative to nutrition, exercise, smoking, alcohol consumption, and hygiene (Pratt 1976). Recognition that lifestyle factors are the single most important determinant of most of our chronic diseases has focused attention on the importance of the family's responsibility to teach its members how to maintain and preserve health, as well as how to actively problem solve when disruptions in health occur.

The family's role as caregiver for the chronically ill, disabled, and aging has been further highlighted by the rapid expansion of home health services and hospice programs. The latter has led to the identification of two distinct caregiving roles that may be assumed by the family, namely care provision and care management. The care provider identifies those services the family member needs and performs them, whereas the care manager identifies the needed services and manages their provision by others (Archbold 1983). In some instances, the two roles overlap.

From the review of literature, five primary health responsibilities of the family can be identified. They include (a) the provision of opportunities for members to achieve a satisfactory sense of personal identity and worth through access to affect, power, and meaning within the family situation, (b) emotional support and cognitive guidance for members experiencing life transition and personal crises, (c) care provision and/or care management for chronically ill, disabled, or aging members, (d) education of members about how to maintain health and when and how to use professional services, and (e) the socialization of members to value health and to accept personal responsibility for its maintenance.

A CONCEPTUAL FRAMEWORK FOR FAMILY ASSESSMENT

A conceptual framework provides direction to the collection, organization, and interpretation of data about the family's health situation. To be useful to a professional engaged in clinical practice, the framework needs to be based on a set of explicit assumptions about the phenomenon of interest, delineate the essential concepts, and specify the interrelationship between and among concepts (Marston and Chambers 1980). The conceptual framework for family assessment advanced here is designed to assist community health nurses in evaluating the extent to which families are able to fulfill their designated health responsibilities. It is based on a systems view of the family and emphasizes those structural and organizational characteristics of families that are likely to foster or impede effective functioning in relation to health concerns. The conclusion reached by the nursing assessment is a judgment that the family is functioning more or less optimally in meeting its health responsibilities, as opposed to a judgment regarding the health status of a particular family member. This does not remove from any one individual family member the responsibility for individual actions and reactions, but emphasizes the contributions of the individual to overall system effectiveness or strain.

Figure 4.1 presents a schematic diagram of the two core ingredients essential to effective functioning of family systems. As illustrated, the pool of energy and consciousness within the family reflects, to a large extent, its health potential. Each has been depicted as an irregular-shaped mass in order to connote fluidity; the family's energy and consciousness may contract or expand according to life situations. Moreover, at times a family may have sufficient energy but lack the knowledge to use its energy constructively to attain desired goals. The reverse also may occur. Thus it is only when energy and consciousness interface and overlap that system functioning is likely to realize its potential. A discussion of the two core concepts as well as those family processes and structural characteristics that influence the level of energy and consciousness within a family system follows.

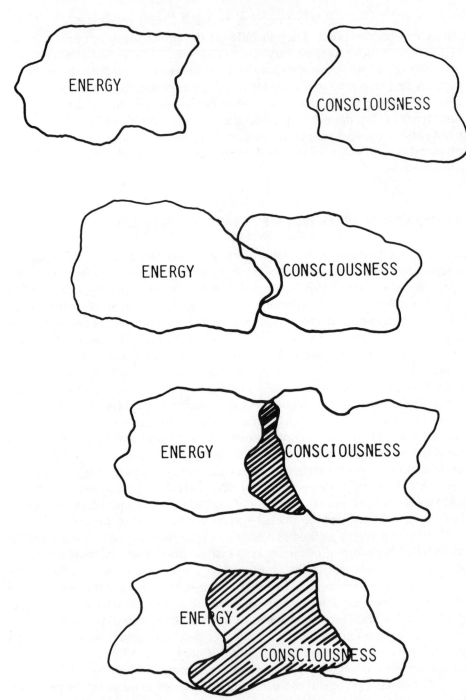

Figure 4.1.   Family potential for effective health functioning

Energy

The family, as do all systems, needs usable energy in order to function effectively. To actively cope with life's stresses, to teach members good health practices, to utilize the professional care system, or to provide members access to affect, power, and meaning all require the investment of energy. The critical issue in family functioning is the regulation of energy flow to attain energetic balance as opposed to imbalance — too much or too little energy (Kantor and Lehr 1976). When energy is depleted, there is an increase in perceptual defensiveness and a narrowing of possible alternatives for action. With overstimulation, behavior is likely to be chaotic and ineffectual. A family experiencing either form of imbalance may have difficulty fulfilling its health responsibilities. Furthermore, when individual energies clash, basic needs and tasks may not be achieved, resulting in a rise in tension within the family system. For example, the stress experienced by new parents coping with the demands of a newborn or by family care providers dealing with ill or aging members may reflect disharmony in the patterning of energy expenditure among family members. By assisting family care providers to utilize available community resources for respite or by helping new parents reorder their priorities, the nurse may be instrumental in restoring energetic balance.

In addition to the regulation of energy flow, a vitally important process for the family is the acquisition and accumulation of energy. The potential sources of energy vary from family to family, from individual to individual. For some, the source may be physical activity, religious beliefs, or social relations. The nature of the source is unimportant, provided the family acquires sufficient energy to meet the demands placed on it. The nurse, however, may find it useful to delineate the sources of energy for a given family, for with a family that manifests a low energy level, intervention may take the form of helping the family identify alternative ways of acquiring energy.

Relevant questions to consider in assessing the family's energy balance are:

Does the family have enough energy to meet the demands placed on it?
Is the family able to gauge its needs and distribute its energy accordingly?
Does it overextend itself, undertaking more demands and expending more
    energy than it can hope to supply?
Are family energies squandered?
Do members have satisfying outlets for their energies?
How does the family replenish its energy (sources)?
Does the expenditure of energy within the family in meeting the demands
    placed on it occur repeatedly at the expense of one particular family member?
    (Kantor and Lehr 1976)

Consciousness

Bentov (1977) defines consciousness as the capacity of a system to respond to a stimulus. Quantity and quality of consciousness are reflected in the transactions of the family. That is, the greater the consciousness, the more options the family will define for itself and the repertoire of choices generated will be more refined. Growth, in essence, is the experience of concepts and percepts being detotalized (reduced to their component parts) and then retotalized (reconstructed) to include new disclosures of the world (Jourard 1968). Growth and change within a family are directly linked to the family's level of consciousness, since knowledge may be translated into experience.

Families store experiences in the forms of images, feelings, and meanings (Kantor and Lehr 1976). Beavers (1977) refers to these shared images and meanings that a family has as its "myths." Family myths reflect its awareness of how it operates as a family. The extent of congruence between family mythology and objective reality has been linked to the health of the family; the more incongruent the mythology, the less healthy the family (Lewis et al. 1976; Beavers 1977). Quite obviously, much of the health teaching and counseling done by the nurse may need to take the form of helping the family to experience new realities and to define alternative solutions to its expressed concerns.

In assessing the family's level of consciousness within the context of the cultural environment, the nurse needs to consider:

What is the family's knowledge with regard to specific health and developmental needs of its members?
Does it hold incorrect beliefs that are likely to lead to unsound health care practices?
Is its perception of how it functions congruent with reality?
What are the sources that the family utilizes in acquiring knowledge?
Does it actively seek to expand its level of consciousness or does it respond only to crisis demands?
How do past family experiences influence its consciousness about health issues?

Boundaries
A family has both system and subsystem boundaries. Auger explains that "a boundary may be defined as a more or less open line forming a circle around the system where there is greater interchange of energy within the circle than on the outside" (Auger 1976). In actuality, family boundaries are spatial (territorial) and conceptual (rules, sanctions) fields of interactional activity. Interchanges between the family, its extended kin, work colleagues, neighbors, and other community groups reflect the openness of the exterior boundaries that the family creates for itself. Having selectively permeable boundaries allows for family growth and change, since the use of resources outside the family is enhanced. The latter can contribute to family functioning by developing awareness of alternative courses of action and by increasing understanding of personal health practices and the value of self-directed action for promoting health (Pratt 1976). Conversely, the amount of information a family can handle adequately is limited, and an excess of information or conflicting information

from the outer environment may amplify and create family disorganization (Friedman 1981).

Markedly restricted interchange with the environment creates a greater reliance upon inner family resources. Relatively closed families may exhibit more energy, in the form of tension, than they can discharge in constructive ways. Studies repeatedly have noted that child abuse clusters in families that are isolated from friends, neighbors, and society (Justice and Justice 1976; Williams and Money 1980). In healthier isolated families, the members tend to believe that all or most of the needs of the members can be met within the family or the family's reference group (Sedgwick 1981). Yet such reliance on internal resources may occur to the detriment of one or more family members in situations involving long-term chronic illness or disability, as evidenced by caregiver fatigue (Archbold 1983).

Kantor and Lehr (1976) describe a number of mechanisms by which families maintain their territory within the larger community, the essential analogy being one of mapping. With mapping the family develops its own "mental picture" of the exterior culture — one that indicates the ways in which the culture resembles and differs markedly from the interior family; it also specifies those people, things, events, and ideas that are safe and worthwhile for family members and those that are not. In some families, the map is quite uniform for all members, and in others each member has a different map.

While the establishment of exterior boundaries regulates the flow of people, resources, and information that enter the family system, the maintenance of interpersonal boundaries is a crucial factor in the differentiation of self within the family system. Differentiation is the process whereby family members evolve a definition of "I" within a "we" (Karpel 1976). The sensitivity of the family to each member's needs and the encouragement of personal responsibility for feelings and behavior serve to delimit areas of autonomy experienced as separateness (Minuchin 1974; Beavers 1977). Differentiation of self, however, cannot occur without a sense of belongingness. Access to love and emotional support in family interactions is critical to the development of self-identity (Kantor and Lehr 1976). The way in which the family uses physical space also has an impact on the experiencing of a sense of separate self. Provision for individual privacy and personal possessions fosters the experiencing of self as separate and distinct from others.

Minuchin (1974) conceptualizes the boundaries within and between subsystems as lying along a continuum from disengaged to enmeshed.

————————————— / ————————— - / ....

disengaged	clear boundaries	enmeshed
(inappropriately rigid)	(normal range)	(diffuse, unclear)

Disengaged boundaries are present when members interact in rigid, undeviating patterns that tend to be unresponsive to changing family needs. Members may feel overly independent and lack a sense of belonging and family support. At the other extreme, family members are overinvolved or enmeshed with one another, resulting in a lack of individuality and a sense of dependence. Such families tend to overact when one particular member responds differently or encounters stress. Because so much energy is channeled toward maintaining the overcloseness that exists, tensions are likely to erupt into conflict at cyclical intervals. Moreover, the repertoire of responses of such families to stress is less refined; feelings tend to dominate logical thought processes (Minuchin 1974; Lewis et al. 1976). Clear boundaries, on the other hand, foster self-identity and promote effective subsystem and system functioning.

Boundaries among subsystems within the family need to be age-appropriate. The parental subsystem must establish boundaries that allow the children accessibility to the parents and yet preserve the integrity of the spouse subsystem. For example, when a small child asks why she can't stay up as late as her parents and is told that children need more sleep than parents, a boundary of the parental subsystem is exemplified and privacy for the spouse subsystem is preserved. Healthy development requires some free choice, but a strong parent-child coalition in which the child possesses the power and freedom of a parent has been observed to be characteristic of severely disturbed families (Beavers 1977).

The sibling subsystem serves as an important training ground for the development of peer relationships. The sibling subsystem boundaries should function in a way that will allow for the development of personal goals and interests without undue parental constraint. Maintenance of the right to privacy and freedom to make mistakes also must be safeguarded by sibling boundaries. When children begin to relate to peers outside the family, they utilize the transactional skills learned in the sibling subsystem (Minuchin 1974).

Because of the differing purposes they serve, nursing assessment needs to examine the adequacy of interpersonal boundaries within the family as well as the permeability of exterior boundaries. Transactions between the family, its social support network, and community groups are indices of the latter. Questions pertinent to each of these parameters are outlined below.

Community transactions: What is the family's territorial complex? To what extent do family members participate in organizations or utilize community services? Is the family aware of community services relevant to its needs? How does the family feel about groups or persons from whom it receives services? How do these groups view the family? What is the family's overall perceptions of the neighborhood/community in which it lives?

Social support systems: Does the family maintain ongoing relationships with relatives, friends, or other social groups? Which of the relationships are more meaningful than others? To whom does the family turn for help or guidance with concerns? How accessible is such help? To what degree do interactions with its support network foster or impede the family's abilities to cope with its concerns? Is the family satisfied with its social support network? Have relationships been added, changed, or lost recently?

Interpersonal boundaries: Are relationships between and among family members age-appropriate? Do they evidence respect and tolerance of individual interests and goals? Are members afforded some privacy and personal possessions of their own? Do family interactions promote a sense of attachment without overinvolvement or overcloseness?

Role Structure

Roles incorporate the goals and actions that are expected to characterize the occupant of a specific position. No role exists in isolation but ideally is patterned to complement the reciprocal role of a partner or partners. The degree of role complementarity that exists is a critical issue in the effective functioning of the family. Discrepancies in role expectations of family members tend to give rise to tension and conflict that, if left unresolved, may deplete the usable energy available to the system (Spiegel 1968). The general energy level of the family will, in turn, influence the extent to which the family can invest itself in the resolution of role conflict.

Roles are learned according to the cultural values of the family and society. Here the family's level of consciousness may facilitate or hinder the choices available to its members. The choices available, in turn, tend to regulate members' access to power and meaning. Flexibility of role definitions provides for greater freedom in members' access to power and meaning and enables the family to deal more effectively with developmental transitions and situational crises (Otto 1976).

Multiple factors may contribute to role conflict among family members. First are cognitive discrepancies in which cues are misinterpreted and misunderstanding reduces complementarity of expectations. Cognitive discrepancy is a characteristic problem between adolescents and parents. It also occurs during transitional phases requiring learning of new roles, such as the birth of the first child, the first severe illness, or death of a family member. Second, discrepancies in goals between role partners may become a source of role conflict, as in the example of the parent who cannot accept the limited intelligence of a retarded child and holds expectations of performance that the child cannot fulfill. A third source of role conflict results from allocative discrepancies: one member assumes or is given a role that the other views as not rightfully assumed. An example is the stepfather who disciplines his wife's child for misbehavior and is challenged for doing so. Fourth are instrumental discrepancies in which role conflict arises because a family member lacks the technical resources to meet his or her obligations. A common example of such conflict is found in low-income families where the male is viewed as the "breadwinner" but does not earn enough money to buy all the possessions family members expect and want. Finally, differing cultural orientations of family members may lead to role conflict as members fail to meet each other's expectations (Spiegel 1968).

In assessing the role structure of a family, the nurse needs to be sensitive not only to the sources of existing role conflict, but also to the ways in which the conflict is handled. Spiegel (1968) identifies two modes that the family system may use to resolve role conflict. The first method, role induction, is effected by means of a unilateral decision. In essence, the stronger member coaxes or coerces the other to submit and take the complementary role. Role modification, the second method, is based on mutual negotiation by both partners and results in the redefinition of their roles in order to achieve a more complementary fit. The way in which a family chooses to resolve role conflict has implications for the flow of energy within the system. Role induction may disrupt the free flow of energy, since much energy may be channeled toward maintaining the coercion. Under such circumstances, members are less likely to direct their attention to health issues.

Specific questions pertinent to an assessment of the family's role structure are

What roles do each of the family members fulfill?
Are these roles acceptable and consistent with the individual's and family's expectations?
If role strain or role conflict exists, what are the contributing factors?
How are role conflicts resolved?
How competently do members perform their roles?
How do past family experiences influence members' role performance?
Is there flexibility in roles when needed?

Communication Patterns
The communication patterns and networks within the family system and with intrafamilial systems in the environment are key dimensions of family behavior. Observation of a family's communication pattern yields an understanding of its structure and organization, as well as the meaning accorded to them by various family members. Communication theorists have articulated a number of axioms that are useful in describing the dynamics involved in family communication (Watzlawick et al. 1967). The first axiom asserts that it is impossible not to communicate. All words or actions have message value. Thus, when a woman responds with silence to her husband's attempts at initiating a discussion, she is communicating, though the message may be unclear.

Second is the principle that every communication conveys both content and a definition of the relationship between the communicants. From the perspective of communication theory, definitional messages connote one or several of the following assertions: "This is how I see myself," "This is how I see you," "This is how I think you see me." The crucial feature in the exchange that follows is the recognition accorded to the other. Responses may confirm, reject, disqualify, or disconfirm the other's self-definition. Disqualification and disconfirmation occur through messages that are self-contradictory, ambiguous, tangential, inconsistent, and/or topic changes (Watzlawick et al. 1967).

Observations of the patterns of acknowledgment among family members provide evidence of the affect, power, and meaning accorded to each member. Feelings of self-worth are developed and internalized through repetitive interactions with significant others (Satir 1972; Lewis et al. 1976).

The third axiom notes that every communication is simultaneously a stimulus and a response (Watzlawick et al. 1967). Disagreement about how to punctuate the sequence of events, namely, who is to blame, is basic to many relationship struggles among family members. Closely related to this axiom is the fourth, which describes the verbal and nonverbal aspects of communication. Both modes are used concurrently and are essential to comprehending the full meaning of messages transmitted between the parties involved. Verbal language conveys the concrete substance of the message, while nonverbal language transmits the more subtle nature of the relationship and describes more fully the true significance and intent of the message. The degree of congruence and balance between the verbal and nonverbal portions of an exchange define the degree of clarity and openness present in a relationship. The dynamic nature of family communication, however, points to the importance of members' developing skills in eliciting feedback and validations of messages in order to further minimize misinterpretation of cues and faulty mind reading (Bandler et al. 1976).

The significant role power plays in communication is reflected in the fifth axiom, which speaks to the symmetrical or complementary properties of interpersonal exchanges. Symmetrical exchanges emphasize equality, whereas complementary exchanges emphasize differences among communicants. Typically, in a complementary situation, one party assumes the dominant position and the other follows. Both patterns may exist within a relationship and may serve useful functions under varying circumstances. A healthy family is able to shift from one mode to another, providing for some degree of choice for all members as appropriate (Kantor and Lehr 1976). By noting the patterns of symmetry and complementarity within family interaction, the nurse may infer the leadership structure of the family.

Covert family rules also have a significant impact on family communication patterns. Satir (1972) defines rules as the "should" and "should nots" of family life. For example, a family rule may be that only positive feelings should be expressed, or that sex is not an appropriate topic of discussion. Rules are the clearest reflection of the value system operating in the family and are often socioculturally determined. Problems arise when rules unduly restrict freedom of expression and growth.

Communication patterns are, perhaps, the most observable manifestations of the family's level of differentiation and consciousness. The use of "I-ness" as opposed to "we-ness" and the extent of mind reading and censorship (e.g., "You shouldn't say that," "You have no reason to feel that angry") present in members' communications with one another provide important clues to the clarity of interpersonal boundaries and the system's level of differentiation (Lewis et al. 1976). In linking communication patterns to the family's level of consciousness, Reiss (1971) notes that when individuals share their ideas and feelings freely and completely, they have a broad and common base of cues and provisional solutions upon which to base their final conclusions. Problem solving is more effective in such families because members contribute to the solution of the concern. Moreover, extreme negativity as a communication pattern limits learning. Members learn what is not expected of them, but are given no clear explanations of alternative behaviors (Harris 1973). Research findings documenting negativity as a characteristic interactional style of abusing families may help to explain why abuse appears in successive generations of families (Justice and Justice 1976).

Questions useful to consider in evaluating family communications include

Who talks to whom?
Are interactions among varying members symmetrical or complementary?
Do members clearly state their needs and feelings (congruence between verbal and nonverbal messages)?
How well do members listen when others are communicating?
Do members elicit feedback and validation in communicating with one another?
What are the predominant patterns of acknowledgment accorded varying members?
Are messages age-appropriate?
Is there much mind reading or censorship of members' messages?
What feelings or issues are closed to discussion?

Decision-Making Processes
Decision making is central to the fulfillment of family tasks and responsibilities (Paolucci et al. 1977). Essentially, it is a process that involves (a) the recognition of a need for a decision, (b) identifying and weighing alternatives, and (c) selecting an alternative and facilitating its implementation. Central to effective decision making is the processing of information; the decision maker(s) must be able to discriminate between what is important and what is not, between what is relevant and what is irrelevant, between actions that will achieve goals and those that will not. Ultimately closure is reached and a choice is made (Paolucci et al. 1977).

The rules used to weigh alternatives and to arrive at a choice are important indicators of family values. Preference ranking involves the original arrangement of alternatives according to perceived advantages and disadvantages. The latter may involve evaluating the alternatives against one or more subjectively defined attributes; the more attributes evaluated, the more complex the decision making. The alternative chosen may reflect the most effective option, the one likely to yield the quickest solution, or the one easiest to implement, or some combination thereof. While family decision making should not consume inordinate amounts of time, immediate closure through the selection of a single option without explicit ranking or elimination of alternatives is characteristic of dysfunctional families. Healthy, functioning families explore numerous options, and if one alternative does not work, the family backs off and tries another, instead of trying to make just one option work (Pratt 1976; Paolucci et al. 1977). Quite obviously, the family's level of consciousness and decision-making competence are integrally related.

Observations about family decision-making processes also help to clarify its power structure. Families tend to reach decisions either by consensus or accommodation (Turner 1970). With consensus, a particular course of action is mutually agreed upon by all concerned. With accommodation, some member(s) assent in order to allow a decision to be reached. Accommodation occurs by use of compromising, bargaining, and coercion. The result of such differentiation is that persons most closely identified with the decision reached come to be defined as dominant. Yet, it is important to recognize that even when a consensus is reached, some family members decided that the suggestions of others are better than their own. Thus, the astute observer, by measuring and locating the direction of system energy flow, can identify power that is exercised covertly (Kantor and Lehr 1976).

Of equal importance to note are those situations in which families arrive at no decision. Discussions finish inconclusively and are then decided by events, as with a couple who argue about what form of birth control to use until the wife discovers she is pregnant. Such an event is called de facto decision making in that things are allowed to happen without planning. De facto decision making is a characteristic of multiproblem families, many of whose members feel powerless and/or lack the energy to actively manage their lives. It also may occur in highly stressful situations when members' abilities to process information is reduced or when problems in communication exist (Friedman 1981).

In assessing family decision making, the nurse needs to examine both process and outcome. Pertinent questions for consideration are

Who makes what decisions?
Are there particular needs/issues that are not recognized or addressed?
Is the family able to discriminate between information that is relevant and that which is irrelevant to the decision?
Are alternative solutions generated?
What criteria are used to weigh alternatives?
Is the selected alternative implemented?
To what extent does family decision making involve consensus, compromise, bargaining, or coercion?
Does the mode of decision making affect the outcome?
Is the family satisfied with the results of their choices?

Temporal Perspective
The family's temporal orientation works as a filter for members' experience in the present. Stresses and unresolved conflicts from past generations can compound the difficulties a family experiences as it progresses through its own life cycle. Families who are unable to acknowledge the passage of time are

likely to experience developmental transitions as more stressful (Lewis et al. 1976; Beavers 1977). Furthermore, the prioritizing of daily activities is dependent on an awareness of a past, a present, and a future. Inappropriate pacing rhythms may lead to energetic imbalance (Kantor and Lehr 1976). The family literally overextends itself, undertaking more demands and using more energy than it can hope to supply. With such imbalance, health needs of members are likely to go unmet.

Individual members of a family also may find themselves out of phase with one another because of widely disparate schedules. Some shared time is essential if members are to gain access to affect, power, and meaning from one another (Kantor and Lehr 1976). Lack of adequate time for communication of ideas and feelings is likely to foster immediate closure in decision making. In addition, the ability to prioritize and effectively manage time facilitates anticipatory planning and minimizes de facto decision making (Paolucci et al. 1977; Friedman 1981).

Questions relevant to an assessment of the family's temporal perspective include

What is the family's orientation to the past, present, and future?
Do individual members emphasize differing temporal perspectives?
Is the family able to acknowledge the passage of time?
Can the family maintain a temporal balance in scheduling activities in order to avoid misuse of its energies?
Do members have opportunities for shared time?

Values
Knowledge of the value orientations of the family provides direction to understanding the why of family dynamics. A family's configuration of values ascribes meaning to certain critical events and suggests ways to respond to them (Friedman 1981). The identification of family values, however, is often compounded by the family's own lack of awareness of how it ascribes worth to people, events, and things. It is important to distinguish both the overt and covert values operative in family behavior.

Kluckhohn (1968) proposes that value orientations of the family reflect their ideas, beliefs, and feelings about (a) the nature of man, (b) the relation of man to nature, (c) the definition of people's relation to one another, and (d) the modality of human activity. Beliefs and feelings about the nature of man may underlie family members' responses to one another. Given the view that people are basically evil and potentially threatening, then relationships are likely to be oppositional. Parent-child interactions, under such circumstances, tend to emphasize control and discipline. Distrust of others also is likely to curtail relationships outside the family, leading to more closed boundaries. On the other hand, if people are perceived as basically good, though subject to mistakes, family relationships are more likely to be open, trusting, and tolerant of diversity.

How a family perceives its relation to nature may be reflective of the extent to which it actively copes with its concerns. The family that feels it has little control over what happens does not take the initiative to seek out new ideas, information, or resources and apply them to the solution of family problems or to minimize health risks. In addition, support systems mobilized during crises tend to be guided by beliefs about people's relationships with each other. Assistance from the extended family occurs more frequently in families that view lineal and collateral ties as important (Kluckhohn 1968). Changing perspectives about family ties, to the contrary, may be manifested in intergenerational conflict. The discrepancies in role expectations that emerge between the elderly and their adult children and grandchildren are illustrative of such conflict.

Kluckhohn subdivides the family's activity orientation according to the relative emphasis placed on "being," "being-in-becoming," or "doing." The being orientation encourages the spontaneous expression of self in the here and now, whereas the being-in-becoming orientation is more of a striving toward self-actualization. The doing orientation emphasizes productivity and accomplishments. Again, discrepancies in role expectations may arise when family members do not share similar activity orientations.

There is a hierarchial nature to family values that gives them a varied priority or potency. The relative ranking of health in the family's hierarchy of values is important in determining the extent to which forces within the family tend to sustain or undermine health care behavior (Friedman 1981). Disparity between values held by the family and nurse can result in divergent goals. An accurate assessment of a family's value system should help to tailor interventions to goals that are important to the family.

A family's values are a reflection of its subculture, as well as the community in which it resides. Obviously the greater the degree of congruence between a family's subcultural values and the community's values, the more the community supports the family's identity. Incompatibility in values between the family and community generates conflict that increases stress within the family as a system. Such stress may disrupt family functioning and negatively affect members' self-esteem (Handel 1972; Friedman 1981).

Key questions to consider in assessing a family's values are

What are the salient values that guide family behavior?
Are the values overt or covert?
How important are the identified values to the family?
What is the relative ranking of health in the family's hierarchy of values?
Are there any value conflicts evident within the family, between the family
    and community?
Do these conflicts impede family functioning?
To what extent do family values foster active coping and mastery of concerns?

FAMILY ADAPTABILITY

The nursing assessment not only provides information about how well the family is able to fulfill its health responsibilities, but also serves as a predictor of the family's adaptive potential. Family adaptability refers to the family's capacity to meet obstacles and shift courses as a family (Beavers 1977). Change is an inherent aspect of family life. Role positions and reciprocal relationships within the family and its suprasystem alter with the developmental changes of members. The family life cycle is described in terms of developmental stages characterized by major family events — in particular, the addition and exiting of members (Carter and McGoldrick 1980). The concept of family developmental tasks, central to the life cycle perspective, refers to changes in the normative expectations for the family at any given stage. Paranormative events, such as divorce, miscarriage, illness, or job loss, may modify the normative momentum of the family unit. Such events, however, do not occur universally to all families (Terkelsen 1980). Key transitions in the family life cycle, as outlined by Carter and McGoldrick (1980), appear in Tables 4.1 and 4.2.

The accomplishment of its developmental tasks assures the continuous functioning and health of the family throughout the life cycle. Bain (1978) advances a theory to predict the capacity of families to cope with life cycle transitions that may serve as a guide for the community health nurse. According to his theory, the capacity (C) of a family to cope with a transition is inversely proportional to its transitional density (TD) and the magnitude of role changes (RC) involved in the particular transition; it is directly proportional to the degree of organization of the formal social container (FSC) it comes in contact with during the transition and the size and relevance of its social network (SN).

$$C = \frac{FSC \cdot SN}{TD \cdot RC}$$

More specifically, transitional density refers to the number of normative and paranormative changes that are taking place within the family at the given point in time. The magnitude of stress created by such changes is cumulative and is equal to the sum of their varying intensities. Bain posits the use of Holmes and Rahe's Social Readjustment Rating Scale (1967) as one means of measuring the cumulative magnitude of role change. In cases of transition where there is institutional contact, the definition of the event by the institution and available services constitutes the social container. Lastly, there is the preparation for the event and help in adjustment that may be derived from relatives, friends, neighbors, work, and other colleagues who constitute the family's social network (Bain 1978).

Based on the preceding theory, one may predict that those families who are likely to have the least capacity to cope with transitional crises, or who are at most risk, are (a) those with a high transitional density involving (b) role changes of a great magnitude, who come in contact with (c) a highly fragmented social container and have (d) a social network that is small and irrelevant to the transition.

CONTRACTING: THE NURSE-FAMILY TRANSACTION

Since family competence in fulfilling its health responsibilities requires self-direction and self-governance, the model for nurse-family transactions should facilitate the family's active participation in dealing with the health concerns or issues that it is experiencing. Indeed, the family's active participation in nurse-family transactions may be a significant variable in determining the effectiveness of nursing intervention. The contracting process provides a vehicle for enhancing family participation in its own health maintenance. Contracting is based on the belief that families have the potential for self-growth and the right to self-determination. It calls for an active participative as well as a collaborative role for both family and nurse. "The essential ingredient in such a model is mutual interaction in which energy can be freely exchanged between the persons involved in the process. In this way dominance and dependence diminish while interdependence, sharing, and trust evolve" (Williamson 1981).

The contracting process may be subdivided into five interlinking, sequenced phases (Sloan and Schommer 1975). As with any relationship, the phases denote an ebb and flow of movement rather than discrete points at which something begins or ends. In the description that follows, each phase is discussed separately.

1. Identification of Health Concerns, Needs, and Problems

This phase begins with the initial contact between the family and the nurse. Knowledge, both subjective and objective, is gained about each other through observation and exchange of information. The use of a conceptual framework for assessing family functioning facilitates a clear identification of the problem(s) and any accompanying concerns or interests. The preferable outcome of this first phase is an agreement between the nurse and family on the definition of the problems, needs, and concerns to be addressed in subsequent interactions. Two other outcomes are also possible: (a) referral to a more appropriate service, or (b) termination because congruence between nurse and family does not exist and effective problem solving is not feasible (Williamson 1981).

In working with the family as the focal unit of service, it is important to establish the perspective that concerns and problems are those of the family rather than that of an individual. Consequently, meeting with as many family members present as possible is desirable, especially early in the process. The usefulness of such family representation lies in a number of reasons. First, by mere physical presence, each family member is demonstrating some concern

Table 4.1. The Stages of the Family Life Cycle

Family Life Cycle Stage	Emotional Process of Transition: Key Principles	Second Order Changes in Family Status Required to Proceed Developmentally
1. Between families: the unattached young adult	Accepting parent-offspring separation	a. Differentiation of self in relation to origin b. Development of intimate peer relationships c. Establishment of self in work
2. The joining of families through marriage: the newly married couple	Commitment to new system	a. Formation of marital system b. Realignment of relationships with extended families and friends to include spouse
3 The family with young children	Accepting new members into the system	a. Adjusting marital system to make space for child(ren) b. Taking on parenting roles c. Realignment of relationships with extended family to include parenting and grandparenting roles
4. The family with adolescents	Increasing flexibility of family boundaries to include children's independence	a. Shifting of parent-child relationships to permit adolescent to move in and out of system b. Refocus on mid-life marital and career issues c. Beginning shift toward concerns for older generation

5.	Launching children and moving on	Accepting a multitude of exits from and entries into the family system	a.	Renegotiation of marital system as a dyad
			b.	Development of adult-to-adult relationships between grown children and their parents
			c.	Realignment of relationships to include in-laws and grandchildren
			d.	Dealing with disabilities and death of parents (grandparents)
6.	The family in later life	Accepting the shifting of generational roles	a.	Maintaining own and/or couple functioning and interests in face of physiological decline: exploration of new familial and social role options
			b.	Support for a more central role for middle generation
			c.	Making room in the system for the wisdom and experience of the elderly: supporting the older generation without overfunctioning for them
			d.	Dealing with loss of spouse, siblings, and other peers and preparation for own death. Life review and integration

Reproduced with permission from: Carter EA and McGoldrick M. The family life cycle: a framework for family therapy. New York: Gardner Press, Inc., 1980.

Table 4.2. Dislocations of the Family Life Cycle Requiring Additional Steps to Restabilize and Proceed Developmentally

Phase	Emotional Process of Transition Prerequisite Attitude	Developmental Issues
DIVORCE		
Decision to divorce	Acceptance of inability to resolve marital tensions sufficiently to continue relationship	Acceptance of one's own part in the failure of the marriage
Planning the breakup of the system	Supporting viable arrangements for all parts of the system	Working cooperatively on problems of custody, visitation, finances. Dealing with extended family about the divorce
Separation	Willingness to continue cooperative co-parental relationship Work on resolution of attachment to spouse	Mourning loss of intact family Restructuring marital and parent-child relationships; adaptation to living apart Realignment of relationships with extended family; staying connected with spouse's extended family
Divorce	More work on emotional divorce: overcoming hurt, anger, guilt, etc.	Mourning loss of intact family: giving up fantasies of reunion Retrieval of hopes, dreams, expectations from the marriage Staying connected with extended families
POST-DIVORCE FAMILY		
Single parent family	Willingness to maintain parental contact with ex-spouse and support contact of children with ex-spouse and his family	Making flexible visitation arrangements with ex-spouse and his family Rebuilding own social network
Single-parent (noncustodial)	Willingness to maintain parental contact with ex-spouse and support custodial parent's relationship with children	Finding ways to continue effective parenting relationship with children. Rebuilding own social network

REMARRIED FAMILY FORMATION

Entering the new relationship	Recovery from loss of first marriage (adequate "emotional divorce")	Recommitment to marriage and to forming a family with readiness to deal with the complexity and ambiguity
Conceptualizing and planning new marriage and family	Accepting one's own fears and those of new spouse and children about remarriage and forming a stepfamily	Work on openness in the new relationships to avoid pseudomutuality Plan for maintenance of cooperative co-parental relationships with ex-spouses Plan to help children deal with fears, loyalty conflicts, and membership in two systems. Realignment of relationships with extended family to include new spouse and children Plan maintenance of connections for children with extended family of ex-spouse(s)
Remarriage and reconstitution of family	Final resolution of attachment to previous spouse and ideal of "intact" family; acceptance of a different model of family with permeable boundaries	Restructuring family boundaries to allow for inclusion of new spouse-stepparent Realignment of relationships throughout subsystems to permit interweaving of several systems Making room for relationships of all children with biological (noncustodial) parents, grandparents, and other extended family Sharing memories and histories to enhance stepfamily integration

Reproduced with permission from: Carter EA and McGoldrick M. The family life cycle: a framework for family therapy. New York: Gardner Press, Inc., 1980.

with the situation. Second, having more than one person acknowledge a problem suggests to all assembled that the complexity of the issue extends beyond the individual and an isolated problem. Third, the nurse can observe pertinent data about family interaction patterns and will be less likely to be drawn into a premature alliance with any one family member (Herr and Weakland 1979). The operationalization of such an approach may necessitate an expanded and more flexible policy concerning the scheduling of family visits during evening hours or on occasional weekends. Though the time investment initially may be greater, when this approach is used the family may achieve its goals in a shorter period of time.

An initial phone contact prior to the visit can facilitate the arrangement of a convenient time for family members and the nurse to meet. For example, a nurse might use the approach "It would help me in working with Michelle's diabetes if I could get together with the entire family to talk this matter over." During the first meeting, the ground rules for future meetings should be negotiated and established. The frequency and length of time for each contact as well as who should be present are items to determine. The environment should be made as free as possible from interruptions and distractions such as the radio or television. The nurse's help in structuring the session allows each person the chance to speak about his or her feelings or ideas. With a particularly chaotic family in which the members consistently talk at once, the nurse may need to take a more directive approach by pointing out this behavior and setting a rule that one person speak at a time (Minuchin 1974).

In the first few sessions, the family members may express their discomfort by frequently questioning the reason for meeting with the nurse. Nonverbal manifestations of this response include canceling meetings or members' arriving late, leaving early or working on "important projects" in other rooms of the home. Their embarrassment and tension may be expressed by disruptive laughing, joking, and fidgeting during early meetings. Frequent explanations of the importance of getting to know everyone and their ideas may be necessary. The normalcy of the members' feelings of discomfort and anxiety, particularly if they have not been communicating well in the past, should be emphasized. Direct discussion about the source of the discomfort also may be beneficial. When family members become more involved and committed to working with the nurse, these behaviors generally diminish. In some instances, however, the nurse may never achieve full family participation. It is still important to recognize that the essential ingredient in working with families is the conception of problems in terms of family systems rather than in individual terms.

2. Mutual Setting of Family Goals

What does the family hope to accomplish? This is a crucial question and one that is not asked often enough. By asking what the family hopes to gain from the intervention, the nurse assists the family to focus on its own goals and priorities. The nurse also can gain a sense of congruency between individual member and family goals, often a source of potential conflict. In essence, this phase involves collaborative negotiations and democratic compromise rather than practitioner goal setting (Williamson 1981). The nurse, however, shares observations and knowledge that can facilitate the family's identification of goals.

The communication style used by the nurse can foster or hinder the family's acceptance of a suggested goal. For instance, "Perhaps we need to work on ways to reduce the distress this situation is causing your family" is likely to be met with a more favorable response than "You need to work on improving your communication with one another." The latter approach will invariably raise the family's defenses, while the former approach fosters its willingness to allow the nurse to enter the family as a change agent. Goals that are drawn from the family's expressed concerns and framed in the language of the family, rather than exclusively from the nurse's assessment of what needs to be changed in the family, are more predictive of success. Helping the family to clarify and set realistic, attainable goals is one of the key functions of the nurse in this regard.

Goals should be stated in a precise manner capable of being monitored and a time frame for accomplishment specified. For example, "Mother will explain to son why his behavior is unacceptable and offer suggestions as to what is acceptable behavior under the circumstances" is a more measurable goal than "Mother will improve discipline techniques." Even when specific goals are set, there may be problems. The family's prioritizing of goals may conflict with the nurse's. The nurse may need to support the family's priorities in order to free its energy for other goal attainment. If the nurse cannot offer such support because of possible injury to a particular family member, she or he needs to inform the family what action will be taken.

3. Delineation of Alternatives

Once the goals are established, the nurse and family need to discuss how they can be best accomplished. This process involves (a) the exploration and determination of the family's strengths and available resources, (b) the steps or methods needed to meet the goals, (c) the negotiation and division of responsibilities, and (d) the establishment of a reasonable time limit for implementing the plan.

Emphasizing the already existing family strengths reinforces the family's belief in its own ability to solve problems and meet goals. In working with a family having difficulty with limit-setting and discipline, the nurse might begin by acknowledging the attempts the parents have made to solve the problem and emphasizing how well they are managing other areas of child care. Such an approach fosters esteem and confidence in the family and may facilitate the

Table 4.3. Determination of Risk by Client and Professional and Probability of Success

Desirability		Probability of Success
Client	Nurse	
High	High	High
High	Low	Possible. May lead to
Low	High	experimental agreement
Low	Low	Low
None	High or low	Minimal to no probability
High or low	None	
None	None	None

From: Williamson JA. Mutual interaction: a model of nursing practice. Copyright © 1981, American Journal of Nursing Company. Reproduced with permission from Nursing Outlook, February; Volume 29, Number 2, page 106.

family's acceptance of the nurse as a helping person. A temptation to be avoided is the offering of numerous suggestions about how to do something better or differently before recognizing and drawing out the family's estimation of its problem-solving abilities and resources. Helping the family to identify its own abilities also will enforce its sense of control and power over the problem at hand. The nurse can then supplement the developing knowledge base by introducing family and/or community resources not identified by the family for its consideration.

Feasible solutions can arise from a mutual brainstorming session in which family and nurse identify as many alternatives as imaginable. The nurse should help the family avoid discussing pros and cons of each idea until the list is completed. Opening the brainstorming to every idea imaginable helps the family to test reality as well as to elicit all members' ideas. The brainstorming process concludes with reviewing the merits of each idea proposed. Each is judged in terms of desirability and probability of success. Desirability refers to an acceptable strategy, although not necessarily one that is equally valued by nurse and family. Probability of success implies a strategy that will meet specific goals; it is directly related to desirability in that it is affected by the degree of acceptance of the strategy by the family (Williamson 1981).

A method for evaluating the risks of alternative strategies appears in Table 4.3. For example, a nurse and young couple discussing methods of contraception may differ in their perception of the desirability of available methods. The couple may prefer to rely on spermicidal foams due to their aesthetic appeal and ease of insertion for the wife. Therefore, they rank this method high. From a more scientific orientation, the nurse may feel the use of a diaphragm would be a more desirable choice because of its greater effectiveness in preventing pregnancy. Therefore, the nurse ranks spermicidal foams low. While the diaphragm, indeed, may be a more effective mode of contraception than spermicidal foams, its unacceptability to the couple may lead to irregular usage and, thereby, mitigate any probability of success in preventing an untimely pregnancy. Thus, after hearing the couple's viewpoint, the nurse may alter her or his judgment and support the couple's choice of a method of contraception in an effort to increase the likelihood of its success.

The last step in the planning process is to decide on the sequence of events and the time frame needed to achieve the goal. The nurse generally plays a supportive role in the planning process, encouraging the family to make specific and detailed plans that clearly and concretely outline each person's responsibilities. Agreement on the nurse's role and ways to monitor progress are crucial outcomes of this phase.

4. Implementation of the Plan

The plan and division of responsibilities mutually agreed upon are tried. The nurse plays particularly vital roles during this phase. First is the anticipation of problems or setbacks that may arise, followed by helping the family recognize and deal with them in as positive a way as possible. A series of minor setbacks can discourage and demoralize the family to the point that the carefully negotiated plan may be prematurely abandoned. Frequent contacts for guidance and support during the implementation phase can help individual family members accomplish their tasks. Second, the nurse has a role modeling function: the carrying out of assigned tasks as agreed, within the given time limit. If problems are encountered, the nurse should communicate them openly to the family and seek help in making alternate plans.

Results range from successful implementation to discovering that the selected alternative is not acceptable to the family. The latter may happen when the family and nurse fail to identify the "real" problem, they select unrealistic solutions, or unforeseen outcomes occur.

5. Evaluation

Evaluation is an ongoing process throughout all phases of the nurse-family transaction as well as being an end-phase. Crucial questions to consider in end-phase evaluation are

Was the goal(s) achieved?
Was the selected solution(s) effective?
Should the nurse-family relationship be terminated or should other goals and
    plans be developed?

As in other phases, the family should be encouraged to participate equally by sharing feelings and concerns about its course as well as about the nurse's role in accomplishing outlined responsibilities. Emphasis on positive strides, though they be small, can bolster the family's sense of competence.

The manner in which the nurse-family relationship is concluded is as vital as the way in which it is begun. The establishment of a plan for continuity of care, if needed, is crucial. Often following a period of intensive nursing intervention, a plan for periodic reassessment of the situation is warranted. This is particularly applicable to families dealing with long-term chronic illness or disability. The family should know how to recontact the nurse should unanticipated changes occur prior to the scheduled interval for reappraisal.

SELECTED FOCI FOR FAMILY INTERVENTION

While the goals for each family are highly individualized, it is possible to outline some general focal areas and possible approaches to intervention. The primary purpose of community health nursing is to enhance the family's coping abilities as a way of raising its level of functioning and overall health. Competent families contribute positively to community maintenance of health.

Facilitation of Family Communication

The community health nurse can design approaches to help the family interact more openly and clearly in accomplishing its goals. Helping the family recognize an interactional pattern that is hindering its progress is a key role. Satir (1972) describes several communication games that can be adapted for use by community health nurses for families. An example follows:

Two members of the family are asked to sit back to back and talk about a particular issue, then face each other and "eyeball" each other without talking. They then hold hands with their eyes closed without talking. Finally, they are asked to talk while "eyeballing" one another.

After each step in the exercise, family members may be asked to share their perceptions. In this way, family members become more aware of verbal and nonverbal behaviors and the importance of congruency between these levels of communication.

The nurse may choose to function as a role model and facilitator of effective communication among family members. In doing so, he or she intervenes in the ongoing process between family members and provides new examples of how to respond. For instance, the nurse might intervene when one family member interrupts another by commenting, "I'm interested in what you have to say, Fred, but I'd also like to finish hearing Mary's point of view." Or the nurse might note that while a family member states he agrees with the solution reached, his tone of voice suggests skepticism. Similarly, the nurse may ask family members to comment on what they think a particular member has said and then elicit the member's feedback on whether the message has been interpreted correctly (Bandler et al. 1976). Taping nurse-family interactions and replaying portions of the tape also may facilitate members' recognition of their own ineffective communication styles.

Some family members may benefit from structured skills training in communication (Guerney 1977). The nurse may encourage a couple to enroll in a parent effectiveness training program or a human relations course sponsored by a community agency. She can then assist family members in applying the knowledge gained to their own situations as they work on resolving health concerns. With families uncomfortable with joining a group program, the nurse may attempt some basic skills training in the home. Tapes and workbooks often can be borrowed from community facilities offering such courses to aid in home education.

Nurse-family interactions can serve as a vehicle for fostering communication channels along appropriate interpersonal boundaries (Herr and Weakland 1979). The exclusion of the identified patient from family discussions and problem solving is discouraged. Often grown children act as if an aging parent cannot contribute solutions for meeting his or her care needs. Likewise, if a mother and daughter have formed an alliance that weakens the marital dyad, the nurse can encourage more direct dialogue and decision making between the husband and wife. By taking a leadership role and redirecting interactions as necessary, the nurse assists in restructuring unclear or inappropriate distributions of power between and among members.

Prevention of Role Conflict and Role Insufficiency

The developmental phases of the family life cycle, along with illness and disability, are the occasions for a number of important role changes. Meleis (1975) outlines a number of strategies for preventive role supplementation. Preventive role supplementation entails "the information or experience necessary to bring the role incumbent and significant others to full awareness of the anticipated behavior patterns, units, sentiments, sensations, and goals involved in each role and its complement." It includes (a) role clarification, (b) role taking, (c) role modeling, and (d) role rehearsal.

Role clarification involves the identification of expected behaviors, sentiments, and goals associated with a particular role vis-à-vis significant others (Meleis 1975). For example, the nurse may help new parents to define expectations for self and other. Asking each partner to write down what they view as their responsibilities, what they view as the partner's responsibilities, and what they consider are shared responsibilities can be a useful exercise. The latter will enable the nurse and parents to identify areas of congruence and incongruence. Incongruities in expectations can then be negotiated and compromises reached. The goal in helping family members resolve role incongruities is to minimize role induction, namely, the coercion of one member to assume responsibilities by the reciprocal role partner.

Role taking is the imaginative assumption of the feelings or point of view of another person (Meleis 1975). Prospective parents can be encouraged to explore their feelings about parenthood with each other. For example, the wife may be asked to imagine how the husband may feel about caring for an infant, what concerns he may experience. Or the daughter anticipating the addition of an aging parent into the home situation may be encouraged to think about how the parent may act and feel in the first few weeks following the move. The nurse can assist family members to share and validate their imaginative perceptions, thus sensitizing members further to the others' views.

Through role modeling, the nurse actually can demonstrate certain expected behaviors, e.g., infant feeding or other caring tasks and responsibilities. Closely related to role modeling is the technique of role rehearsal. The nurse can employ role rehearsal in assisting a family member to plan a call to a relative to request assistance with transportation to clinic. How the request will be phrased, how the family member will respond if the request is refused, and alternative courses of action can be reviewed and role played prior to the actual call (Meleis 1975).

Each of the preceding strategies can be employed with individual families or in a group context. Meleis notes that the organization of reference groups composed of families with similar concerns can foster role learning. Reference groups serve as forums for obtaining knowledge and exploring alternatives so that individual participants have a basis for formulating their own expectations. For instance, a postcoronary discussion group for patients and their spouses can facilitate adjustment to diet and activity limitations imposed by illness.

Promotions of Effective Decision Making and Problem Solving

The supportive, teaching, and nurturing roles of the nurse relative to this area of family functioning cannot be understated. Helping family members discuss and clearly identify the concern or problem to be addressed is crucial. During the discussion, the nurse needs to be alert to the family's ability to discriminate between relevant and irrelevant data. Obvious and underlying factors contributing to the problem should be explored (Paolucci et al. 1977).

For example, in the T family, Mrs. T was experiencing severe pain associated with the terminal phase of cancer. The pain was most severe in the early morning hours; other times it was well controlled with pain medication. In spite of the severe morning pain, Mrs. T refused to ask for or take a dose of pain medication at night, claiming that she didn't need it at that time. Her husband and two teenaged sons were becoming increasingly alarmed by the degree of pain she experienced in the morning. Discussion of the problem in a family meeting revealed that (a) Mrs. T did not wish to disturb family members' sleep, was fearful that the medication might make her go to sleep "forever," and did not want to die alone at night; (b) Mr. T had stated many times that "as long as he could get his six hours of sleep, he could manage her care at home" and had taken to sleeping in the guest room; and (c) the youngest son was hardly sleeping because he could hear his mother's restlessness at night, and yet, when he would go to her room to check on her, she would appear to be asleep. Quite obviously, the problem was not simply one of pain, but Mrs. T's fear of dying alone during the night. Mr. T's move to the guest room and his repeated statement about needing "a good night's sleep" were contributing factors influencing Mrs. T's behavior.

Once the problem to be addressed has been identified clearly, the nurse can assist the family in generating alternative solutions. As noted previously, it is important to list all possible alternatives before rejecting any. Immediate closure by considering only one or two alternatives may result in ineffective decision making and problem resolution. Once all conceivable alternatives have been listed, the nurse should aid family members in identifying the criteria to be used for weighing the advantages and disadvantages of each alternative. For instance, with a couple choosing a form of birth control, is the choice to be made on the basis of the method that has the highest percentage of effectiveness in preventing conception? Or are aesthetic appeal or the potential side effects of the various methods important considerations for the couple? Specifying the criteria to be used in reaching the decision enables the nurse to help family members select the most desirable (acceptable) alternative for them (Paolucci et al. 1977). Since desirability has been related to probability of success in implementation, the latter is particularly crucial in meeting identified goals for the family (Williamson 1981).

The nurse can also be facilitative in helping the family recognize the interrelatedness of some decisions. The family encounters many situations in which a strategic choice is the basis for making other choices. For example, the decision of a couple to have a baby may necessitate later choices, such as the need to move to a larger home, whether the wife will continue to work following the birth of the baby, child-care arrangements if the wife desires or needs to work. Often families fail to recognize the multiple choices that follow a central decision (Paolucci et al. 1977). Families with a predominant present-time orientation especially may benefit from nursing guidance in this area. Anticipatory guidance may prevent future crises.

Enhancement of the Family's Sense of Competence

Family members' self-esteem and sense of mastery are critical elements in the family's overall feeling of competence to deal with change. The nurse can assist the family to feel more worthwhile and in control by using approaches designed to raise individual and family self-esteem. The previously discussed interventions aimed at improving communication, role performance, and decision making of the family inherently have the effect of raising family self-esteem by involving members in working out their own problem using their own resources. In *Conjoint Family Therapy*, Satir (1964) outlines numerous therapeutic approaches designed to increase the family's sense of value, self-control, and tolerance of differences between members. As in the other approaches, the core technique is one of role modeling behaviors that project a sense of respect for each family member. Efforts directed at increasing the clarity of communication by validating meanings of statements underscore the value the nurse places on each member.

The nurse needs to guard against giving the impression of having all the answers. Encouraging members to seek clarification when they don't understand his or her messages helps them to acknowledge the nurse's fallibility. Accentuating the mutuality of the interventive process and responding positively to the family's attempts at problem solving will foster their self-esteem. Statements such as "I wonder if you realize how really well you are communicating with one another right now" or "You really know how to work hard in this family" are examples.

Labeling is also useful in raising self-esteem. Families with low self-esteem frequently attach negative labels to one another. The nurse can redirect this process in an esteem-building way by creating positive labels. For example, the youngest son is labeled the "baby" of the family by his parents and siblings. During the history-taking process, the nurse learns that he is a talented pianist. Later, she refers to him on several occasions as the "musician" in the family and praises the self-discipline he possesses in adhering to his daily practice sessions. In this way, the positive features of a berated member are brought to the attention of the family, with the additional effect of nurturing and elevating the status of the individual.

A pivotal aspect of interventions designed to raise self-esteem lies in setting expectations that are realistic, attainable, and highly productive of success. Success begets success, while failure often results in more failure. Asking questions the family is capable of answering is one way to encourage success. Setting small, concrete tasks and goals that the family is likely to accomplish will help them feel more in control and less frustrated. Making "homework" assignments between family meetings that the family may work on together perhaps will re-introduce a sense of family competency. For example, a nurse was visiting two elderly sisters living together. The identified patient, diagnosed with congestive heart failure, complained that her sister was afraid to let her do anything. Further exploration revealed that she particularly missed cooking the meals, formerly in her domain. Their negotiated homework assignment was for the sisters to cook a meal together by the time of the next meeting. The sisters planned a simple menu that was carried out with considerable ease, much to the delight of the patient. By the following meeting, the sisters were planning other meals. Small, successful gains often evolve gradually into major accomplishments when underpinned with a rising self-esteem.

Asking family members to describe themselves using only positive terms or to write down all the things they like about themselves can be a useful exercise. This can be done individually, then shared with the rest of the family, or the family can work together on describing each other in positive ways. The nurse must first set a norm that it is okay to compliment oneself occasionally and give the family permission to brag a little. These parameters can be set when introducing the exercise. The nurse could say, "I'll start. For instance, one of the things I like about me is my ability to get my point across." This approach achieves two objectives. First, it role models the norm. Second, it communicates that it is all right to speak directly about what one thinks and feels. Most families find this exercise embarrassing at first, but later find it fun and refreshing to focus on something good again. The exercise helps the family to shift its thinking and helps the members to recall pleasurable experiences and feelings. A similar, but more anxiety-provoking exercise can be used to reinforce the strengthening features of the differences between members. The family members are asked to list the ways in which they differ from one another. During the ensuing discussion, the nurse can emphasize how these differences may make the family better equipped to cope with various situations.

Strengthening Family Support Systems

The family that appears to need multiple supports and has few or none poses a serious concern for community health nursing. Often a thorough assessment of the structural and interactional processes in the family will help the nurse to gain insight as to why the family lacks an effective support system. An absent or poor support system is more likely a symptom than a cause of dysfunction. Consequently, finding the cause rather than dealing with the symptom may be the first priority.

A family's low sense of self-esteem, coupled with a need to be in complete control, may be one reason why external supports are not utilized. Poor communication may make past associations with supports less than satisfactory. Referring such families to multiple agencies or resources will likely end in failure due to the family's increased resistance. Rather, helping the family to work on underlying issues develops positive feelings toward nurses as helpers that can facilitate the family's referral to other resources in the future.

It is equally important to assess the family's attitudes toward using help. Exploring past utilization of external supports helps a family recognize similarities between the situations and clarify its need to engage external systems. Society tends to place high value on self-sufficiency, sometimes making it difficult for a family to reach out for help. Additionally, the stigma associated with certain health concerns may make it even more difficult for the family to seek help. Families unwilling to seek professional services may be encouraged to join self-help groups with similar concerns. Often peer support from others in a group will promote family readiness for further intervention.

With some families who find it difficult to accept help from external supports, the nurse might attempt a simple game or exercise. She can have the family members pretend that they are running a small business (e.g., restaurant, grocery store). Each member is assigned a specific role (e.g., owner, manager, clerk) to play. Problem situations are written on cards and then given to the individuals to solve. For example, a clerk could go on disability following an illness. Those family members assigned decision making roles must then arrive at solutions for operating the business in the interim. Roles can be exchanged, allowing each family member to experience several types of roles. The game allows the family to look at an analogous problem in a more objective and less emotionally laden way. The need to compensate for jobs that must continue becomes clear, and often the need to seek external resources seems logical and clear. As a result, the family may more clearly understand its own need to restructure internal resources and utilize external supports during certain life changes.

The nurse also can work together with the family to identify whether the need exists for enhancing the quantity and/or quality of its day-to-day support systems. As necessary, the nurse can help the family explore more comfortable ways to communicate needs to relatives, neighbors, and friends. Brainstorming can lead to the identification of new sources for social contact and support. However, it is most important that the nurse respect the family's desire and values concerning the use of supports. She or he must remain a resource regarding possible sources of support rather than impose unwanted supports on families. No referrals or contacting of relatives and friends should be undertaken without the family's expressed consent.

Reduction of Environmental Stress

The home environment may be an additional source of stress for families. Environmental alterations in the use of space often are necessary in the management of an extended illness in the home. The need for personal space and comfort, the integration of the ill member into family routines and activities, and the convenience for the primary caregiver are important considerations in space reallocation. The nurse can make feasible suggestions regarding arrangement of space in the home, considering family members' feelings and values about their environment. He or she also may need to encourage caregivers to reserve time and space to meet their personal needs, thereby minimizing role strain and fatigue. In fact, helping family caregivers recognize and accept their own needs without feeling guilty may be one of the most significant contributions to maintaining home care.

SUMMARY

The primary health responsibilities of the family are (a) the provision of opportunities for members to achieve a satisfactory sense of personal identity and worth, (b) emotional support and cognitive guidance for members experiencing life transition and personal crises, (c) care provision and/or care management for chronically ill, disabled, or aging members, (d) education of members about how to maintain health and when and how to use professional services, and (e) the socialization of members to value health and to accept personal responsibility for its maintenance. Conceptual models are used to assess family functioning relative to these health responsibilities. The model proposed here suggests that the pool of energy and consciousness within the family reflects, to a large extent, its health potential. Many family processes and structural characteristics may influence that level of energy and consciousness within a family system. Nursing approaches for enhancing the family's capability to fulfill its health responsibilities must be evaluated within the overall framework of the nurse-family contract. Through the promotion of family competence and adaptability, a community's health can, indeed, be advanced.

REFERENCES

Ackerman N. The psychodynamics of family life. New York: Basic Books, 1958.

American Nurses Association, Community Health Nursing Division. A conceptual model of community health nursing. Kansas City, Missouri, 1980.

American Public Health Association, Governing Council. Definition and role of public health nursing practice in the delivery of health care. Am J Public Health. 1982; 72:210.

Archbold P. Impact of parent caring on women. Fam Relations 1983; 32:39.

Auger JR. Behavioral systems and nursing. Englewood Cliffs, N.J.: Prentice-Hall, 1976.

Bain A. The capacity of families to cope with transition: a theoretical essay. Hum Relations 1978; 8:675.

Bandler R, Grindler J, and Satir V. Changing with families. Palo Alto, CA: Science and Behavior Books, 1976.

Beavers WR. Psychotherapy and growth: a family systems perspective. New York: Brunner/Mazel, 1977.

Bentov I. Stalking the wild pendulum. New York: Dutton, 1977.

Carter EA, and McGoldrick M, eds. The family life cycle: a framework for family therapy. New York: Gardner Press, 1980.

d'Abate L. Understanding and helping the individual in the family. New York: Grune and Stratton, 1976.

Friedman MA. Family nursing: theory and assessment. New York: Appleton-Century-Crofts, 1981.

Guerney B. Relationship enhancement. San Francisco: Jossey-Bass, 1977.

Handel G, ed. The psychosocial interior of the family. 3rd ed. Chicago: Aldine-Atherton, 1972.

Harris SE. Negativity as a major communication pattern in a family. In: Smoyak S, ed. The psychiatric nurse as a family therapist. New York: Wiley, 1975.

Herr JJ, and Weakland JH. Counseling elders and their families: practical techniques for applied gerontology. New York: Springer, 1979.

Holmes TH, and Rahe, RH. The social readjustment rating scale. J Psychosom Res 1967; 11:213.

Janosik EH, and Miller JR. Theories of family development. In: Hymovich DP, Barnard MU, eds. Family health care. Vol. 1. New York: McGraw-Hill, 1979.

Jourard SM. Disclosing man to himself. New York: D. Van Nostrand Rheinhold, 1968.

Justice B, and Justice R. The abusing family. New York: Human Sciences Press, 1976.

Kantor D, and Lehr W. Inside the family. New York: Harper & Row, 1976.

Karpel M. Individuation: from fusion to dialogue. Fam Process 1976; 15(3):67.

Kluckhohn FR. Variations in the basic values of family systems. In: Bell N, Vogel E, eds. A modern introduction to the family. New York: Free Press, 1968.

Lazlo E, ed. The relevance of general systems theory. New York: George Braziller, 1972.

Lewis JM, Beavers WR, Gossett JT, and Phillips VA. No single thread: psychological health in family systems. New York: Brunner/Mazel, 1976.

Marston MV, and Chambers BM. Development of family conceptual frameworks. In: Miller JR, Janosik EH, eds. Family-focused care. New York: McGraw-Hill, 1980.

Meleis AI. Role insufficiency and role supplementation: a conceptual framework. Nurs Res 1975; 24:264.

Minuchin S. Families and family therapy. Cambridge, MA: Harvard University Press, 1974.

Otto H. Criteria for assessing family strength. Fam Process 1976; 2:329.

Paolucci B, Hall O, and Axina N. Family decision making: an ecosystem approach. New York: Wiley, 1977.

Parsons T. The normal American family. In: Skolnick AS, ed. Families in transition. Boston: Little, Brown, 1971.

Pratt L. Family structure and effective health behavior: the energized family. Boston: Houghton Mifflin, 1976.

Reiss D. Varieties of consensual experience: a theory for relating family interaction to individual thinking. Fam Process 1971; 10:1.

Ryder NB. The family in developed countries. Sci Am 1974; 235(9):123.

Satir V. Conjoint family therapy. Palo Alto, CA: Science and Behavior Books, 1964.

Satir V. Peoplemaking. Palo Alto, CA: Science and Behavior Books, 1972.

Sedgwick R. Family mental health: theory and practice. St. Louis: Mosby, 1981.

Sloan MR, and Schommer BT. The process of contracting in community health nursing. In: Spradley BW, ed. Contemporary community nursing. Boston: Little, Brown, 1975.

Spiegel JP. The resolution of role conflict within the family. In: Bell N, Vogel E, eds. A modern introduction to the family. New York: Free Press, 1968.

Terkelsen KG. Toward a theory of the family life cycle. In: Carter EA, McGoldrick M, eds. The family life cycle: a framework for family therapy. New York: Gardner Press, 1980.

Turner R. Family interaction. New York: Wiley, 1970.

von Bertalanffy L. General systems theory. New York: George Braziller, 1968.

Watzlawick P, Beavin J, and Jackson D. Pragmatics of human communication. New York: Norton, 1967.

Williams GJ, and Money J, eds. Traumatic abuse and neglect of children at home. Baltimore: The Johns Hopkins University Press, 1980.

Williamson JA. Mutual interaction: a model of nursing practice. Nurs Outlook 1981; 29:104.

INDIVIDUAL AS CLIENT 5

Cheryl L. Cox

Care of the individual across the age span, across the health-illness continuum, and in a variety of environmental settings has always occupied a significant part of community health nursing practice. This "generalist" role has traditionally emphasized the integration of individual client care within the context of the family and the larger community. The last two decades, however, have witnessed both a shift in and expansion of this emphasis. Care of the individual as client is exploding in kind, quality, and quantity. While the context of community health nursing practice is still individuals and their social and structural environment, the depth and breadth of the generalist practice with individual clients have been significantly extended. Many of today's community health nurses are competent in providing primary care for adults and children with acute self-limiting and chronic illnesses. With fewer resources for in-patient care, more emphasis is being placed on home care; as a result, community health nurses are dealing with more serious illnesses in the home than has been the tradition. There is no apparent end in sight for the extent to which this practice will be further expanded in the future.

Accompanying this tremendous diversification of community health nursing practice to meet individual client needs is the simultaneous explosion of knowledge about individual health behavior, approaches to effecting lifestyle changes, and the impact of various environmental factors on the individual's health status and utilization of health care services and resources. This knowledge is derived from the basic sciences, the psychosocial sciences, and the synthesis of these sciences with the practice arts of nursing. In order to more fully utilize this knowledge to develop sound community health nursing interventions in diverse practice settings, it must be organized and systematically related within some type of practice conceptual framework. At the same time, this organized knowledge should provide direction for testing the impact of community health nursing practice on outcomes relevant to the individual as client. The systematic organization and subsequent testing of this extensive knowledge base clarifies exactly who the client is in need of community health nursing services and just how nursing interventions can be developed to address his or her needs.

This chapter focuses on community health nurses' care of individuals. The scope and nature of community health nursing practice as it relates to the individual is explored; then a conceptual framework derived from the concepts and constructs within the psychosocial sciences and nursing relates these characteristics of practice to individual client health outcomes. Finally comes a

129

discussion of the significance of this conceptual framework for community health nursing practice and research.

THE SCOPE OF COMMUNITY HEALTH NURSING PRACTICE WITH INDIVIDUALS

Current economic, social, and political trends occurring within the health care system have demanded that community health nurses expand their skills and responsibilities to include the evaluation and management of individual client illness at the primary, secondary, and even tertiary care levels. At the same time, community health nurses continue to carry major responsibilities for the promotion of individual clients' health-generating behaviors aimed at achieving higher levels of wellness. A few of the public and political determinants that have forced this tremendous practice expansion in caring for individuals ar considered in this discussion.

Two areas that have contributed significantly to the expansion of the community health nursing role with individual clients are (a) the political and professional concerns with the organization, delivery, and financing of health care, and (b) the public's increasing demands for the general availability, accessibility, and acceptability of health care. The cost issue in health care is paradoxical to the availability and accessibility issues. As political and health professional efforts are increased to provide health care services more extensively and equitably to all members of American society, the reality of cost containment in health care seems to grow more elusive.

These problems are not new to community health nurses. The elderly, minorities, poor, and residents of geographical locations unserved by physicians have in the past borne and still today bear the brunt of the high cost and inaccessibility of health care services. It is the community health nurse who has traditionally addressed the health care needs of individuals comprised by these groups. Recently, through expansion of their physical assessment and illness management skills, community health nurses have been able to demonstrate their exceptional capabilities in providing direct primary care to clients (Runyan 1972, 1975; Sullivan 1982) and their ability to address effectively the cost containment issues in the delivery of this care (Yankauer and Sullivan 1982). (See Chapter 6 for a more detailed review of community health nursing research in primary care.)

Another major determinant of community health nursing's role expansion is the proliferation of home health care. The exorbitant costs of hospital care and the reduction of hospital beds, together with the increasing availability of financial resources to cover the expense of home care, have led to the earlier hospital discharge of seriously ill clients than has been customary in the past. Local health planning agencies are putting pressure on hospitals to transfer clients more rapidly from acute care beds to extended care beds and eventually to home care with skilled nursing intervention.

Additionally, home health care increasingly represents an appealing health care alternative for the elderly. While those 65 years of age and older comprise only 11 percent of the total population, they account for nearly 30 percent of the national health expenditures (HEW 1979). The largest single expenditure for this group is hospital care, which comprises 45 percent of their health care costs; nursing home care represents an additional 23 percent.

The decreased emphasis on hospital care, the increased demand for home health services, and the increasing number of elderly who are already home-bound or who would elect to stay in their homes if home health care were available has clearly had an impact on the community health nursing role. Community health nurses have become skilled in the assessment and man-agement of more morbid conditions. Equipment and technological interven-tions that were at one time only to be found in institutions providing secondary and tertiary levels of care are now common occurrences within the home. Dialysis machines, respirators, and cardiorespiratory monitors are increasingly becoming the kinds of equipment with which community health nurses must routinely deal. They must not only be familiar with this advanced technology but also with the client responses and problems associated with such technology.

Additionally, community health nurses have become skilled in the labora-tory assessment of clients in the home. Often, medications and specific inter-ventions are initiated or discontinued on the basis of the clients' laboratory findings. Because some clients are not able to get to the appropriate facility for laboratory evaluation and because the effective management of their health care is dependent upon these data, the community health nurse has had to become familiar with and skilled at the collection of specimens and, in some cases, even the performance of the laboratory procedure itself. Routine urin-alysis, prothrombin times, serum digitalis and potassium levels, other clinical chemistries, and throat, blood, and urine cultures are but a few examples of the laboratory evaluations being done for home health care clients (Runyan 1975).

Once the data are obtained, then the community health nurse is faced with making judgments about specific management techniques based on the results of the laboratory procedures. These judgments are frequently made indepen-dently, either based on a specified protocol or based on phone consultation with a physician. In either case, this level of decision making is a departure from the traditional community health nursing role and has appreciably ex-tended the scope of the practice.

Another contribution to the expanded scope of practice is the emphasis on the provision of health care through the use of preventive and environmental measures and the increased assumption of responsibility for health care by individuals themselves. Health care consumers are demanding wellness care (Preventive Medicine 1976; Levine et al. 1979; Hingson et al. 1981), preventive care in addition to curative care, and greater individual responsibility for their own health care (Preventive Medicine 1976; Knowles 1977; Gussow and Tracy

1978; Butler et al. 1979–80). Health professionals and those in the political arena are advocating the cost-reducing potential of preventing or controlling disease or illness by focusing on attaining, maintaining, and regaining health (Lee and Franks 1977).

Again, community health nurses have led the way in emphasizing health and self-care in contrast to illness and technical professional intervention. Kinlein (1977) demonstrates the viability of an independent nursing practice that focuses on self-care within the community. Sullivan (1979) documents the effectiveness of community health nursing interventions in defining self-care assets and in increasing the use of preventive and promotive health practices. Pender (1982) captures important and manipulative variables and constructs relative to health promotion and self-care.

Community health nurses have extended their functional roles and enlarged their knowledge base to meet the changing needs and serve the interests of the larger society. Economic and social pressures have called for expanding the community health nurse's clinical diagnostic and management skills across the age span. Political and social needs have necessitated their learning and implementing interventions that address the important sociopsychological determinants of client health behavior, which affect the assumption of increased self-care and long-term lifestyle changes.

With the advancement of these clinical skills and the increasing use of intervention principles derived from the psychosocial sciences, the community health nurse's depth and breadth of knowledge about the individual as client is more expansive today than ever previously. This knowledge potentially allows for a more precise description of what community health nursing is and does, and who and what constitutes the individual as client.

THE NATURE OF COMMUNITY HEALTH NURSING PRACTICE WITH INDIVIDUALS

Community health nursing practice with individuals as clients has advanced to the point that its extensive knowledge base can be used to clarify the nature and focus of its practice. Through organizing and systematizing this accumulated knowledge into contextual wholes that describe the focus, process, and outcome of practice, community health nurses will not only more effectively utilize this knowledge in practice, but they will begin to develop the discipline as a scientific field of inquiry.

The first charge issued to any would-be scientific discipline is to identify and describe the object, event, or phenomena that will comprise that scientific discipline's interest and investigations (Hempel 1965). In general, the phenomena of interest to community health nurses caring for individuals as clients are (a) the individual, (b) the environment, (c) the health state of the individual, and (d) community health nursing interventions that maintain or promote the individual client's health state.

Going beyond simple identification is the need to clarify the nature of these phenomena. The description of the inherent or basic constitution of the identified objects or events should have universal meaning to everyone in that particular scientific field of inquiry. For community health nursing this descriptive clarification is derived from the general philosophy of nursing practice and from the specific principles of community health nursing practice. How nurses perceive the nature of health, nursing, the individual, and the environment as well as the role of theory affects this clarification.

The Nature of Health

As a concept, health has generated extensive discussion and debate. Examples of the range of descriptions of health include (a) the antithesis of disease, (b) complete psychological and social well-being, and (c) functional mobility and adaptive mental status (Hingson et al. 1981). These descriptions are not fully reflective of nursing's concept of the nature of health.

The American Nurses Association's (ANA) definition of health (1980) captures the underlying philosophical tenets of the profession:

Health is a dynamic state of being in which the developmental and behavioral potential of an individual is realized to the fullest extent possible. Each human being possesses various strengths and limitations resulting from the interaction of environmental and hereditary factors. The relative dominance of the strengths and limitations determines an individual's place on the health continuum; it determines the person's biological and behavioral integrity, his wholeness.

This description of the nature of health demonstrates its fluidity; it further presents health as a relative state for each individual. Because of its fluidity and relativity, health has an abstract nature and defies description in the strict scientific sense.

The Nature of Nursing

Nursing, as a field of scientific inquiry, cannot have at its core a phenomenon that is not objectively identifiable and capable of being described. Therefore, while health may defy scientific rigor and description, the phenomena of *human responses* to health, as proposed within the recent ANA Social Policy Statement (1980), do not. Human responses to health are categorized into two types: (a) health restoring, which includes reactions to actual health problems (physical, emotional, social, cognitive), and (b) health supporting, which includes concerns about potential health problems (need for health education, identification of risks, skill development, and behavioral changes). Human responses are directly or indirectly observable and thus capable of being scientifically described. To this end, then, they meet the standards of what constitutes scientific phenomena. The nature of nursing is to diagnose and treat human responses to actual and potential health problems (ANA 1980).

The Nature of the Individual

In accordance with the historical and expanded scope of community health nursing practice and the outlining of scientific interest in two types of human response, the nature of the individual as client for community health nursing can be described. First of all, clients whose human responses to health are restorative include the recovering ill, the adapted well, and the terminally ill. The *recovering ill* have been previously assessed as manifesting responses to a health problem, but treatment has been initiated and recovery from the negative health state is imminent. Clients in this category seek out the community health nurse to assist them in their recovery through the development of self-care activities and specific interventions directed at their health needs. The *adapted well* clients have specific health problems, but those problems are controlled and stabilized (e.g., the diabetic). Nurse-facilitated client self-care is implemented to maintain this stability and control. The *terminally ill* client is apprised of the condition and looks to the community health nurse for maintenance of comfort and assistance in sustaining as high a level of functioning in the final days of life as may be possible.

The second type of response — health-supporting — involves two categories of clientele. The *well* client has no specific health problem. He or she may not, however, be practicing preventive health behaviors or be aware of risk factors that are a potential threat to the current wellness state. The *very well* client is functioning at a high level of wellness; usually he or she wishes to maintain or even further maximize that high-level state of health, well-being, and self-actualization. The nurse functions as an information provider for these categories, offering specific inputs on health risks as well as on behaviors that will significantly advance wellness.

The Nature of the Environment

The environment is particularly important to the practice of community health nursing. It represents the contextual setting in which nursing interventions take place and cannot be underestimated in its impact on both client and nurse. The environment is pervasive: it includes physical setting and cultural/social milieu; negatively, it is a reservoir for potential physical, social, and psychological threats to the health and well-being of the client. The ever-expanding scope of practice of community health nursing carries with it a multitude of environmental settings and the need to adapt nursing interventions to accommodate the changing environments.

Theory

Through theory and its subsequent empirical validation, the true — not speculative or rhetorical — nature of a phenomenon is captured and utilized in meaningful ways. Once some descriptive clarification of the phenomena concerning a field of scientific inquiry has been attempted, the next step is to relate or link together these phenomena. Concepts, principles, and processes derived from a discipline's knowledge base are related to one another within a theory or within a conceptual framework that will lead to theory in an effort to explain and in some cases predict the phenomena under investigation.

Table 5.1 presents a comparision of the early nursing theorists' views of the individual, nursing, society/environment, and health. Each theorist subsumes within her theory a set of philosophical assumptions about each of these phenomena and their relationships. At the same time each theorist reflects the level of nursing knowledge current in her era (the latter theories evince a particular clinical emphasis). There are remarkable similarities and distinctive differences between these various theoretical formulations. Relative to the individual, an overwhelming consensus is presented of holism, uniqueness, and the capacity for choice, self-determination, and adaptation. Environment, on the other hand, is differentially viewed as the primal phenomenon (Nightingale), as a co-extension of man (Rogers), and as something to minimize as much as possible (Hall).

Nursing as a phenomenon is similarly regarded in all the frameworks. An interpersonal and facilitative process, nursing addresses the broad spectrum of client needs. The process is one by which a professional strives to maintain the integrity and holism of the client while attempting to meet the multiple demands of the health care need or problem.

Health emerges in these theoretical formulations just as variably as it does in the general literature. Some of the theorists have not defined health at all; others have related it strongly to the absence of disease and functional limitations. Still others have treated it as a dynamic concept that is to be regarded abstractly.

Many aspects of the community health nursing practice related to individuals are represented in these early nursing theories; however, community health nursing goes well beyond these conceptualizations. Because of its tremendous scope of practice, a theoretical/conceptual framework for community health nursing must be conceptually broad enough to apply to the multiple and diverse practice situations. Further, it must demonstrate specificity in its choice of concepts and variables to reflect the depth of knowledge on individual health behavior that has accumulated in the last decade and a half.

Out of the challenge to meet the diversity of client needs has come an expanded scope of practice for community health nursing; together with this extended practice has come an expanded knowledge base. This extensive knowledge base must be placed within an organizing and clarifying frame of reference. This framework should facilitate an orderly use of the multiple facts

(text continues on page 145)

Table 5.1. A Comparison of the Early Theorists' Views of the Individual, Nursing, Society/Environment, and Health

Author	Individual	Nursing	Society/Environment	Health
Florence Nightingale (1860)	The individual is viewed as having vital natural powers for the reparative process.	Nursing is viewed as a noncurative process that depends on placing the individual in the best condition for nature to act, particularly by providing an environment conducive to the reparative process. Communication with the person is considered to be vital and should be unhurried and free from interruption. Communication with physicians and family members should occur in the client's environment. Observation and specific data collection for individual clients are essential to prevent health problems. The goal of nursing is to assist the reparative process. The same principles apply for keeping the well	Environment is the central concept. It is viewed as all external conditions and influence affecting life and development of the organism. The major areas of concentration are ventilation, warmth, effluvia (odors), noise, and light.	Disease is viewed as a reparative process, and the disease is not always the cause of suffering that occurs with disease. The cause of suffering is more often factors like poor environmental conditions, poor diet, or lack of spiritual strength. The laws of health are viewed as the same as the laws and nature of nursing.

Hildegard Peplau (1952)	The individual is viewed as an organism who strives in its own way to reduce tension generated by needs. Each individual is viewed as unique, having learned perceptions and pre-conceived ideas that are important to the interpersonal process.	Nursing is viewed as a significant therapeutic interpersonal process. The interpersonal process is a maturing force and educative instrument for both the nurse and the client. Self-knowledge in the context of the interpersonal interaction is essential to understand the client and to reach resolution of the problem. There are four sequential phases of the interpersonal process: (a) orientation, (b) identification, (c) exploitation, and (d) resolution.	Culture and mores are factors to consider in dealing with the individual.	Health is defined as forward movement of the personality and other ongoing human processes in the direction of creative, constructive, productive, personal community living.
Ida Jean Orlando (1961)	Individuals are viewed as unique. It is the individual who initiates a nursing situation by exhibiting or expressing a need. The individual changes in relation to time and space.	Nursing is viewed as a process of interaction with an ill individual to meet an immediate need. The nursing situation consists of (a) patient behavior, (b) nurse's reaction, and (c)	Setting can cause an unmet need to occur.	Nursing action is only needed when an unmet need occurs, generally in one of three categories: physical limitations, adverse reaction to a setting, and experiences that prevent

Table 5.1. (Continued)

Author	Individual	Nursing	Society/Environment	Health
		nursing action appropriate to the patient's need. The nurse is accountable to the individual receiving care.		communication of needs. Nursing serves only the ill, but health and illness are not defined.
Ernestine Wiedenbach (1964)	Individuals are holistic human beings who possess unique potential and strive toward self-direction and needs stimulation.	There are three components of nursing: (a) identification of a patient's need for help, (b) ministration of the help needed, and (c) validation that the help provided was indeed helpful. The nursing process begins with an activating situation that exists among certain realities, arousing the nurse's consciousness. Clinical nursing has four components—philosophy, purpose, practice, and art.	The environment is viewed as one of the realities comprising the nursing situation.	Promotion of health and conservation of life are professional goals. The nature of the goal of health is defined by the nurse and the individual mutually at each encounter and depends on each person's values, attitudes, and abilities.

| Lydia Hall (1966) | Motivation and energy for healing are within the individual. Motivation is discovered by bringing feelings into awareness, making it possible for individuals to make conscious decisions on their own behalf. | Nursing is viewed as three interlocking circles. The care circle represents intimate bodily care and nurturing. The core circle represents nondirective reflection and therapeutic use of self to help the patient gain self-identity and develop toward maturity. The cure circle represents carrying out medical, surgical, and/or rehabilitative prescriptions made by the physician. Professional nursing occurs when learning is possible. | In order to provide a nondirective setting for recovery, the environment should have no routines, schedules, or demands that interfere with the motivation and energy needed for healing. | Framework deals with health after an acute stage of illness. Self-actualization and self-love are considered to be the goals to be attained. |

Table 5.1. (Continued)

Author	Individual	Nursing	Society/Environment	Health
Virginia Henderson (1966)	Mind and body are inseparable. No two individuals are alike. The individual's basic needs are reflected in the 14 components of basic nursing care.	Nursing is viewed as a unique function independent of physicians' roles. Nursing involves assisting individuals sick or well in performing activities contributing to health and helping individuals gain independence in these tasks as rapidly as possible. The activities contributing to health are stated in the 14 components of basic nursing care, for example, helping the patient with such activities as breathing normally, eating and drinking adequately, playing or participating in various forms of recreation, etc.	Cultural background affects health, and the family always has a role in health care.	Health is based on the individual's ability to function independently in the 14 components

| Myra E. Levine (1967) | The individual is viewed as a holistic being who exhibits organismic responses to attempt to adapt to the environment. | Nursing is viewed as supportive and therapeutic interventions based on scientific or theoretical knowledge. Supportive interventions are designed to maintain a state of wholeness as consistently as possible with failing adaptation. Therapeutic interventions are designed to promote adaptation that contributes to healing and restoration of health. All nursing actions are based on conservation of energy, structural integrity, personal integrity, and social integrity. | Society is viewed as the total environment of the individual, including family, significant others, and the nurse. | The balance normally present in the individual is disrupted by illness. The goal of nursing is to restore a holistic balance. Health practices are considered as they relate to illness. |

Table 5.1. (Continued)

Author	Individual	Nursing	Society/Environment	Health
Martha E. Rogers (1970)	Unitary man is viewed as an energy field, the boundaries of which extend beyond the discernible mass of the human body. There five general characteristics of unitary man, or the life process upon which the unifying principles of nursing are based: (a) unified wholeness, (b) openness, (c) unidirectionality, (d) pattern and organization, and (e) sentience.	The science of nursing is viewed as a science of humanity—the study of the nature and direction of human development. It is directed toward describing and explaining man in synergistic wholeness. Life processes of humanity are the core around which nursing revolves. Emergent nursing science, which will guide nursing practice, is based on the principles of homeodynamics: (a) reciprocity, (b) synchrony, (c) helicy, (d) resonancy.	Environment and man are energy fields coextensive with the universe.	Pattern and organization of the human energy field, evolving along the space-time continuum, have relevance for the integrity of the field. Growing complexity of organization occurs as a result of multiple interactions over the life span. When patterns or organization no longer exist, the integrity of the human field is destroyed and death occurs. Death is viewed as a transformation of energy
Dorothea E. Orem (1971)	The individual is an integrated whole composed of the internal physical, psychologic, and social nature with varying degrees of self-	Nursing is a human service, an interpersonal process, and technology (formalized methods or techniques) required for specific action. These	Environment is viewed as the elements external to the individual interacting with the individual to affect the self-care system. Culture is	Health is viewed as a state of wholeness or integrity of the individual. Universal self-care is the basis for optimal functioning in six areas:

Theorist	Individual	Nursing	Society/Environment	Health
	care ability. Self-care is preceded by reflection to assess needs and deliberate choice of how to meet these needs.	nursing actions are directed toward enhancing self-care ability and therapeutic self-care ability. The goal of nursing is optimal wellness.	viewed as the context within which self-care behavior is learned. Society specifies the conditions that make it legitimate for individuals to seek services for self-care.	(a) air, water, food, (b) excretions, (c) activity and rest, (d) solitude and social interaction, (e) hazards of life and well being, and (f) being normal. Health deviation self-care is the response to illness, injury, or disease.
Imogene M. King (1971)	Individuals are viewed as (a) reacting beings, (b) time-oriented beings, (c) social beings, with the ability to perceive, think, feel, choose, set goals, select actions to meet goals, and make decisions. The individual's perception of reality is a major concept upon which the nursing process is based.	Nursing is viewed as an interpersonal process of action, reaction, interaction, and transaction. This process provides assistance to individuals in meeting basic activities of daily living and to cope with health and illness.	Social systems are central in that individuals function in social systems to achieve common goals. Interactions in social systems are influenced by standards or norms set by the group and are based on a system of values. The internal environment consists of organ systems, cells, hormones, and inner thought processes in all their unique interaction. The external environment consists of all things that influence the person from the outside.	Health is viewed as a dynamic state in the life cycle that implies continuous adaptation to stress in the internal and external environment through use of resources to achieve maximum potential for daily living.

Table 5.1. (Continued)

Author	Individual	Nursing	Society/Environment	Health
Sister Callista Roy (1976)	Individuals are viewed as biopsychosocial beings who must be considered as a whole. There is constant interaction with the environment, and the individual copes with environmental change through biopsychosocial adaptive mechanisms. The individual's adaptation level is determined by the focal, contextual, and residual stimuli that result in the need for adaptation. There are four modes of adaptation: (a) physiologic, (b)self-concept, (c) role function, and (d) interdependence. Adaptive modes are activated when need excesses or deficits occur.	Nursing is viewed as an interpersonal process that is initiated by the individual's maladaptation to change in the environment. Nursing actions are directed to reducing or removing stimuli and to enhancing the adaptive level of the individual.	Environment is a central concept in that it constantly interacts with the individual, providing matter, energy, and information to the individual. Stimuli originate in the environment.	Health is a state of human functioning whereby continual adaptation occurs. Health is viewed as a continuum from death to peak wellness, with normal health being in the middle. Poor health is considered to be the result of maladaptation to environmental change.

Reprinted with permission from: Chinn P, and Jacobs M. Theory and nursing: a systematic approach. St. Louis: CV Mosby Co., 1983.

and principles now at our disposal and help to advance a scientific explanation of the nature of our practice. The newest challenge is to create a conceptual framework that accomplishes this organization — not an abstract organization as has been the tradition in nursing theory, but rather a specific framework that allows for the definitive testing of the relationships that exist between individuals as clients, their responses to health problems or needs, community health nursing interventions, and health outcomes. Through testing these relationships, community health nursing can establish its practice focus and process (nature) as a science as well as an art.

The following section of this chapter presents a conceptual framework of individual health behavior and community health nursing intervention. The framework is a conceptual model, not a theory. Only with extensive testing and confirmation of the relationships described by the model will it become a theory. This model proposes to address the nature of the phenomena (individual, environment, health, nursing intervention) of community health nursing through the identification and specification of variables and concepts derived from nursing as well as other disciplines.

A CONCEPTUAL FRAMEWORK FOR COMMUNITY HEALTH NURSING

As with the earlier theorists' frameworks, the framework presented here has certain inherent philosophical assumptions that represent world views, beliefs, and values about the objects and events addressed in the framework. Not only do these assumptions represent personal views but they reflect the more general philosophical assumptions held by nursing as a profession and by community health nursing as a discipline within the profession.

Just as commonalities and differences were noted for the theories just reviewed, so too will certain assumptions, variables, and concepts within this model be seen as similar to and yet different from those of the earlier frameworks. The similarities are reflected primarily in the common philosophical assumptions shared by most nurses. The differences are demonstrated primarily in the depth, breadth, and specificity of variables and concepts that reflect the current era of nursing knowledge and the practice of community health nursing.

Philosophical Assumptions

The primary assumption of this framework is that individuals as clients are not reducible to component parts. Sick or well, the client is a holistic being — at any one given time the body, mind, and spirit are functioning as components that make the whole operative. Certainly there are those times when one component may need to dominate the attention of the health professional, but the health assessment and planned interventions for that client should habitually take into consideration the dynamism of the other components.

A second assumption is that clients have the ability to make choices about their behavior; they are capable of making many relevant decisions about their health states and intervention or nonintervention to maintain or promote that health state. Where once the primary health problems facing both the client and the clinician were acute illnesses, the majority of today's health care problems are the result of chronic and degenerative illnesses and detrimental lifestyle factors. The treatment of acute illness, of necessity, requires the client's dependency upon the decision-making powers of health professionals. The treatment of chronic illness and the institution of more health-promoting lifestyle behaviors, on the other hand, require the client's acceptance of responsibility for his or her own health care and an increased reliance upon individual decisions about health behavior. Today's health care problems demand an informed, active, independent role for clients in contrast to the uninformed, passive, and dependent role assumed in years past.

Many of today's health care clients are asking for the opportunity to assume increased decisional control over their health behavior. Clients are no longer willing to be passive recipients of health care; rather, they are asking what alternatives in treatment are available and, in many cases, are electing no treatment at all (Annas 1975; Cox 1981). One has but to look at the explosive self-care and self-help movement to realize that active client-participation — not passive, mandated compliance — is fast becoming a norm (Waitzkin and Waterman 1974; Levin 1975; Marieskind and Ehrenreich 1975; Schnert and Eisenberg 1975; Butler et al. 1979–80).

A third assumption basic to nursing and this framework is that each client is unique. We all share the presence of common background characteristics (demographical/social), personality attributes, physiology, motivation, emotions, and world views; but the extent to which these characteristics are operative and the way in which they interact within a particular individual are singular.

These assumptions suggest that clients are capable of making informed, independent, and competent choices about their health behavior, and that these choices are differentially affected by various aspects of the client's singularity (demographic, physiological, sociobehavioral characteristics) and by specific aspects of the client-provider relationship. Additionally, these assumptions imply that clients should be given the maximal amount of control within the limitations of their internal and external environments in determining the quality of their health state and the actions taken to preserve that health state.

An Interaction Model of Client Health Behavior

The object of this model or framework is to identify explanatory relationships between the individuality of the client, client–community health nurse inter-

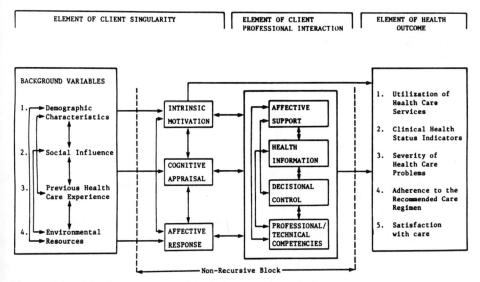

Figure 5.1.   The interaction model of client health behavior. Reprinted with permission of Aspen Systems Corporation, from Cox CL. An interaction model of client health behavior: theoretical prescription for nursing. Adv Nurs Sci 1982; 5:41–56.

action/intervention, and subsequent health outcomes. The environmental settings for health care are not limited by the model and include general clinics, hospitals, schools, industry, home care, and independent nursing practices. Further, this model allows the making of predictions about health outcomes because it incorporates an extensive set of client factors that address psychological, environmental, and sociological determinants of behavior, as well as short-term behavioral processes that may arise during the client-nurse encounter. The variables, concepts, and processes described by the model are grounded in nursing practice and research as well as in empirical data from the psychosocial sciences.

Figure 5.1 is a representation of the Interaction Model of Client Behavior (IMCHB) (Cox 1982). It identifies the major categories or elements within the model (client singularity, client–community health nurse interaction, health outcomes), and the factors that comprise these elements. The model demonstrates a multidirectional flow (depicted by the arrows) to suggest the mutual influence of one set of elements and factors upon another. Table 5.2 defines the major elements, their factors, and the postulated relationships among them.

Element of Client Singularity
Client singularity is the term used to describe the unique configuration of the client's background variables, expression of intrinsic motivation, cognitive appraisal of the health care concern, and the affective response to that concern.

Table 5.2.   Elements of the Interaction Model of Client Health Behavior

Elements	Variables
Background profile	Demographic characteristics Amount and consistency of social influence Previous health care experiences Environmental resources
Motivation	Competency Self-determinism
Cognitive appraisal	Cognitive representation of the health concern
Affective response	Degree of fear/anxiety associated with health concern
Client singularity (equals the client's configuration of these four elements during the health care encounter)	Background variables Motivation Cognitive appraisal Affective response
Client-nurse interaction (equals the client's configuration on these four elements during the health care encounter)	Affective support Decisional control Quantity, quality, approach to provision of health care information Professional/technical competencies of the provider
Health outcome	Utilization of services Clinical health status indicators Severity of health care problem Satisfaction with care Adherence to the recommended care regimens
Hypothesis:	Health outcome is determined by the fit of the interaction configuration with the singularity configuration.

The model suggests that individuals can be uniquely assessed as to the way in which these multiple factors are expressed and interact with one another. It is this unique combination of personal and environmental characteristics that must be attended to by the community health nurse in determining an intervention. Each of the components of client singularity will be reviewed below.

Background variables.   The background variables include the client's demographic characteristics, the influence of the client's social group, previous health care experiences (inclusive of current physiological state), and environmental resources (e.g., personal financial resources, availability and accessibility of health care facilities, interventions). All the background variables interact cumulatively, simultaneously, and often interdependently with each other to produce a specific health behavior. For example, knowledge of (a) the client's socioeconomic status, (b) his or her social group values (social influence) relative to a certain health care issue, and (c) the financial and geographic accessibility of health care to the client is more likely to predict a certain set of health behaviors than if one of those variables is examined in isolation from the others.

Similarly, the background variables operate over time within each client to produce a specific health behavior. For example, social group values relative to a particular health care problem may become less significant after the client has had repeated experiences of symptoms, pain, or inconveniences in the treatment related to that problem (previous health experiences).

Background variables are temporally prior to other factors in the model. As such, they can be seen as contributing to the later variables or constructs. For example, what clients know about a certain health issue (cognitive appraisal) may be a function of their previous experience with the problem or of the social value placed on that issue (e.g., dental hygiene) by the cultural group. A client may not know that brushing her teeth is a sound preventive practice if it is not valued by her culture.

Through an understanding of the temporal order and mutual interaction of these background variables with one another and health behavior, specific management or intervention approaches can be tailored to address selected configurations of these variables (e.g., guidelines for community health education programs can be developed according to the values of the group that is the target of the program).

Intrinsic motivation.   Drawing from Hall's theory (Chinn and Jacobs 1983) as well as nursing's commitment to clients' self-determination (ANA 1980), intrinsic motivation is portrayed as a primary factor within the model. This model recognizes choice, desire, and the need for competency and self-determinism as causal factors in behavior.

Human beings are dynamic organisms in constant interaction with and adaptation to their environment. They demonstrate a need to experience themselves as competent and self-determining in this interaction. These positive feelings provide an intrinsic reward for the individual and are a prerequisite for physical and psychological well-being (Deci 1975). This reward or feedback, then, serves to reinforce the motivation to continue to engage in the behavior.

Where other theories of motivation have claimed basic drives as the source of energy for the operation of the will, the theory of intrinsic motivation (Deci 1975) views the process of choice or deciding as the primary source of dynamics. It is the human need to be competent and self-determining that provides the energy source to oppose the drive forces, to control emotions, and to hold competing or conflicting motives in abeyance (Deci 1980).

Intrinsic motivation is related to other factors within the model. Certain sociocultural variables (e.g., ethnicity, socioeconomic status, environmental resources, cognitive appraisal, and affective response all contribute to and interact with the degree and expression of motivation. Through specifying these relationships, the theoretical base for nursing interventions is made clearer and stronger. A client's motivation to engage in a certain behavior may be decreased owing to certain sociocultural influences, an increased affective response, or an unreliable cognitive appraisal. The intervention, then, should be specifically directed at the primary source of the decreased motivation. For example, if the client is anxious about being a new diabetic, then the general intervention of patient education should be very concrete, spaced over a period of time, and limited in depth (initially) in an effort to reduce the anxiety. Were the nurse to supply the client with information about the diagnosis, the complications, and medical regimen in a more highly cognitive way and in a less client-centered way, anxiety would increase, the client's feelings of competency to deal with the problem would decline, and the motivation to pursue therapeutic behaviors might be compromised.

Cognitive appraisal.   Cognitive appraisal is responsible for the client's interpretation of an existing health state, the choice of behavior that will influence that health state, and the character of the relationship that exists with the nurse. Health and illness not only generate cognitive representations of well-being but also those that involve self-concept, belief systems, social and occupational functioning, values, commitments, and emotional state (Lazarus and Laumier 1978).

Clients act in accordance with their perceptions of reality. These perceptions may or may not be congruent with objective reality. Client perceptions of health and illness are characterized by many of the factors that have been discussed as background variables. For example, Lipowski (1969) has pointed out the many different ways individuals view illness and how these varied interpretations can influence the choice of coping and adaptational responses that clients make in dealing with their health care problems. Various personality characteristics, sense of self-confidence, religion, and attitudes as well as personal resources all affect the cognitive appraisal or representation of the health care problem (Lipowski 1970).

The IMCHB depicts the background variables as having a direct impact on the individual's cognitive appraisal. For example, in certain cases religion will significantly affect the client's cognitive appraisal of abortion and subsequent behavior related to that appraisal (e.g., abortion is wrong and therefore not an intervention option). Similarly, the client may well value prophylactic dental care, but the availability of financial resources will mediate the effects of this cognitive appraisal on subsequent behavior. By specifying those factors that are potential antecedents to the cognitive appraisal, a broader explanation for the sources of variation in client interpretations of the health problem is offered and a theoretical base for the development of interventions to enhance more accurate health appraisals is formulated.

The model emphasizes the relationships that exist between cognitions and the affective response to the health concern. To be certain, this relationship is exceedingly complex, but it must be explored if a greater understanding of client health behavior is to be advanced.

Emotion (affect) can disrupt or interfere with cognitive activity and thus substantially affect behavior. For example, the stress emotions of anxiety, fear, guilt, anger, sadness, envy, and jealousy can interfere with the cognitive representation of an issue by serving as distractions or producing selective attention, thereby narrowing the range for receiving informational input or cues (Lazarus and Laumier 1978). Similarly, a cognitive appraisal can generate emotional arousal. A client's distorted cognitive appraisal of the pelvic examination may lead to an affective response of fear of pain — which, in turn, may result in failure to obtain the recommended annual Pap smear.

Affective response. It should be obvious that health behavior cannot be explained purely on the basis of rational thought; cognitions must be viewed simultaneously with affect or emotion. The IMCHB posits that the background variables and the cognitive appraisal of the health care problem or concern act both as contributors to and mediators of the client's affective response to the health care issue. As a result, variance in health behavior (human responses to health or health threat) will be more fully explained through the consideration of the interrelationships between these factors and their combined effects on the health outcome.

Although the cognitive appraisal and affective response may be derived from the same antecedents (previous experience, selected demographic characteristics, social influence), they have a different impact on behavior. It must not be assumed, therefore, that even though two clients hold similar cognitive appraisals of a particular health problem, their behavioral responses will be the same. For example, where both clients outwardly appraise a situation as one that carries a low threat (Pap smear), one client may use denial to arrive at that appraisal and the other may have at her disposal specific information that contributed to that perception. Conceptually subsuming these clients' affective responses under the cognitive appraisal might be misleading in terms of developing interventions for problems that do not require further health information, but rather require the management of anxiety. A single intervention may have very different effects on cognition and affect.

In keeping with this example, a fear-arousing intervention designed to change the cognitive appraisal from one of low threat to one of mid-level threat (warning of the hazards and dangers inherent in not securing the test) will affect the two clients differently. For that client whose affective response is low anxiety about the procedure, the intervention may well be beneficial: it prompts the client to get more information or take some direct action. For the client who is already so fearful about the exam that she is forced to use denial to reduce her anxiety (her mother died of uterine cancer), such an intervention approach will contribute to the exacerbation of denial.

The affective response to the health concern, therefore, must be viewed as a conceptually separate construct from cognition. Not only do emotions affect behavior differently from cognitions, but health care interventions will have very different impacts on these two behavioral determinants.

An individual is uniquely characterized by demographic factors, previous health and illness experiences, the amount and consistency of social influence, and the availability of environmental resources. These factors are interrelated; they enter into both how each person cognitively appraises a health care concern and how he or she affectively responds to a health care event. The motivation to engage in certain behaviors is affected by environmental characteristics as well as by emotional arousal, the cognitive appraisal, and background characteristics.

All of these factors are initially prior to and independent of the client-nurse encounter. Clients enter the care system with specific demographic, social, and motivational characteristics; associated with these characteristics are cognitive and affective responses to the health concern. Collectively these characteristics can provide informational signals to the nurse and challenge her to structure the encounter/intervention to fit the client's needs and individuality.

Element of Client–Community Health Nurse Interaction

This model identifies the client-nurse interaction as a major influence on health behavior. It suggests that there are four components that define the interaction and that the strength of these components will vary according to the client's singularity and the health care need that is expressed. In keeping with the continuous care offered by the community health nurse, the model further describes the relationship between client and nurse as a continuous reciprocal interchange between aspects of the client's singularity, the interaction, and the health care outcomes. The client's behavior, the relationship with the nurse, and external and internal personal client factors all operate as interlocking determinants of each other. Each of the four components that define interaction as well as their interrelationships is described below.

Affective support.   Affective support within this model refers not only to attending to the client's level of emotional arousal but also to the process of building an affiliative bond with the client. These two aspects of affective support are related in complex ways.

Emotional arousal has been demonstrated to be a significant mediator of the cognitive appraisal of the health care need or problem and of the motivation to engage in specific behavior. Interventions that focus only on cognitions (the provision of health care information) are ineffective: clients are often not ready to assimilate information if their affective state is too high or too low. That state may seriously hamper the client's ability to process information or to assume any degree of control in effecting behavior.

Emotional arousal is related to motivation in that the higher the degree of emotional response, the less the degree of motivated or goal-directed behavior. Schacter (1959) demonstrates that when emotional arousal (stress) is high, there is a greater need for affiliation; because of the stress-producing nature of many health concerns, clients are often highly affectively aroused, and thus their need for affiliative bonding is increased (Cohen and Lazarus, 1979).

Janis and Rodin (1979) suggest that when health care providers fail to build and maintain a strong affiliative bond with their clients, they lose a source of major social power—referent power. Referent power applies to those individuals who are perceived by others to be likable, benevolent, admirable, and accepting. Referent power would appear to be a strong motivating factor initially in effecting positive health behaviors; if clients do not like the provider, their motivation to continue the therapeutic behavior is substantially reduced.

In order to build referent power, community health nurses must emphasize the similarities between themselves and their clients with regard to beliefs, attitudes, and values. By reducing the clients' sense of status inequity, nurses reinforce their sense of competency and self-determination in the health care setting. Further, nurses should praise and reinforce client behavior that is consistent with positive health care goals. This effort serves to help clients identify the relationship that exists between their behavior and subsequent outcomes, as well as to reinforce a sense of self-efficacy in health care (Leventhal et al. 1980).

In addition to affiliative bonding with clients or establishing referent power, nurses must consider clients' need for affective support in keeping with their singularity. If the affective response of the client predominates over the cognitive appraisal of the health concern, then the intervention must be directed at reducing that level of emotional arousal to a level where the cognitive appraisal might be altered (e.g., providing information that facilitates coping and assists the client to develop a more accurate representation of the need or problem; this will, in turn, serve to further reduce the degree of emotional arousal).

The preceding discussion should serve to point out the complex interrelationships that exist among the components of the interaction element as well as those that exist between the components of client singularity and interaction. Information is often essential to reduce anxiety and increase the client's control over the health care problem; however, providing information without effectively dealing with the client's anxiety can further exacerbate that problem, thus decreasing the potential for the client to assume cognitive and decisional control over it.

In sum, denying affective support to clients for whom that need is paramount results in client dissatisfaction, withdrawal, or perhaps even aggressive behavior (Christman 1978). Conversely, lavishing affective support on clients for whom that need is not the most salient also results in client dissatisfaction;

affective support in lieu of useful information for the more cognitively focused clients is as inappropriate an intervention as not providing reassurance and anxiety-reducing interventions for the highly emotional clients.

Approach to the delivery of health care information: Information is an obvious necessity for adaptive behavior in any setting. Given that (a) the amount of information provided is neither too small nor too great, (b) the nature of that information has meaning for the recipient, and (c) the internal and external conditions of the individual are amenable to the processing of that information, then action leading to adaptation should follow.

The quantity of health information has an impact on health behavior in two ways. First, if clients are given information above and beyond their capacity to process, fewer positive health behaviors are generated. Information overload can result from a nurse's attempts to provide information when the client's affective response to the health concern is high; a client simply cannot attend simultaneously to both cognitive issues and a charged emotional state. Further, the nurse may be giving information that is not in keeping with the client's singularity; previous health experiences and the level of the client's understanding significantly dictate how much and how quickly information can be processed.

Second, too little health information can alter a client's health behavior. Without sufficient information, a client cannot formulate accurate cognitive appraisals, set health care goals, or decide upon a course of action.

Health information varies in both type and function. Some health information is useful in generating and understanding a cognitive representation of the health problem; other information is designed to generate a plan of action (Leventhal et al. 1980). Similarly, different forms of health information have different functions. Johnson et al. (1978) and Fuller et al. (1978) demonstrate that specific sensory information is superior to abstract information as a means of fear or distress reduction. If coping and adaptation are to be facilitated, then information specific to coping techniques and responses must be given to a client. Other researchers underline the effectiveness of information that is specific to a client's problem, concrete and simplified, in eliciting positive health behavior (Ley 1976).

The approach to the delivery of health information can also have an impact on health behavior. Some approaches to the provision of health information are intended to be threatening or fear arousing. The results of studies that have examined fear-arousing communications are not consistent. Some studies demonstrate that strong threat messages result in less adherence to health recommendations than do milder communiqués. Others suggest an increase in adherence behaviors when strong fear messages are conveyed. Yet others conclude that the effect of fear-arousing communications varies according to the type of threat, type of recommended actions, and type of personality (e.g., client singularity) (Janis and Feshbach 1953).

The IMCHB acknowledges that information and knowledge are necessary conditions for effecting positive health behaviors; however, they are not sufficient conditions. The relationship that clients have with the nurse, the amount of control clients perceive themselves to have in the health care setting, and aspects of the clients' singularity together influence what health information is processed and how that information is used.

The information that is given to clients affects their cognitive representation of the health concern, their affective response, and their motivational state. The relationships of affect and cognitive appraisal to the provision of health information were outlined in the preceding section (see Affective support). The relationship of information to motivation warrants further consideration.

Information imparts knowledge to the client about the threat of the health care problem, as well as details about what can and cannot be done to deal with this threat. This knowledge can then be utilized to formulate goals for action or to identify motives for behavior, reduce anxiety, and provide feedback about the sense of competency and self-determinism. If the information that is presented is clear in depicting the nature and substance of the threat and potential plans for action, and if it avoids both positive and negative effects of fear, then it will be a powerful determinant of behavior (Leventhal et al. 1980). On the other hand, if the information exceeds the client's capacities, is not matched to the singularity presented, and arouses excessive fear, the client will not feel competent and self-determining and probably will not assume the most adaptive behavior.

Decisional control.   The third client-nurse interaction factor is decisional control, which refers to the individual's expectation of having the power to participate in making decisions in order to obtain desirable consequences. In keeping with the notion of intrinsic motivation, decisional control involves the freedom of choice, being aware of opportunities to select goals and the behaviors essential to meet those goals. Providers often limit clients' sense of perceived control through their failure to provide clients with useful information and their use of coercive authoritarian tactics (Francis et al. 1969). These factors contribute significantly to the clients' decreased sense of competency and self-determinism relative to health matters and a decreased sense of responsibility for their own health care (DiMatteo et al. 1979).

Again the IMCHB suggests a number of complex and interrelated relationships between decisional control, the other interaction factors, and aspects of a client's singularity. Increased cognitive control facilitates adaptational responses (e.g., the provision of specific sensory information assists the client to feel competent and self-determining in dealing with an aversive medical procedure); decisional control increases the client's sense of self-efficacy and facilitates commitment to health relevant behaviors (e.g., by being allowed to choose between treatment alternatives, the client's sense of commitment to that approach is enhanced and the behavior is viewed as self-determined). Thus control is related to the cognitive representation of the problem, the motivational state of the client, and the informational and affective factors of the interaction.

The model emphasizes the tailoring of decisional control to the client's singularity. A client should be offered the maximal amount of decisional control, given the constraints of his or her internal and external environments. This includes consideration of the client's affective state and cognitive appraisal. If the client is anxious, it would be inappropriate indeed to expect a high level of client decisional control. Similarly, if the client's cognitive appraisal of the health problem is inaccurate due to the lack of information about the issue, decisional control is again limited.

Decisional control is integral to the amount of intrinsic motivation the client may or may not exhibit. Goal selection is the heart of self-determination; it emphasizes the freedom to behave as one chooses, in accord with one's thoughts, motives, and feelings as well as in accord with the constraints of the environment (Deci 1980). By emphasizing active client participation in the decision-making process, the nurse is fostering self-determination from the very start of the relationship; this support strengthens a feeling of self-efficacy and will lead eventually to the internalization of responsibility for health-generating behaviors.

The nurse's role is one of supplying clients with information about the predictable consequences of various behaviors in order that they may be in a position to make more informed choices/decisions. Further, the nurse should direct his or her efforts at strengthening the clients' sense of competency and self-determinism; this is accomplished through five interrelated efforts: (a) helping the clients to bring into awareness what they do and do not do to maintain their health; (b) helping the clients to formulate standards against which to compare their behavior and set goals; (c) fostering a sense of self-efficacy in clients that emphasizes their capacity for making choices and decisions about their health care; (d) assisting the clients to see the relationship between their behaviors and specified health care outcomes: and (e) helping the clients to see what can and cannot be changed in regard to their health states.

Professional-technical competencies: A final issue that completes the list of factors operative in the client-nurse relationship is the professional-technical competence of the nurse. The technical skills and general competencies of the nurse are an important part of the comprehensive evaluation and confirmation of a client's physiological and psychosocial needs. The greater the client's need for technical tasks (monitoring vital signs q4h, IV therapy), the less the need for client decisional control: and thus the need for affective support is increased and the need for information varies according to the client's health state and ability to process the information. As the need for technical intervention decreases, then the client's own abilities and competencies should be brought into play in an effort to increase his or her sense of decisional control, competency, and self-determinism.

Elements of Health Outcome

Throughout the presentation of the IMCHB, the implied outcome measure has been health behavior or health state resulting from that behavior. The model describes five broad health outcomes. They are (a) the utilization of health care services, (b) clinical health status indicators (blood pressure, well-being, glucose levels), (c) severity of health care problems, (d) adherence to the recommended care regimen, and (e) satisfaction with care. Each of these outcome measures can vary as to its meaning. For example, increased clinic utilization might be assessed as a positive health behavior in the preventive realm of care and as a negative health behavior when the objective is to increase self-care capabilities. In general, positive health behavior within this model refers to those conditions that are considered to maintain or promote the health state of clients. Negative health behaviors are those activities that place clients at risk and decrease their capacity for self-actualization, physical, and psychosocial well-being.

Summary

The Interaction Model of Client Health Behavior depicts those factors that define the individual client as unique. It describes the factors that define the client-nurse relationship and specifies the general outcome measures critical to the evaluation of client-nurse interaction/interventions. The behavior of the client and nurse, as evidenced in this model, is reciprocal. Thus as more successes in health care are met, health behavior becomes more rational and directed than emotional and haphazard. Clients begin to internalize what they have cognitively processed; the new knowledge gained and the realization that they are capable of performing health behaviors on their own behalf begin to develop or reinforce a sense of competency and self-determinism in regard to health care. This response, in turn, increases the client's motivation to continue to engage in these behaviors. The nurse should continually reinforce the client's independence in health care activities. Possible methods for the nurse are helping the clients to identify new goals, expand their self-care options, and realize that what they are doing to take care of themselves is important.

The model is designed for application to a variety of health care decisions and behaviors, and the strength of the elements varies according to the issues under consideration. For example, attitudes and values are posited to play a far more important role in the decision on abortion than they would in a decision about the use of a hospital emergency room. For this reason, the model must be specified in accordance with a particular community health nursing problem.

Using such a framework to guide community health nursing practice and research achieves holism and avoids the fragmentation of community health nursing concepts into such parts as (a) phase of the illness (prevention, acute, chronic), (b) locale of practice (school, outpatient department, industry, home), (c) medical or nursing specialty (surgery, maternal-child health), or (d) type of relevant theory (decision making, learning, nurse as change agent). This conceptual model demonstrates how the philosophy and practice principles of a discipline, which represent its art, can be organized and systematized to scientifically describe its nature — a nature portrayed as conceptual variables that represent both the discipline's knowledge base and its practice principles. Finally, holism of the individual, adaptation of the nursing intervention to the uniqueness of the client, and the promotion of individual responsibility for health care can be presented conceptually, but because these elements are grounded in knowledge, they may in addition be operationalized and tested empirically.

THE APPLICATION OF A THEORETICAL FRAMEWORK TO COMMUNITY HEALTH NUSING PRACTICE

The Interaction Model of Client Health Behavior (IMCHB) just presented has two purposes: (a) to organize and relate the extent of community health nursing knowledge relevant to practice with individuals, and (b) to demonstrate how this framework can guide the development of nursing interventions based on knowledge in contrast to interventions that are based on "trial and error." The model is a blueprint that describes how to construct a situation in which the individual client's health state can be maintained or promoted. The following sections of the chapter address how this blueprint can be used by community health nurses to facilitate individual clients' health states.

Goals and Objectives

The overall community health nursing practice goal emphasized by the model is the maximization of positive health outcomes for the individual client at each encounter and over time. While all the health outcomes specified in the model may not be relevant for all clients all of the time, a nurse should be able to identify the most salient outcomes on the basis of the particular client's needs. The effort to meet this overall goal involves a number of nurse objectives that are implied by the model. The nurse should be able to

1. identify those factors constituting the client's singularity that will have the greatest significance for the health outcome.
2. identify those factors constituting the client's singularity that will have the strongest implications for interaction and intervention approaches.
3. identify those factors constituting the client-nurse interaction that will be most useful to effect positive client health outcomes.
4. determine how those factors constituting the client-nurse interaction best can be tailored and matched to the client's singularity configuration to produce the desired health outcome.

While the content of these objectives would appear to be discrete, the nurse is accumulating these data simultaneously and continuously. Information necessary to meet these objectives is in multiple forms, and the nurse's attention must be multifocal. For example, before the first word between client and nurse is ever exchanged during a home visit, the nurse should already be gathering information on important background variables: sex, age, relative socioeconomic status, immediate environmental and social support resources. Certain posturing and nonverbal gestures provide insight on other important client singularity factors. If the client is comfortably settled in posture, maintains direct eye contact, and does not manifest those mannerisms typically associated with anxiety, strong cues about affect and even sense of competency and self-determinism (intrinsic motivation) in this situation are being manifested.

Activities to Meet the Goals and Objectives

The IMCHB is a general blueprint designed to fit the full range of client needs and community settings involving the community health nurse. While the nurse objectives implied by the model will fit any community health nursing situation, the activities to meet these objectives must be specified in accordance with the client's particular health care need or problem. Each of these objectives relative to nursing activities is addressed separately below.

Client Singularity and Health Outcomes
Two major mechanisms assist the community health nurse to identify those client singularity factors that potentially will have an impact on health outcomes. The first mechanism is general and is derived from the nurse's experience and knowledge base. For example, let us assume that the health care issue being addressed is the client's decision to have an amniocentesis. The health outcome is utilization of services. The nurse knows from experience and a general knowledge base that the client's acceptance of amniocentesis and perhaps abortion will be tremendously influenced by attitudes and values (affect) in contrast to purely rational thought or knowledge. Therefore, of all the client singularity factors, affect and cognitive appraisal are apt to have the most important impact on health outcome.

The second mechanism through which the nurse will identify important client singularity factors is derived from his or her specific interaction with the client. Using the example above, the nurse would take into consideration all the client singularity factors specific to that client and abortion. Perhaps the client's value system does not forbid abortion; instead the client is frightened of the procedure because she doesn't really understand what is involved. Another possibility is that the client does not have the financial resources necessary to pay for the procedure. Either client singularity factor, without intervention, is apt to result in nonuse of services. Knowing, in general, what cluster of client singularity factors is likely to have an impact upon a specific health outcome alerts the community health nurse to explore these factors with the client. Approaching a client encounter with this objective not only systematically utilizes the nurse's knowledge base but further maximizes the time spent with the client. The intervention then naturally follows from what the nurse has learned about the client's singularity.

The example used above emphasizes the role of attitudes and values in influencing a particular health outcome. Again, the nature of the model demands that the relationships specified by the model be in accordance with a particular health problem or issue. We could have just as easily utilized the example of adherence to an antihypertensive regimen. The health outcome would be adherence to a recommended care regimen; the general client singularity factors that would lead the nurse in initial explorations with the client would more than likely be the client's level of motivation and perhaps cognitive appraisal (knowledge). Other client singularity factors would, no doubt, come into play, but these factors would play a central role.

Client Singularity and Interaction/Intervention Approaches

The second nurse objective implied by the model is the identification of those client singularity factors that have the strongest implications for interaction/intervention approaches. While most nursing interventions are multifocal, clients often manifest certain aspects of their singularity that should alert the nurse to some prioritizing of the foci within the overall intervention. For example, for the new diabetic, the general intervention is health education to acquaint the client with new information and new skills sufficient for him or her to assume self-care. If the nurse fails to address the complexity of the client's singularity and proceeds on the basis of the required general intervention, compromise of the client's health and well-being may result.

Assume that a client's affective response to the newly diagnosed diabetes is one of fear, an emotional arousal preventing her from processing any highly cognitive information. The client's singularity is clearly dictating the intervention necessary here. An exacerbated affective response is taking precedence over the need for health information about diabetes. If the nurse proceeds with an intervention of health education without first dealing with the client's fear and anxiety, more than likely the client will not understand what she is to do and may even refuse care altogether.

This example may seem like so much common sense when addressed in isolation from an actual client-nurse encounter. Numerous studies, however, have documented that health professionals fail to attend to the affective needs of their clients in an effort to accomplish certain agency goals and objectives or to meet certain personal needs for routine (Francis et al. 1969; Freeman et al. 1972). Through approaching community health nursing practice under a framework that emphasizes the multiple factors comprising the unique needs of a client, we are more likely to be alert to the affective needs of our clients and will more vigorously pursue interventions that address these needs. When applied to practice, the model forces us to systematically consider the complexities of clients and the array of complex interventions at our disposal.

Client-Nurse Interaction and Health Outcomes

A third nurse objective is to identify those factors within the client-nurse interaction that will be most useful in bringing about positive health outcomes. Certain outcomes demand an emphasis on certain intervention/interaction approaches. While all the factors comprising client-nurse interaction have an impact on each health outcome, one factor usually dominates.

The activities related to this objective are less specific to the client and more specific to the health outcome desired. Thus, this objective assists the nurse in developing a general intervention plan that is problem specific. This general plan is useful in situations where information about a client's singularity may not be available or will not be assessed until some time in the future. For example, if the objective is to increase the utilization of a screening clinic for hypertension, then specific information about that service should be targeted at the social values and educational level of a particular group. Affective/affiliative support for using the service from both strong community groups and professionals is needed.

Client-Nurse Interaction, Client Singularity, and Positive Health Outcomes

The primary conceptual objective of the IMCHB is the ability of the community health nurse to match her interaction/intervention approach to the singularity of the client in an effort to produce the maximal health outcome for that client. Several examples (Table 5.3) will follow to demonstrate the nursing activities.

The first example illustrates a client with no previous experience with diabetes. If the client is frightened over the new diagnosis, then indeed this affect will be reflected in speech and body language. The nurse's primary objective is to assist the client in reducing that anxiety through affiliative bonding and support and through deliberate and concrete information that would point out the possibilities of controlling the disease and the avoidance of problems. Issues the nurse should leave for a later discussion include the relevancy of blood glucose monitoring, the specific action of the oral agents or insulin, the multiple complications, and the hereditary implications of the disease. Nor should the nurse expect high-level decision making from the client relative to a type of antidiabetic therapy, employment, and family lifestyle changes at that time. The first goal of intervention in such a case is to supply the client with the basics sufficient to reduce anxiety and to begin the therapeutic regime. Another clinic or home visit within two or three days would provide the client with the needed affective support and reassurance; the nurse could then re-evaluate the client's anxiety and gradually step up the patient education program and the client's evolvement toward self-care.

The second example is an executive with hypertension. She reflects a self-assured, nonemotional level of responding, along with the need to know as much as possible about the diagnosis, the treatment, complications of the dis-

Table 5.3. Predicted Community Health Nursing Activities Based on Selected Aspects of the Client's Singularity and Components of the Client-Nurse Interaction

Aspects of Client Singularity	Client-Nurse Interaction Factors	Requisite Community Health Nursing Activities
1. The new diabetic client a. ↓ Experience	1. a. ↑ Affective support	Able to identify cues that would suggest need for supportive explanations to reduce anxiety associated with limited information
b. ↑ Affective response	b. → Need for client decisional control	Able to identify cues that suggest that client has little cognitive information that would facilitate decision-making and as a result feels less competent and self-determining
c. ↓ Feelings of competency and self-determinism (intrinsic motivation)	c. ± Informational input	Able to identify educational and comprehension level of client that would suggest amount, type, and approach to the provision of health education information
2. Executive with hypertension a. ↑ Intrinsic motivation	2. a. ↓ Affective support	Able to identify postural and verbal cues that suggest self-esteem, feelings of personal control, self-assuredness, competency, and self-determinism
b. ↓ Affective response	b. ↑ Need for client decisional control	Able to identify through the health history the amount of information that the client has at his/her disposal that will support decision making relative to intervention approach
c.	↑ Informational input	Able to offer specific, advanced information that will facilitate adaptation to the health need/problem and that will increase self-care capabilities

3. Anxious client with chest pain a. ↑ Affective response	3. ↑ Affective support	3. a. Able to determine that client's affective arousal is increased due to the inaccurate cognitive appraisal of the problem (if the client is extremely anxious because she associates her chest pain with an MI, then nursing efforts must be directed at reducing the affect)
b. ↑ Inaccurate cognitive appraisal	→ Decisional control	b. Able to assess the degree of inaccuracy in the cognitive representation to ascertain client's capacity to make health care decisions
	→ Informational input	c. Able to adjust the quantity, quality, and approach to health care information to client's level of comprehension/education and in accordance with the affect displayed
4. Obese client a. → Intrinsic motivation	4. ← Affective support → Need for client decisional control initially	4. a. Able to identify source of increased affective response
b. ↑ Affective response		b. Able to structure the health care encounter in order that need for client decisional control is reduced; client relies on structured environmental support in the absence of a social support system
c. → Social support	→ Informational input	c. Able to offer specific and limited concrete information that will reduce the affect and provide a beginning level of cognitive control over the health care problem

ease, and her options for self-care. In all probability, this client will be quite verbal about her knowledge and will identify perceptual gaps with little to no prompting from the nurse. This client expects sophisticated answers from the nurse: answers that address drugs by their generic or trade names, the role of the drug in reducing hypertension, the current blood pressure readings, and the desired levels for control. She expects to have a choice of therapy relative to her lifestyle. If lethargy and slowed thought processes are associated with one drug, will a substitute drug suffice or can an alternative medication schedule be developed? This client wants control; she has those singularity factors that should suggest to the nurse that complete client control is an option. The role of the nurse becomes that of information provider and technical advisor. To deny this client control will surely result in client dissatisfaction and perhaps a complete withdrawal from the prescribed regimen.

A third example is a client who has an inaccurate appraisal of the health problem. If the client associates a recurring chest pain with a myocardial infarction, he may present as extremely anxious. As in the first example, information that will reduce that anxiety is in order, coupled with affective support and efforts at affiliative bonding. On the other hand, in the case of the client who does not perceive his compliance with a diabetic diet to be of importance, this affect may need to be heightened through the provision of concrete fear-arousing communication in order to promote action. In both cases the objective of the nurse is to give the client a more accurate picture of the immediate problem. The interventions, however, are different in that they are aimed at decreasing the affect in the first client with chest pain, and increasing the affect in the second client who defaults on his diet.

The final example is the client who is responding primarily affectively to the health concern (obesity), lives alone, and who is undirected as to health care goals and their implementation. Again, the nurse must respond in an affectively supportive way. She or he must provide the client with a structured, but supportive milieu and prescribe concrete and assumable tasks for the client to accomplish (e.g., lose 1½ pounds in 10 days). This type of intervention begins to assist the client to reduce the affect through participating in the structure prescribed and lays the groundwork for the development of a sense of competency and self-determinism through the achievement of tasks.

These examples are clearly oversimplified. Clients must be addressed in accordance with all aspects of their singularity — not in response to one or two aspects in isolation. Nevertheless, the reader should be able to grasp from these illustrations the approach to a conceptual framework "thinking process" in planning community health nursing care interventions. These strategies demonstrate how to create conceptually based interventions that recognize the singularity of clients and the interface of that singularity with nursing interventions and health outcomes.

There has been a virtual knowledge explosion in community health nursing practice with individuals as clients. Further, this knowledge can be organized and systematically related within a conceptual framework of individual client health behavior and community health nursing interaction/intervention. This organizing framework could be applied in a number of ways in practice to enable a more systematic evaluation of an individual client's needs and a more deliberate development of nursing interventions to meet these needs.

An additional charge to any scientific field of inquiry is the test of its conceptual formulations in order to demonstrate their predictive validity and their potential to become tested theories. While most of the variables, concepts, and processes included in the framework presented have been tested in the psychosocial sciences, they have not been definitively applied in the health sciences. Grounding this framework scientifically implies testing through rigorous research. The next and final section of this chapter will examine how the IMCHB may be used in community health nursing research to study issues of individual client care.

APPLICATION OF THE FRAMEWORK TO COMMUNITY HEALTH NURSING RESEARCH

The IMCHB can guide community health nursing research in multiple ways, including (a) further confirmation of the relationships among the elements and factors within the model, (b) exploration of specific model constructs and concepts, (c) the development and testing of specific nursing interventions in accordance with the conceptual content of the model, (d) exploration of the longitudinal effects of time on the relationships described by the model, and (e) the investigation of the process of nursing care.

Confirmation of the Relationships Posited by the Model

Additional exploratory research utilizing the model is crucial to further substantiate the general structure of the model as well as to take detailed looks at specific model components. For example, the collection of observational data on client-nurse interaction will add greater substance to the interaction element of the model. Qualitative data collected utilizing video/audio-taped interactions or the use of participant observers of client-nurse encounters will enable the researcher to code and analyze the interaction according to the four components of the interaction element and prospectively demonstrate the impact of these components on subsequent client health behavior.

Further, the relationships described by the model differ in strength according to the health care setting and broad categories of health care problems. The model needs to be applied to community health educational campaigns. Are mass screening and educational programs addressing the singularity of their target groups? Will the relationships posited by the model hold consistently in school health and hospice settings? Will the role of the various factors within the interaction element differ from that in a neighborhood health center encounter versus a home health visit?

In terms of the model another area of research of interest to community health nurses is the stability of the relationships within various population subgroups for the same health care problem. Are the client singularity configurations for the adolescent diabetic vastly different from the singularity configurations for the elderly diabetic? Do the relationships posited by the model hold for ethnic and cultural subgroups, or is the model biased to a more limited cultural perspective in its view of client health behavior?

The Development of Specific Model Constructs

Intrinsic motivation or competency and self-determinism have not been developed as specific constructs within health care research. Presently, most of this work has been done in experimental psychology or applied in educational settings with school-age children. Because motivation is so inseparably linked to health maintenance and promotion behaviors, this construct should be studied in depth by community health nurse researchers in relation to the health care problems that they encounter. What are the important correlates and antecedents of motivation in behavior that promote high-level wellness? Does intrinsic motivation in one area of self-care extend to other areas of self-care within the same client? What role does intrinsic motivation play in clients' utilization of health services (educational programs, preventive health care programs)?

The Development and Testing of Nursing Interventions

If a major objective of the Interaction Model of Client Health Behavior is to serve as a conceptual base for intervention development, then it follows that these interventions themselves should be tested. For example, the model implies that health outcomes will be improved if the client-nurse interaction configuration fits with the client singularity configuration. Such a hypothesis can be subjected to test in quasi-experimental and/or experimental designs (see Chapter 7). One test might be to randomly assign clients to an experimental intervention emphasizing self-determinism and choice of their health care regimen; a control group would receive the traditional approach controlling for as many extraneous factors as possible. Clients who were not highly self-determined and who did not want decisional control relative to their health problem and subsequent intervention might be expected to demonstrate different outcomes between the two groups. Studies that examine the other interaction factors and components of client singularity could be similarly designed.

The Effect of Time on the Relationships Described by the Model

The conceptual content of the model implies that as more health care goals are achieved, health behavior becomes more rational and directed than emotional and haphazard. Appropriate nursing intervention fosters an increased sense of competency and self-determinism; the clients increase their self-care and decrease their dependency on the nurse. Longitudinal studies are needed to examine what happens to the various elements in the model and to client health behavior over time. For example, what are the long-term effects of health care interventions that foster self-determinism? Do clients more readily participate in health promotive behaviors if the nurse has consistently provided support for their self-determinism in health care?

Another time-relevant issue in regard to community health nursing practice concerns the effects of various interventions at different stages (longevity) of chronic illnesses. The study of how the relationships described by the model hold for the new diabetic versus one who has had diabetes for 2 years or 10 years would be of enormous significance in the planning of general health education interventions. For example, one might expect the affective components to be the strongest determinants of health behavior early in chronic illness, whereas later the strength of the client's self-determinism would be the crucial predictor of behavior.

The Investigation of the Process of Nursing Care

The ultimate personal objective in developing the framework presented is to demonstrate conceptually what has heretofore been the intuitive base upon which nursing care interventions have been implemented; that is, to match specific intervention factors to aspects of clients' singularity. It is this process of care that the author believes to be uniquely within the domain of nursing practice.

The structure, content, and flexible context of the model can guide community health nurses in their process investigations in three primary areas: (a) the exploration and documentation of nursing intervention and its subsequent impact on client health behavior, (b) the investigation of the role of self-care practices in health and illness, and (c) the examination of the efficacy of care approaches that subscribe to holistic client-centered care. Each of these areas is of current concern to community health nursing.

The Interaction Model of Client Health Behavior can be used to verify what community health nursing is and what community health nursing does. The majority of the documentation of nursing intervention has occurred within the acute care settings. Community health nurses can now assume leadership positions in the exploration of client behavior and intervention in the preventive/promotive and chronic disease arenas. For example, the model could be used to address the following concerns:

1. Is the client's perceived threat in chronic illness of less immediacy than that associated with acute illnesses and surgical procedures?
2. Does this reduced threat influence client behavior?
3. Should intervention in chronic illness focus more on the cognitive response in contrast to the affective response as in acute illness?
4. To what extent are the client singularity variables predictive of care outcomes in chronic illnesses?
5. Will the internally focused and highly self-determined individual be more responsive to a high level of decisional control?
6. Will the dependent client require more affective support and environmental planning from the nurse to maintain the standard of self-care in chronic illness?

These are but a few of the intervention questions that are based in the process of care and thus directly address community health nursing concerns.

Perhaps in no other area of nursing is the concept of self-care and maximal autonomy in maintaining and promoting health of more relevance than in community health nursing. Our clients are in their own environments and not under the protective health care supervision in which acute care clients find themselves. Self-care interventions by their very definition demand that the community health nurse be skilled in the identification of the client's holistic needs and singularity in order to prescriptively tailor individualized plans of care. The model can guide community health nursing research to answer such questions as: (a) To what extent are the client singularity variables predictive of an individual's ability to assume expanded self-care health practices? (b) Are there levels of self-care with respect to singularity, and if so what is the role of the nurse within each level? (c) Would the issues of decisional control and cognitive/affective responding determine the extent to which one would choose to be active in his or her own health care?

Finally, the model may offer community health nurses the opportunity to test a system of health care based on a holistic philosophy of health care. For example, such issues as these could be addressed through research directed by the model: (a) Does a care system that views the body–mind–spirit as one significantly alter the client's behavior and relationship with the nurse? (b) How will a system that emphasizes health — not illness — impact upon the current epidemiologic and economic patterns associated with health problems in this nation? (c) Will a system that negotiates decisional control relative to client singularity in matters of quality and quantity of life find itself serving a more responsive client who is willing to assume his or her share of responsibility in maintaining and promoting health?

The implications for further community health nursing research relative to the Interaction Model of Client Health Behavior seem limitless. Those areas of inquiry that hold the greatest interest for this author as a community health nurse researcher have been advanced, but clearly the list presented is not exhaustive. The model can be applied in any community health setting, to multiple client subgroups, and to any health care issue of concern to community health nurses. With each subsequent test of the model, new insights will be illuminated and new theoretical notions will be generated. These advances then can be returned to the clinical practice setting, where client and nurse alike will benefit from the new knowledge gained.

SUMMARY AND CONCLUSION

It is an immutable given that community health nursing will continue to develop and expand its practice with individuals as clients. Unlike any other area of nursing practice, community health nursing sees individual clients across all age spans, all categories of health care needs and problems, and in a multitude of environmental settings. Because of the multifocal nature of their practice, community health nurses are in a position to meet the major practice challenges presented by individual clients and the larger health care system.

These practice challenges stem directly from the individual client's problems in health care. The problem of client noncompliance, the lack of client responsibility for his or her health state, and the inattentiveness to risk factors and preventive measures that would address these factors are all issues that are manifest at the individual client level. Further, interventions that address issues fundamental to health maintenance and promotion must be examined and tested at the individual level. The determination of the best intervention approaches to the problems of client nonadherence to therapeutic regimens, the fostering of increased individual responsibility in health care, and the promotion of increased preventive self-care activities would begin to approach some of the nation's health care problems at the most basic level possible.

It is also an immutable given that community health nursing knowledge will continue to expand to meet the demands of its extending practice with individual clients. The complexity of this knowledge necessitates that it be approached in a highly organized and specific fashion. These data must be related in ways that are capable of directing community health nursing practice.

Finally, community health nurses must begin to demonstrate that their interventions do have an impact on individual client health outcomes. Economic, political, and social pressures are such that professional efficacy can no longer be assumed because the practitioners are well intentioned. Specific and measurable interventions must be derived from sound conceptual bases, and once developed, they should be tested through rigorous empirical analysis.

New practice horizons and new knowledge go hand in hand. There must, however, be some linking mechanism that will effectively blend the practice and the knowledge in ways that are mutually reinforcing and potentiating. The development of conceptual frameworks that can be empirically tested represents such a linking mechanism. By approaching individual client practice and research under the directives of a conceptual framework, such as the one just presented, practice-oriented investigators will move the discipline of community health nursing well beyond the state of being an art and into being a scientifically based practice discipline.

REFERENCES

American Nurses Association. Social policy statement. Kansas City, Missouri. 1980.

Annas G. The rights of hospital patients. New York: Aron Books, 1975.

Butler R, Gertman J, Oberlander D, and Schindler L. Self-care, self-help, and the elderly. Int J Aging Hum Devel 1979–80; 10:95–117.

Chinn P, and Jacobs M. Theory and nursing: a systematic approach. St. Louis: Mosby, 1983.

Christman L. Assisting the patient to learn the patient role. Nurs Digest 1978; 3:53–56.

Cohen F, and Lazarus R. Coping with the stresses of illness. In: Stone GC, Cohen F, Adler NE, eds. Health psychology—a handbook. San Francisco: Jossey-Bass, 1979.

Cox CL. The choice. Am J Nurs 1981; 81(9):1627–1628.

Cox CL. An interaction model of client health behavior: theoretical prescription for nursing. Adv Nurs Sci 1982; 5:41–56.

Deci EL. Intrinsic motivation. New York: Plenum Press, 1975.

Deci EL. The psychology of self-determination. Lexington, MA: Lexington Books, 1980.

Di Matteo M, Prince L, and Taranto A. Parents' perceptions of physicians' behaviors: determinants of patient commitment to the therapeutic relationship. J Comm Health 1979; 4:280–290.

Francis V, Korsch B, and Morris M. Gaps in doctor-patient communication: patients' response to medical advice. N Engl J Med 1969; 280:535–539.

Freeman B, Korsch B, Negrete V, and Mercer A. How do nurses expand their roles in well-child care? Am J Nurs 1972; 72:1866–1871.

Fuller S, Johnson L, and Endress P. The effects of cognitive and behavioral control on coping with an aversive health examination. J Hum Stress 1978; 4:18–25.

Gussow Z, and Tracy G. The role of the self-help clubs adaptation to chronic illness and disability. Nurs Digest 1978; 2:23–31.

Hempel C. Aspects of scientific explanation and other essays in the philosophy of science. New York: The Free Press, 1965.

Hingson R, Scotch N, Sorenson J, and Swazey J. In sickness and in health: social dimensions of medical care. St. Louis: Mosby, 1981.

Janis I, and Feshbach S. Effects of fear-arousing communications. J Abnormal Soc Psych 1953; 48:78–92.

Janis I, and Rodin J. Attribution, control and decision-making: social psychology and health care. In: Stone GC, Cohen F, Adler N, eds. Health psychology—a handbook. San Francisco: Jossey-Bass, 1979.

Johnson J, Rice V, Fuller S, and Endress P. Sensory information, instruction in a coping strategy, and recovery from surgery. Res Nurs Health 1978; 1:4–17.

Kahana R, and Bibring G. Personality types in medical management. In: Zinberg NE, ed. Psychiatry and medical practice in a general hospital. New York: International Universities Press, 1964.

Kinlein L. Independent nursing practice with clients. Philadelphia: Lippincott, 1977.

Knowles J. The responsibility of the individual. Daedalus 1977; 106:57.

Lazarus R, and Laumier R. Stress-related transactions between person and environment. In: Pervin LA, and Lewis M, eds. Perspectives in international psychology. New York: Plenum Press, 1978.

Lee P, and Franks P. Primary prevention and the executive branch of the federal government. Prevention 1977; 6:209–226.

Leventhal H, Meyer D, and Gutman M. The role of theory in the study of compliance to high blood pressure regimens. Washington, DC: National Institutes of Health, 1980.

Levin A. Talk back to your doctor. New York: Doubleday, 1975.

Levin A, Katz A, and Holst E. Self-care: lay initiatives in health. New York: Prodist, 1979.

Ley P, Jain V, and Skillbeck C. A method for decreasing medication errors made by patients. Psychol Med 1976; 6:599–601.

Lipowski A. Physical illness, the individual, and the coping process. Psychiatry Med 1970; 1:91–201.

Lipowski, A. Psychosocial aspects of disease. Ann Intern Med 1969; 71:1197–1206.

Marieskind H, and Ehrenreich B. Toward socialist medicine: the women's health movement. Soc Pol 1975; 6:34–43.

Pender N. Health promotion in nursing practice. Norwalk, CT: Appleton-Century-Crofts, 1982.

Preventive medicine USA: health promotion and consumer health education (John E. Fogarty International Center for Advanced Studies in the Health Sciences). New York: Prodist, 1976.

Runyan J. The public health nurse as a practitioner in chronic disease. South Med 1972; 60:15–19.

Runyan J. The Memphis chronic disease program: comparisons in outcome and the nurse's extended role. JAMA 1975; 231:264–267.

Schacter S. The psychology of affiliation. Stanford, CA: Stanford University Press, 1959.

Sehnert K, and Eisenberg H. How to be your own doctor sometimes. New York: Grosset and Dunlap, 1975.

Sullivan J. Research on nurse practitioners: process behind the outcome? Am J Public Health 1982; 72:8–9.

Sullivan J, and Armignaccio F. Effectiveness of a comprehensive health program for the well elderly. Nurs Res 1979; 28:70–75.

U.S. Department of Health, Education, and Welfare. Health United States 1979. Publication No. 80-1232. Washington, DC: Government Printing Office, 1979.

Waitzkin H, and Waterman B. The exploration of illness in capitalist society. Indianapolis: Bobbs-Merrill, 1974.

Yankauer A, and Sullivan J. The new health professionals: three examples. Ann Rev Public Health 1982; 3:249–276.

RESEARCH AND EVALUATION IN COMMUNITY HEALTH NURSING PRACTICE

II

Planning and implementing effective interventions depends upon the collective capacity within a discipline to rationalize and evaluate its work. Community health nursing investigators' successful performance of that role follows from an understanding of the cumulative development of knowledge available for application in the field and the major methods used to study it effectively. In addition, they must learn to plan and implement effective interventions.

Chapter 6 begins with a review of recent research in community health nursing, with a commentary on its status. Chapter 7 provides direction for increasing methodological rigor in research in this field. Finally, Chapter 8 outlines general principles of program evaluation.

Collectively, this section covers the research base of the recent past, from which we can, by specific methods and strategies, design the research and program evaluation of the future. The references will prove invaluable for nurse-investigators who accept the challenge of research and evaluation in this field.

OVERVIEW OF COMMUNITY HEALTH NURSING RESEARCH AND EVALUATION 6

Judith A. Sullivan

INTRODUCTION AND HISTORICAL PERSPECTIVE

Research in community health nursing has received a great deal of attention recently, almost as if it were a recent phenomenon. True, a great deal more work is needed, but research in the field is far from a recent phenomenon. The beginning stages of evaluation research in community health nursing occurred before 1900, when summary descriptions were given of the nature of this new field of practice, presented at the early conventions, and published in the early nursing journals. Over the next 60 years, research in community health nursing consisted largely of classifying and collecting information on the activities of the public health nurse. This information was used largely for reports of service activities during an expansionary period, albeit with little emphasis on using the data for research and none on theory development.

We are fortunate in public health nursing that in 1958 Hortense Hilbert, a public health nursing leader with extensive experience both in the United States and abroad, directed a project funded by the U.S. Public Health Service to compile all studies in the field to that time. She included in her search "all studies of public health nursing in any of its phases, studies of nursing that include public health, studies of public health in which nursing is explicit, studies made and reported by public health nurses and those in which public health nurses are represented in the population studied" (Hilbert 1959). She found that the earliest one of the 232 studies meeting these criteria was published in 1924, and she extended the search through 1957.

During this period of rapid growth in community health nursing there was so much more to be done than could be accomplished that as much effort as possible was given to developing and administering the service programs rather than to researching the effects or evaluating the practice beyond the descriptive level. Clearly, the emphasis was placed on matching nursing services to the public demand. Studies of nursing utilization, cost to administration, and organization dominated the first 60 years of research in community health nursing.

Hilbert abstracts and classifies the studies she reviewed into ten categories. The largest category is called "special field," suggesting a *clinical* focus present in the research question. This interesting observation belies the previous assumption that clinical focus was lacking in early research efforts. One explanation may be that 50 percent of the studies occurred within the last six years of the survey, since around 1951. At approximately that same time, major federal support for graduate education in nursing became available, including support for nursing research emphasizing clinical practice areas.

A glance through the list of investigators shows that the majority were public health nurses — a surprising finding in light of the lack of research training in this group and the competition for research funds. Across the categories reported, the designs were generally developed for program evaluation purposes, largely concerned with counting nurses providing services by kind, units of service delivered, and numbers of patients and families served. As a result, these studies may have been largely funded by sources internal to the work setting.

Gradually greater numbers of community health nurses began to engage in research activities. Their involvement grew in proportion to the support for graduate education in nursing. In her review of research in the field of community health nursing between 1972 and 1976, Marion Highriter (1977) identifies 115 published papers on research in community health nursing. Similar to Hilbert, she includes those either written by community health nurses or involving them or their activities. She, however, classifies the studies by *purpose* and groups them into six categories. By this time emphasis had shifted to evaluations of process or outcomes of services, which comprise the largest number of studies (42 percent). This category was followed by client need assessment studies (17 percent) and service description studies (14 percent). Community health nursing education studies (13 percent), attitude studies (8 percent), and study reviews and papers on methodology (4 percent) comprised the remainder.

Following her analysis of the studies in each of these categories, Highriter concludes that they represent a broad range of interests. She also adds insightfully that while the average number of studies published in this field has increased steadily over the past ten years and probably longer, few authors to date have demonstrated much consideration for theory. Given the state of the literature with regard to theory development and the unavailability of research machinery to community health personnel, this trend is not altogether unexpected. In fact, the practical need for most of the studies and their frequent sponsorship by the agencies where the research was conducted understandably resulted in studies highly relevant to problems of the practice field and addressed to applied topics. Highriter cautions present-day researchers to retain this relevance (focus on actual problems) even if funding becomes more readily available from other sources or motivation for initiating studies should change radically.

Concern about the importance of theory is well taken. Descriptive studies will certainly continue and remain important in the exploration of new areas and problems. However, as the training and experience of community health researchers continues to develop, we can expect to see a larger percentage of studies being directed at theoretical issues that help to explain pragmatic practice questions; such work will furthermore be conducted with increasing methodological sophistication. The advancement following this theoretical push will serve well to both clarify conceptual underpinnings of the profession and increase the efficacy of the practice that continues to be the bedrock of the discipline.

To add to the general fund of knowledge from the unique perspective gained from practice, nurses experienced in delivering services in community-based settings *must* be involved in defining concepts, developing hypotheses, developing propositions, and conducting the research to test their ideas. To be sure, some of the clinically oriented experiences and insights gained by community health nurses are similar to concepts used in other disciplines. Interchange and co-investigation with researchers from other disciplines will facilitate the discovery of universal principles as well as isolate those unique to the community health nursing experience. This research will be mutually beneficial as long as the research into community health nursing practice is conducted by a nurse theorist researcher with a strong background in some form of community health nursing practice.

The objective of this chapter is an examination of all studies completed during the decade of 1970–1980 that could be located and that were either conducted by community health nurses or about their practice. In addition, selected studies were reviewed from the prior five years (1965–1970) that are mentioned frequently in more recent research and seem to have had an important influence on the direction of study in this specific field. The reviews are undertaken with an eye toward critical evaluation of past and present research and as a documentary of important and relevant investigative activities in the profession. Depending upon the purpose of the reader, further studies may be sought in the same practice areas prior to 1965, or studies using theories or methods developed in the fields that relate to the practice under review may be sought.

In this review, studies were listed that had a direct reference to the practice of the community health nurse. As many studies were reviewed as could be found by an extensive library search, using the standard major library search methods. The bibliographies of each of the articles reviewed have also been culled for additional citations of community health nursing research. Still some studies have probably been neglected; the reader is encouraged to examine other reviews of research, such as *The Annual Review of Research* in which Highriter presents an update of her earlier presentation in *Nursing Research* (1984).

PURPOSE AND ORGANIZATION OF STUDIES

Two skills highly desirable for the completion of significant research are (a) developing an understanding of the research that has been done in the field and a vision of the gaps needing to be filled, and (b) mastery of the techniques and methods commonly used in the particular area of study. This chapter presents material useful for acquiring the former skill, while Chapter 7 discusses guidelines for the latter. Also developed here is a broad overview for general understanding of the research in community health nursing. For those who plan to study the material very closely for commonalities among the research presented, emerging concepts across subareas of study, and analytic methods that can be applied to data available to them, a bibliography is presented as a roadmap to the original sources. The extent to which it is dwelt upon, turned over in the mind of the reader, and used as a bridge to new ideas is a function of the reader's interest and ingenuity. In other words, the complexity of the content is in the application by the practitioner and researcher and not so much in the manner of presentation.

Presenting research on community health nursing practice can be approached from a number of perspectives. As was done by Hilbert and Highriter, the studies need to be grouped to allow for general description by category. While each of these authors selects categories that in some way separate studies of practice from other areas of investigation, their distinctions are different from each other. The organization chosen for use in this chapter is by functional area: practice, administration, education, and research and ethics. Further, the practice category is subdivided into studies that deal with identifying those at risk, caring for those with minor illness, and providing services for families with an ill member at home. In this way, topical areas of research can be traced cumulatively over a period of time, as each study contributes to general understanding of a particular type of practice; no attempt has been made here to trace generalized concepts as applied across several areas of practice. Generalities of method and theory, however, do exist.

RESEARCH INTO PRACTICE

In general, studies of public health nursing practice are focused either on the client's health state or on the delivery of services to the client. The former are likely to include physical, psychological, and social indicators of health and often deal with the impact of the client's actions, beliefs, and behaviors on his or her health. The latter include finding the risk group, determining the type and number of services to direct toward the risk group, and measuring the effectiveness of the various ways of providing the service. In other words, research in community health nursing practice can be classified into the study of health promotion behavior of clients and the study of delivery of health services to clients. To provide an overview of the research in comunity health, both kinds of studies are discussed within each of the areas of investigation outlined below.

Studies of Health Screening and Wellness Care

Screening and wellness studies are focused on detecting those at risk for a health problem, screening specific populations for early detection of a particular disease or correctable condition, and primary prevention programs such as health teaching to promote health status. The methods commonly used are mass application of individual health assessment techniques, individual and group teaching, and counseling — either in groups or on assessment visits in the home.

Program areas in this category are organized by developmental stages and largely reflect studies of the types of programs offered for each developmental stage. Infant and well-child or preschool programs provide health evaluations, health counseling to parents, and prevention of specific diseases by the administration of immunizations. For the school-age child, activities in health evaluation, teaching, and prevention tend to center around the early detection of abnormalities, teaching of good health habits, the avoidance of maladaptive practice such as smoking and substance abuse, and the continuation of the immunization program. With the emphasis on mainstreaming handicapped children, future studies of providing health care to children in schools may also include health maintenance of chronic illness, but at this time no studies in this area exist. In a few settings, primary care is being offered to children in school.

The remaining areas of research covering this level of care include college health programs, occupational health programs, and wellness-oriented programs for the elderly. Each of these program areas, while primarily focused on improving and maintaining health, may include some aspect of secondary prevention, such as teaching and counseling on a particular disease condition or health state (e.g., pregnancy, the correction of or adaptation to common problems such as vision and hearing deficits, or the control of a health condition such as hypertension or diabetes). These programs are included here because of their focus at the primary prevention level.

Infants and Young Children

Few areas of health programming can attract the nearly universal interest of policy makers than the care of infants and young children enjoys. While many questions remain unresolved (the usefulness of anticipatory guidance and health counseling for mothers, even the expected yield of conditions identified from physical assessments), support for these services has been a constant, if fluctuating, program area since the turn of the century (see Chapter 1). Yet only three studies were found in this category: one study of health teaching, one of screening evaluations, and one report of a family assessment tool.

Each of the studies reveals a different aspect of practice with well infants, which is an interesting point in itself. Any one of them would bear replication to increase the confidence of clinicians in the presented findings. It is by the repeating of work of earlier studies that issues, instruments, and methods are further refined and the conceptualization of practice interventions and their outcomes are clarified. Several points made in these studies are noted below and should be replicated in future studies.

McNeil and Holland (1972) present an excellent example of applied quasi-experimental field research in a nursing context. Comparisons of two methods of providing health teaching to mothers about infants and children (individual home visits and group teaching) are developed. The methods were painstakingly applied and reported so clearly that replication in another setting is possible. This study asks: should group teaching replace individual home visiting? The results indicate some advantages to that course and also point to the importance of finding other means to reach those who do not attend group sessions. Replication will begin to build the cumulative knowledge that will provide direction in our selection of interventions tailored to client objectives.

The screening study reports on the effectiveness of public health nurses using the Denver Developmental Screening Test in identifying deviations from normal in healthy children (Bryant 1973). The screening outcomes of the nurses' exams compare favorably with those of general practice physicians, and the yields of both are reported. Regardless of the examiner, 7.3 percent of the children were selected for follow-up by a pediatrician.

The follow-up component of a screening study is essential, where possible. Data should be gathered on how many of those found "at risk" actually were further evaluated and how many needed treatment. Comparing findings of nurses with another group (usually physicians) provides information on the potential number of cases missed (false negatives). Data on follow-up of cases found provides information on how much "overtreatment" was recommended (false positives). Both pieces of information are critical to the understanding of the effectiveness of a screening program. When it is not possible to build both phases into the same study, replication of the first phase at another time or in another setting can be planned. Because of the prior development of the study methods and evaluation guides, the second phase can then focus on building the data-gathering mechanisms for documenting the often protracted *outcomes* of follow-up.

The parenting tool is reported here because it was developed by a nurse, for use in assessing parenting skills in a home setting (Bishop 1976). She drew from her observations in working with parents — primarily mothers — and developed categories of criteria for assessing satisfactory mothering, signs of difficulty in adapting to an infant, and deterrents to adequate mothering. This qualitative guide could be used as a structure for a clinical interview or could be quantified and tested as a measurement of mothers' relative risk of having difficulty adapting to parenthood. As is true in the case of the development of any tool, it must be used again and again, thus being checked for reliability before incorporation into general use.

The first two studies of well infants and children concentrate on the delivery of services, whereas the parenting tool focuses on the measurement of a parent behavior in relation to the healthy development of the child. Taken together, they address the investigation both into health behaviors and delivery systems.

School-Age Children and Youth

Of all the areas of practice, research in school health produced the largest number of studies. Beginning school, a universal phenomenon, is an ideal time to conduct mass screening of 3- 5-year-olds — both to correct any conditions found and to plan for dealing with these problems subsequently in the school setting.

The first four studies in this group actually focus on health evaluations conducted before the children started school. Attendance at mass screening sessions is usually very good (over 80 percent); and the yield has been measured in terms of numbers of problems referred for follow-up (usually a high yield between 21 and 48 percent) and the cost per child assessment. The key factor here is follow-up — not only in the accuracy of problem identification, but in the methods used to encourage the adequate investigation of problems.

Parents face several dilemmas in achieving optimal health care for their children in school. First, they often are not present during the evaluation and therefore may not identify as closely with the need to initiate action. Second, to seek care, they must frequently take the child out of school (and leave work themselves) for the further investigation of the problem. Further, for many parents, sources of health care for their children, especially medical subspecialties, are new and unknown: guidance is needed for them to proceed with confidence. Evaluation of the importance of these factors to effective follow-up and of the interpersonal techniques used by the nurse in working with parents could be incorporated into almost any follow-up study.

For children who have begun school, problem-specific screening programs are more likely to be reported. Screening of 791 fourth-grade children for heart problems yielded 11 who were referred for further evaluation, 1 of whom was diagnosed with an actual heart problem (requiring surgery) after examination by a cardiologist (Dennison and Fenimore 1971). In a strabismus screening program of 2619 first-grade children, 118 cases of manifest strabismus were detected and later confirmed, yielding a prevalence rate of 4.5 percent. Forty-nine of these cases were newly diagnosed, while the remainder were already under care (Kornder et al. 1974).

Two studies of scoliosis screening were found. Again, the school nurse had had special training to carry out the procedure. After screening 19,000 children between 11 and 14 years old, the nurses in one study (Abbott 1977) referred 657, or 3.4 percent of the children, to a physician; 63 (0.3% yield) were eventually treated (exercise, braces, or surgery). The other study (Benson 1977) involved 7815 students, of whom 17 percent were reexamined by a physician, and 1.5% were found to have scoliosis confirmed by radiography.

One study (Humphrey 1979) reported that 40 percent of 1953 children ages 5 to 11 from 12 schools in one city had height/weight disproportion (27 percent were overweight). Of 410 10, 11, and 12-year-old children receiving a general screening exam by a nurse and then a physician, about 20 percent required follow-up for additional treatment. In fact, the nurse identified more significant health problems than did the physician. These studies recommended that screening programs of this kind should be continued — or even started at an earlier age. In still other studies reporting comparisons with physicians on yield and cost per unit of service, the nurse is usually documented as a highly effective case finder, when well trained on assessment skills, and as a provider of a more cost-effective screen than the physician (Robertson et al. 1976; Asbed et al. 1977; Henzell 1977; Sahin 1979).

From the array of screening program evaluations presented, a number of observations on the state of the art can be made. First, even in populations of healthy school children, incidence and prevalence rates of common health problems have not been established. As a result, the nurse and physician evaluators do not know the "expected" yield with which to compare their results. In this age of rapid manipulation of data by computer, population-specific rates are easier to develop and should be calculated at the school-wide or system-wide level. Judgments made about use of resources can then be associated with yield, cost, and relative effectiveness of the various personnel used for problem identification (nurses, physicians, and others).

Second, the investigators in these studies were careful to report when the nurses had had additional training in some specific screening technique, but they did not as carefully document the methods that were used to engage the child and parents in the problem solving related to the follow-up activities. Several models of health-seeking behavior have been advanced (Suchman 1967; Anderson and Newman 1973; Rosenstock 1974; Cox 1982) that could be used as conceptual frameworks upon which to base study of these aspects of client behavior and nurse effectiveness. Further research must draw from models such as these and contribute to further theoretical advancement by testing the relationships posited within them.

Third, none of the studies address the impact of the false positive effect on the children and families alerted to a potential problem that later proved inconsequential. This phenomenon could be the source of iatrogenic anxiety, causing at least temporary change in self-concept and varying amounts of family disruption. Relatively simple measures could be routinely taken if this response proved to be an identifiable and widespread occurrence (e.g., statements of reassurance and interpretation, increased accessibility to the nurse).

Within the actual follow-up phase itself, six studies were found focusing on a variety of aspects of pursuing problems detected in the school setting. One emphasized cultural aspects and compared types of follow-up methods and their effectiveness in stimulating parental action (Bryan and Cook 1967). This study also measured the effect of introducing a school health aide to the follow-up program. Another study also confirmed the effectiveness of the home visit versus telephone methods in stimulating the parents to follow up on detected problems; it showed that the telephone call yields as high results as the more time consuming home visit. Both these oral forms of communication are su perior, however, to the written note (Cauffman et al. 1969a). A second study by the same authors examined the effect of nurse characteristics and attitudes on children and parents already engaged in follow-up care. Variations were found, with implications for the kinds of learning experiences necessary for nurses to relate to clients and thereby achieve higher levels of follow-up for the children (Cauffman et al. 1969b).

Checking the administrative pattern (health department or board of education) found this factor to have negligible effect on the percentage of children receiving follow-up. When SES was examined, however, significant differences were found (Patterson 1969). Brophy (1970) indicates that 72.8 percent of 320 previously detected but uncorrected defects received attention during an intensive program emphasizing contacting parents at home. In a descriptive case study of six families visited at home, background on visit content, time, and perceived effectiveness is outlined. This descriptive information is useful for the further identification of theory that affects the interaction and outcomes achieved (Callan and McGray 1972).

While many gaps exist in the study of screening and process of follow-up, these investigations show that many strides have been made during the decade in question. The accomplishments are especially high in (a) establishing the importance of researching screening yields and end-results differentially by type of problem(s) sought, (b) viewing the evaluation of mass health assessments in two phases: the investigation of both screening and follow-up activities, and (c) identifying multiple variables — contextual, process, intervening, and outcome in the study of the follow-up phase.

Turning to another element of the school nurse's role, the issue of provision of direct care in the schools has also been addressed. A total of eight studies in school nursing examine direct care provided to elementary and high school students. The first is a program designed to test simultaneously the role of a nurse practitioner functioning with a health aide in a school and that of a physician consultant from a nearby neighborhood health center. This team approach was found to be successful in the selective use of the nurse practitioner role; the rate of follow-up for the children referred for care was superior, but overall the program was a little more expensive than the traditional method (Nader et al. 1972).

A second direct service program addresses the concept of child-initiated care, looking at the rates of utilization of the school nurse's office when children determined what problems to seek care for and when that care was needed. The office was staffed by a school nurse practitioner, who responded to the child's initiation of, and participation in, his or her own care (Lewis et al. 1977). Two additional studies quantified the nature of problems children brought to the nurse's office: one used an instrument developed for systematic collection of data (Rice 1978) and the other evaluated the types and frequency of complaints according to whether the child came from a broken home (Snyder et al. 1980). Absenteeism follow-up is the chief intervention tested in another intervention study (Long 1975), and in still another (Vernon et al. 1976), three techniques for improving immunization levels are evaluated.

The last three studies in this group are directed toward health services delivered to students in high schools: two papers show the description and effectiveness of prenatal care delivered in a public high school (Edwards et al. 1977; Bey et al. 1979), and one demonstrates the problems the nurse dealt with when providing mental health consultation (Coejic and Smith 1979).

One of the major underlying issues within the study of direct care in the school is the divided responsibility for the promotion of a child's health. As a growing and developing individual, the child can use the interaction with the health personnel to increase understanding of self-responsibility for health. Simultaneously, because the child is a minor, the parent or guardian has responsibility and therefore must be involved. It would appear that this fundamental issue should be addressed in the development of interactive components of a nurse's role and in the evaluation of the role's effectiveness. More important, the identification of the child-family dyad as the unit of service may offer new conceptualizations of methods for future studies.

The development of the *role* of the nurse in school is the subject of seven studies between 1970 and 1980. Addressing the familiar problem of different interpretations of the school nurse role is the "Illinois Study of School Nurse Practice." Superintendents, principals, teachers, and school nurses were polled. Recommendations supported standardizing and improving school nursing by state certification and better education for school nurses at the university level (Fricke 1967). Teachers' and administrators' perceptions were sampled (Forbes 1967; Greenhill 1979), nurses' time was recorded on specific functions (Lowis 1969), and communication about the role between nurse and teacher was studied (Smiley 1975). School nurses' knowledge about a specific pertinent disease area (venereal disease) was tested (McGrath and Laliberte 1974). After the introduction of nurse practitioners into schools, role evaluations were conducted including the new functions (Lewis et al. 1974; McAtee 1974).

One instrument was found to be useful to assessing a family with a school-age child. This tool could lead to the enumeration of issues to be dealt with in a way that would establish priorities among family situations, or to the clustering of types of common problems that might lend themselves to a group solution (Holt 1979). Another study dealt with the comparison of nursing functions among elementary, middle, and high school nurses (Gilman et al. 1979).

College Health Services

Wellness-oriented services in college health settings address even more fully the responsibility of the student for his or her own health care. While parents are sometimes involved on the periphery, particularly in episodes of illness, wellness care is virtually the responsibility of the students. For this reason, the participation and response of the student are critical elements in the successful implementation of a college health program. The two studies found in this area emphasize the nurse practitioner role as an influence on client *response* to health problems rather than only as a means of identifying the problems themselves.

One study presents the results of giving a self-administered health instrument followed by discussions with the student about its interpretation and any plans for intervention (Caldwell 1977). The other reported on the highly favorable responses of college women to gynecologic services provided by nurse practitioners (Wagener and Carter 1978). At a period of maximal learning, in many cases simultaneous to the assumption of self-care, the importance of finding the best ways to influence and intervene toward health promotion cannot be overestimated; and extensive research opportunities remain largely untapped in this area.

Community Family Planning and Maternal Care Services

Family planning is a part of the general health services offered to women by nurses in a variety of community settings, including public clinics, schools, adult classroom settings, and the home. The objectives differ in each of these settings, and therefore the focus of studies conducted in these settings differs as well. One characteristic of this area of study is that the process and outcome variables are surprisingly underdeveloped. A partial explanation may lie in the unresolved problem of whether to include the spouse, family, and eventually the offspring in the factors considered, or only the client herself.

In considering the decisions to be made, the attitudinal component takes on greater significance than in most other types of service; as a result it is itself an important factor to measure in the effectiveness of care. None of the studies found describes the attitudes or knowledge level expected of the clients involved, although there is clearly specialized content implied in the programmatic offerings presented.

The general family planning needs of women are addressed in one study through the offering of services by experienced public health nurses trained in family planning, which resulted in a great improvement in the follow-up of clients (LeSueur et al. 1972). In a study of knowledge and attitudes of public health nurses about family planning, age was shown to be a chief factor. However, a majority of nurses felt that they should provide counseling for clients regardless of their personal beliefs (Howard et al. 1972). One study reported on the outcomes of a training program for nurses, including those from community health agencies (Manisoff 1976). Expectant parent classes were also evaluated during a postpartum visit, relating the effect of the classes to the health outcomes of the babies (Thordarson and Costanzo 1976). In a study of 64 maternity patients intended to enhance maternal care, number of immunizations, family planning, and knowledge of growth and development, the issue of family-centered care is examined. This study stresses the importance of instrument development and measurement of variables and raises several critical issues in the design of public health nursing studies (Yauger 1972).

Occupational Health Services

Many evaluation studies have been conducted by nurses in occupational health settings, but they have not been published. Sometimes the studies so conducted are available as government documents or in the literature under someone else's sponsorship, such as a physician or administrator.

Four clinical studies by nurses in this field were found. Evaluation of nurse-conducted pre-employment health assessments indicates that the nurses and technicians they supervised performed 85 percent of the health assessment. Of the remainder that were referred to a physician for further work-up, about half required work restriction (Flight and Schussler 1976). Another study considers the type of communication used with clients to increase compliance in using hearing protective devices (Esler 1978). This study is one of the few to base an intervention on a theoretical position and then to test it.

Nurses specially trained to deliver worksite hypertension treatment constitute another program evaluation with highly successful results (Logan et al. 1979). Tailoring the preparation of the nurses to the management of hypertension as an occupational hazard involved the treatment skills of a primary care provider, psychosocial and counseling skills, and an understanding of occupational health nursing.

A study examining the role activities and responses of nurses in industry to the nurse practitioner role, (Bridges 1976) documents varying responses. With the introduction of this role into the setting, however, together with the advanced education increasingly available in occupational health nursing, this field is in a position to contribute significantly to the growing literature on risk assessment and primary health care.

Older Adult and Elderly

Because of the sharp increase in the elderly population, a great deal of attention has been focused on this group within the past yen years. The majority of studies found in this category are designed to screen or survey various elderly populations for the prevalence of health problems needing attention. First is a two-part survey reporting on the needs of the elderly in Canada followed by a study of services by public health nurses available to meet those needs (Schwenger and Sayers 1971a). The comprehensiveness of these reports provides a clear picture of the health situation of the elderly population upon which to plan service offerings.

Including the general survey reported above, a total of ten surveys of health status of the elderly were found from 1971 to 1977, representing four countries, urban and rural populations, and populations in both private homes and subsidized housing units. The findings can be summarized as follows. Among the major concerns were foot problems, hearing deficits, vision problems, unsatisfactory dentures, and — less often reported but of importance — urinary incontinence. A sizable number had housing problems, and many included an enumeration of accident hazards in the home.

The major psychological problem was loneliness and social isolation, and in one study (Heath and Fitton 1975) 18 percent of the sample were found to have at least one symptom of emotional distress. Nutritional status was also found to be problematic (Barber and Wallis 1976). In terms of carrying out activities of daily living, the major areas of difficulty were in doing laundry, cutting toenails, and walking outside (presumably including shopping and doing errands).

The epidemiology of these problems is suggested by a follow-up to the Canadian study reported above (Schwenger and Sayers 1971b). The authors characterize the greatest proportion of problems as occurring among rural populations, among women, and among the "very old" (over 80 years). In this study the initial survey was conducted by a mailed questionnaire, followed by a selected sampling of both respondents and nonrespondents with an interview and physical examination. Interestingly, nonrespondents evidenced greater physical and mental deterioration, inferior living conditions, and accident hazards than respondents. The high-rise apartment complexes were found to have a lower proportion (68 percent) of residents with minimal or no difficulty than those in a general suburban sample (89 percent). The authors suggest that this difference could be due either to different scoring procedures or to the attraction of high-rise dwellings for the elderly with limitations in physical functioning. Between 10 and 12 percent of the elderly do not have access to medical care.

On the brighter side, the same study showed that over half the sample received regular help with personal care and housekeeping from family members, and many received help from other health service sources where available. Women over 80 living at home in urban settings reported fewer symptoms, better health, and less loneliness and isolation than others. No explanation was advanced as to the reasons for this finding.

In another study, those over 75 had more health problems, were more physically disabled, and were more socially isolated than younger groups (Currie et al. 1974). While the number of symptoms per client varied from one to eight, a very high percentage were fully mobile and independent (89 percent and 95 percent, respectively). The consensus among the investigators was to identify and treat the small and minor problems before they grew to major disabling functional impediments.

In summary, most of the investigators state that the services of the public health nurses are validated in terms of their accuracy in health assessment, their ability to provide on-site treatment and referral services, and their flexibility in working with other health workers in the community (e.g., physicians and health educators) to plan and provide health services according to assessed needs. Additional observations in England deal with the advantages in the attachment of community nurses (health visitors) to physicians' offices and health centers. As liaisons, the nurses can provide easy access to health services for the clients and help promote the use of uniform records for cross-disciplinary recording.

Two studies describe aspects of client care. The first seeks to disclose the factors of greatest concern to elders by interviews and open-ended discussion (Managan et al. 1974). Many reported being lonely, fearing death, and identified problems requiring physical, social, and family-oriented solutions. Considerable descriptive background is provided to illustrate the bases of the authors' recommendations for intervention. The second described three different modes of supplying public health nursing services to the elderly and compared the effects on the health and health perceptions of the subjects in all three groups six months later (Sullivan and Armignacco 1979). The fact that the services provided were helpful was evidenced by the improved health perceptions, the greater response to a preventive program, and the higher proportion of those who had received the highest level of public health nursing services who could identify a source of primary care. This report, too, provides a description of the specific nursing intervention that was carried out.

Two studies report on questionnaires developed to assess the elderly. The first questionnaire was administered by a public health nurse in the home of the subject and was validated by the physician's records (Powell and Crombie 1974). The second compared the client's answers with clinical ratings of physicians and health visitors. Agreement was high for the less complex functions (dressing, walking indoors), but less so for functions such as preparing meals, housework, and shopping (Kaufert and Green 1979).

Of all the groups toward whom health screening and wellness programs are directed, the elderly have recently been one of the more intensively studied groups. Further, the research conducted in this area is more developed in design and methodology than for the other groups. Because the aging are a continually growing population, they will account for increasing proportions of professional attention. The research presented here serves as a base for the breakthroughs that can be expected in delivery of nursing care in the future. The theory development expected through the testing of models of health behavior could well be generated within the future research in this field.

Studies of Nursing in Primary Care

By participating in community assessments and basing the programming of health services on the general health needs of the population, primary care personnel function within a community-oriented definition in the provision of personal health services. The nurses using this approach to providing primary care are the ones selected by the research reported here. Nurse practitioners/clinicians account for the majority of the nurses in primary care, and most of the research in this area focuses on this role and its comparison with that of other providers, especially physicians, physician assistants, and other nurses. The research reported in this section represents clinical studies carried out by primary care nurse clinicians with a community health nursing orientation.

In nursing the most recent advances in providing health care to all the population have come in the expansion of primary care nursing. Until 1965, nursing in primary care was practiced on a limited scale in public health centers and in physician offices and clinics. After 1965, graduates of nurse practitioner/clinician programs began to assume direct responsibility for the primary care of clients. Within a 10-year period, nurses were making an important contribution to the primary care of clients in private offices, hospital and public health clinics, school and occupational settings, and many other institutional and nontraditional settings as well.

The factor probably most responsible for the tremendous upsurge in research in this area is the role autonomy associated with functioning as a primary care provider. Could nurses be as accountable in quality and quantity of care as physicians? Included in this autonomy was decision making and judgment about which clients to see, how to take care of them, and how and when to consult with physician partners. Within the decade, nursing in primary care had undergone a role change, involving an increase in responsibility and a change in educational pattern. The extensive research on the role of the nurse practitioner focused upon the types and content of the programs; the demographic characteristics of the nurses and their practice; the attitudes and acceptance of nurses in this role by physicians, clients, and others; the impact on the quality and type of care delivered; and the personality factors and autonomy issues involved in assuming the role (Sultz et al. 1979; ANA 1980).

Unlike the evolution of most professional roles, this role growth was generously funded by both federal and foundation sources. Support was granted for the development of training programs together with evaluation components. Evaluation researchers across the country focused their attention on the development, acceptability, and viability of this "new" health care provider. Reviews have been written summarizing the findings of these studies, and the reader is referred to these to pursue specific issues within this vast research effort (ANA 1980; Yankauer and Sullivan 1982).

Here the focus is on the research that relates to direct practice of the primary care nurses in community health settings. Fourteen studies and two reviews researching some aspect of direct practice were found. While many of the more general studies were conducted by non-nurses, half of the studies on practice were authored by nurses. More of the research in this field in the future will be reported by nurses focusing on their practice. At this time the field is in a newly emerging stage.

Four of the studies early in the decade describing nursing in primary care refer to outreach and follow-up services by public health nurses/health visitors who served in a liaison capacity. Results of one study are reported in terms of reduced hospital stays for patients with heart disease (Hanchett and Forrens 1967). An important point included in this report is the quantification of issues, such as adherence problems, and emotional and supportive maintenance, that were handled by the nurses in achieving their success. Results of the second study are reported in greater numbers of referrals and communications generated among the physicians, nurses, and social workers (Allen and King 1968).

For successful interdisciplinary practice, raising the opportunity for contact is an important component. In a rural setting, outreach clinics were opened and staffed by local community nurses who saw clients between their specialty neurologic clinic appointments. Client improvements both medically and socially were noted (Haerer et al. 1974). In southwest England, responses to a poll indicated that 90 percent of the physicians had a health visitor and district nurse attached to their office practices. Although many improvements in the system could be made, this high a percentage of practices with nursing personnel in place provides a first step toward effective continuity of care (Forman 1974).

Within the clinics, nurses were beginning to make important contributions as well. In addition to the advantage of additional personnel enabling higher numbers of patients to be seen at lower cost, the nurse practitioners' style of practice included greater attention to the lifestyles and individual characteristics of their clients. In a study of nurse clinicians' practice in a county hospital medical clinic, nurses reportedly placed greater attention than did physicians on the patients' diets and recommended more changes in daily activities and exercise. In addition to having more frequent contact in clinic, they visited their patients at home (Flynn 1974). Another study in a similar setting further substantiates reports of the advantages in the introduction of nurse clinicians into a program. Mentioned there are greater continuity of care, more patient education during clinic visits, and decreased multiple clinic visits (Bessman 1974).

In a study of a nurse-managed triage system in a neighborhood health center, the problem of high "walk-in" rates is addressed. Using this system, more patients were seen with less waiting and with higher satisfaction from their care (Mechaber et al. 1974). One ironic factor identified in a study of the nurse practitioner in a pediatric practice is that while the parents consulted the nurse on a wide variety of issues, they did not see this as a professional consultation (Breslau 1977). Thus, while acceptance was high, definition of the professional service received was not automatic. Another well-controlled study in pediatric practice shows that the nurse practitioners assigned to weekend call handled their telephone consultations better than house officers or practicing pediatricians (Goodman and Perrin 1978). The authors conclude that nurse practitioners can effectively provide weekend coverage for a pediatric practice and that house officers need better training for this aspect of practice (Perrin and Goodman 1978).

In an evaluation of the practice of a primary care nurse in the Philippines, the patient problems and the rates of resolution are described (Ortin et al. 1978). These data provide a valuable baseline against which to trace developments over time. The advantage of running a single program that can handle screening, treatment, and community follow-up services is also reported (Komrower et al. 1979). The effectiveness of these linkages is largely due to the communication and client contact by the nurses. The results show a large savings in early treatment of phenylketonuria (PKU) over the cost of caring for untreated PKU patients. In another study involving children, a nurse practitioner managed a clinical program of "nontreatment" follow-up on children who had high reported blood lead levels. By an aggressive program of communicating directly with parents on the condition, including providing them with the reports on the blood levels and the environmental and child care steps to take to reduce contact with lead, the nurses were successful in reducing the blood lead levels (Klein and Schlageter 1975).

The studies comparing actual performance of nurse practitioners with physicians on patient care activities and outcomes were carefully analyzed by Prescott in 1980 (Prescott and Driscoll 1980). After summarizing the data from a large number of studies in which she classified differences in process and outcome of patient care, she states that the important features of future studies of the work of nurse practitioners are to

1. use process variables with a known relationship to desired outcomes.
2. use a wide range of structure, and outcome variables that reflect the full range of activities within the nurse practitioner role.
3. use outcome variables with adequate sensitivity to detect differences among providers.
4. compare nurse practitioner's practice against explicit criteria and standards rather than comparing nurse practitioner practice with physician practice of unknown quality.

Recent studies are beginning to be designed to demonstrate the factors called for by Prescott. In an editorial in the *American Journal of Public Health*, Sullivan (1982) cites two studies that report on client care in which nurse practitioners managed some of the patients. In these studies, comparison of neither the care nor outcomes between the nurse and physician is the focus. Instead, groups of clients under different care regimens are compared on objective and "hard" evidence, such as blood pressure, weight, and serum chemistries. Sullivan recommends that future studies include *both* hard and soft measures of client outcomes to validate effectiveness of the care provided. She notes the differences in educational services as one factor in the success of the effective interventions by nurses; furthermore, she suggests that the theories involved in the development of the interventions be identified in the explication and implementation of the interventions.

With the advance in research on nursing practice in primary care, all forms of community health nursing are the immediate beneficiary. Many of the process and outcome variables that have been delineated are applicable across nursing practice. Factors related to continuity of care, communication with clients, patient teaching and health counseling, among others, have been identified as key components of the successes nurse practitioners are achieving. Because of the opportunities for studying this practice, many nurses have gained experience in conducting practice research, and others have become sensitized to the important contributions to practice to be made by nursing research.

Studies of Nursing in Home Health Care

One of the most durable roles of community health nursing is the family-centered care of an ill member at home. Because the family serves as the primary caregiver, yet is often disrupted and inexperienced in this role, the nurse needs to address the issues of the family as a whole and not be limited to providing direct care only to the ill member. Just as in primary care practice, community health nursing is practiced in home health care when the families and problems selected for care are based upon a community assessment approach. Rather than serving the population with the greatest voice in demanding service or those most able to pay, the community-oriented home health care program bases its programs upon assessment of populations at risk, level of health care need unmet by other providers, and interventions shown by outcome studies to be most effective. Research on community health nursing with these characteristics is included here.

Home health care includes programs commonly offering care of the ill at home. Because this level of care involves recuperation from an acute illness, maintenance of health during a chronic illness, or rehabilitation after some permanent change in health, it is viewed here as largely aimed at tertiary prevention — although elements of prevention at other levels are often included in the care. The importance of family and other support systems is greater in this group because of the necessary involvement of others in care of the ill. As a result, the prominent factors studied are likely to include family members, social milieu of the home, and the relationship of the family with the community.

One study was found that focused on assessment criteria by which the likelihood of patient progress could be judged (Mayers 1972). The author used participant observation in accompanying 16 nurses on 37 home visits. She reasons that while nursing care at home is highly individualized, there must be observable commonalities among criteria nurses use in assessing patient status. Unexpectedly, upon examining situational phenomena of the "coping" and "noncoping" families, she found additional criteria that could be used in assessment of patient progress. This type of study serves to isolate the factors thought to be important in a given situation. These factors must then be incorporated into a study that quantifies and/or compares them in different circumstances to verify and test their effects. The factors offered in this study remain to be explored in further research.

Three studies were found describing home care programs for children. The first (Hyman 1974) seeks criteria associated with child battering. Health visitors to families where children had been involved in household accidents were asked to complete a questionnaire that collected data on such factors as age of parents and child, size of family, age of the last child, and types of stress in the family. The factors appearing most prominently among the families suspected of child battering are recommended as assessment criteria for casework selection for health visitors.

Hospital versus home care is reported in the other two studies of children (Shah et al. 1975; Hally et al. 1977). In both studies, outcomes of health care are compared among the children cared for in both kinds of programs; and the advantages of care at home are found to be so significant that hospitalization of nearly every child is brought into question. Perhaps further research should focus on the essential criteria for admission to hospital rather than the safety of care at home. More important for nursing in home health care, reaching satisfactory levels of home care of children must be preceded by research directed toward parent coping strategies, the mutual influence of the social group mores with the prescribed health care regimen, and the effects of the interaction between the provider and family.

Of the three studies found on care of adults using home health care services, all validate the need for, and effectiveness of, public health nursing services. The first queried patients one year after discharge about their met and unmet health care needs (Bergman and Hellman 1969). While only 14 percent stated they had not received the medical care they needed, 47 percent claimed they needed nursing care and had not received it. Four years later, a study in the same setting reported on the effectiveness of public health nursing care to discharged patients in comparison treatment and control groups (Epstein et al. 1973). The investigators reported significant differences in the ability of the clients to follow instructions on diet, medication recommendations, and follow-up appointments to physicians.

The third study on general impact of service on adults involves comparisons of clients referred for rehabilitation services for long-term disabilities (Ford et al. 1971). When a client had the physical or mental capacity to respond to rehabilitative efforts, the services of a public health nurse made the significant difference in patient progress. Furthermore, the study reports that even when the client could not improve, the public health nursing services were essential for coordinating other services for the client and family. Primarily because of the linkages between the process of the nursing care and the outcomes of care, these studies constitute an important advance in the nursing component of home health care research. Perhaps the inclusion of measures of family ability to cope with the client, satisfaction with lifestyle, or other quality-of-life indices would illuminate other outcomes of care that are of value to the client, family, and society at large.

More specific process variables are identified in five studies of particular *diagnostic* groups for whom services were delivered. In an attempt to identify the elements of care provided, or the specific treatment issues to address, the studies in this category focus on care to clients with stroke or fractures, schizophrenia, and colostomy; in addition, two report on care of patients suffering myocardial infarction. Each study contributes a unique perspective on ways to examine a particular element of a home care program. One examines the effects of service organized by nursing teams on patient outcome (Christensen and Lingle 1972). A second evaluates the effects of specific visiting patterns on stabilization of schizophrenia (Davis et al. 1972). Another seeks qualitative responses of patient and family to colostomy care, by which method nursing care was to be designed (Davis and Eardley 1974). A fourth describes subjective versus objective signs reported in follow-up of discharged myocardial infarction patients, while differentiating those who survived from those who died (MacIntyre and Haywood 1975). The last describes the elements included in a follow-up program for patients with myocardial infarction and reported qualitatively the nurses' evaluation of the impact of the program on the health of the clients (Hengstberger 1976). The elements of this program were so clearly delineated that qualitative measures could be used to estimate relative contribution to client outcomes.

One final study was found that focused entirely on describing the impact of parent caring on middle-aged offspring (Archbold 1980). From the findings of this study, variables related to many of the dimensions cited above can be identified and later quantified for further research and analysis. For example, the changes in routines of interaction within families is described, including the impact of these changes on the feelings and attitudes among the members. Each new problem added strain to the remaining caretakers, whether the source was an additional problem of the elderly parent or a new problem of the offspring or grandchildren. After sufficient accumulation of problems, the resulting effect was deterioration of the health of the remaining caregiver. This study marks the first attempt found to isolate specific variables not only of the client and immediate significant others, but also of the extended family in the form of care-giving offspring. For community health nursing research on practice in the home, these factors will provide direction toward identifying the relevant outcome variables to include in future studies. With the isolation and study of variables such as these, the impact of the nursing care provided should be better documented within the larger context of the family as client.

Because of the nature of home health care, the interventions are highly individualized. Nurses are involved for different intensities and lengths of time, depending on the wishes of the family and the severity of illness of the ill individual. Many variations in the problems are presented, given the different family constellations, role structures, patterns of activities, attitudes and beliefs, and resources. Only recently have identifiable problem clusters been defined, let alone interventions designed to deal with them systematically. More descriptive research is needed to clearly conceptualize family problems treated by community health nurses. At present, the ANA Cabinet on Nursing Practice is working on the content validation phase of a study to define classifications of nursing practice phenomena (ANA 1983). Several of these phenomena deal with the family and community level of practice. If classifications are validated, critical elements within the intervention will than have to be specified, followed by testing in controlled intervention studies.

Taken together, the preceding studies represent important documentation of the general effectiveness of public health nursing to the ill at home, and of the specific activities and procedures that constitute this care. Upon this base, further research is crucial to the advancement of practice of home health care nursing, especially as the high cost of this type of service demands pragmatic and observable results. More specific delineation of interventions is needed, including the environmental and family factors so integral a part of this practice. Further, outcome measures are needed that specifically reflect nursing care in such areas as teaching, socialization, and self-help-oriented interventions. Measures of functional status appropriate to specific conditions would be an appropriate measure of physical and mental progress of individuals, and family coping and functional status measures could be used to effectively capture the effects of service on the clients' significant others.

RESEARCH IN FACILITATING PRACTICE

The following sections deal with the research on the associated functions that represent *facilitations* to the practice of community health nursing. Specifically, the administration of practice and the education of clinicians are vital to the provision of services and are themselves subject areas to research. Studies are reported here that were found to illustrate aspects of practice that are of prime interest to an administrator or educator, although selected factors within these studies undoubtedly have a bearing on clinical practice as well.

Following this section are a few studies that report on a particular research method or use of data from the point of view of community health nursing. Basic methods, categorizations, tools, and the like also need to be researched to refine, validate, and establish reliability before they can be trusted for broad usage. Last are included studies dealing with issues and attitudes from an ethical perspective.

Research on Administration of Community Health Nursing Practice

Research on community health nursing administration is actually better referred to as evaluation research, in that the emphais is not upon developing new concepts of administrative practice or theories of administration; instead, this research evaluates the *effectiveness* of what is being done and tries to point the direction toward ways to administer this practice more efficiently, effectively, and with less cost, using current administrative strategies.

In an attempt to define the general topic of evaluation of practice, Bergman (1978) discusses the elements to be included from an agency point of view. She summarizes the evaluation of practice, posed here as administrative research, in this way:

Evaluation consists in establishing a relationship between goals and achievement. It is an expression of accountability by agencies and professions. Evaluation of nursing services must be seen within the context of total health status. Questions related to effectiveness are: reality of goals, population coverage, availability, adequacy, accessibility, timeliness, comprehensiveness, continuity, coordination, satisfaction. Those related to efficiency are duplication of programmes, composition of staff, flexibility, utilization of facilities, cost-effectiveness. Impact of the service on practitioners and the profession is another component in evaluation. Staff morale, continued learning, expanding roles, colleague relationships, enrichment of educational programmes, development of standards and models are elements for examination. Strategies are the evaluation of structure, process and outcome. Time, activity and patient progress studies; nursing audit; cost-accounting; use of reports, opinion studies and consultants are some of the methods developed for evaluation in nursing.

A few studies of general issues are included here on the broader concerns of administration, as opposed to practice-focused investigations. One review of patient classification strategies presents a method of indexing the staffing needs by the classification of patient problems (Regnery 1977). Four "levels of care" are established, tested, and found reliable. The objective of this study is to "provide a more comprehensive mechanism for staffing and resultant fiscal management in effective use of nursing manpower (Regnery 1977).

Another common issue that is usually settled by administrative policy is the wearing apparel agreed on as the appropriate garb for work (Rye et al. 1973). One study reports on this topic from the nurses' and clients' points of view and recommended flexibility in administrative policy.

One argument for home health care that has remained somewhat ambiguous is the comparative cost of service versus the cost of hospital admittance. In a study of the economics of home care, comparison of similar diagnoses manifests basically no difference in cost between treatment in the hospital and at home (Gerson and Hughes 1976).

Several programs of posthospitalization care were studied on the premise that the quality of care would be improved, discharges would be earlier, fewer visits to ambulatory care would be needed, and costs would be reduced. The advantages to the patient and family were projected in less disruption, quicker recovery, and greater individual attention (Schimmenti 1973; Strong, and Sandland 1974; McCarthy 1976; Ruckley et al. 1980). Each of the studies presents data supportive to these points, yet none is designed to test the patient classification scheme with the outcomes in cost, quality, time of discharge and frequency of posthospital visits, and family coping and satisfaction. More comprehensive evaluations are needed if wholly different styles of practice are to be compared definitively. In the meantime, these evaluations provide the descriptions of practice needed to determine whether goals are being reached and to establish cost and staffing patterns.

The overall practice activities of the community health nurse are described in several studies (Clark 1976; Watts 1976; Hughes et al. 1979; Brown 1980; Worrall and Goldstone 1980). When multiple programs compete for time and personnel, the first step toward modifying the use of resources according to priorities is to determine the actual practices in effect. Other purposes for conducting descriptive studies of practice are to (a) document the content of the work, (b) attribute effort to a funding source, (c) justify the need for more staff, (d) clarify the effects of expanding a role definition, (e) establish the average workload in different categories of practice, and (f) determine inequities in workload among nursing groups. Closer examination of these studies is warranted when one or more of these areas are to be considered in a future research project.

Research on Education in Community Health Nursing

Systematic research in this field has been conducted, but not in large quantity. The assessment of learning is commonly done in classroom tests and clinical evaluations, but only in selected situations has the educational process been reported in a research format.

The effectiveness of student education is the subject of two studies. One reports on an evaluation tool developed for the assessment of baccalaureate students in a clinical experience (Shaffer and Pfeiffer 1978). Presumably the tool can be validated and used in the evaluation of the clinical experience. The second study examines the effectiveness of a videotape feedback method of teaching interviewing skills to nurse practitioners (Sullivan et al. 1975).

Two studies were found in the evaluation of graduates of continuing education programs. One reports on the ability of the nurses to identify and work with emotional problems of clients and their families after a training program by mental health workers (Lyall et al. 1972). Another documents the use of the course content of a practitioner program for clients by use of a chart audit (Cox and Baker 1981). Despite the time spent debating the use of mandatory continuing education and money invested in its acquisition, many questions related to short-term education of nurses are left unanswered.

Many other areas of student education could be tested. One, for example, would be the understanding of community health nursing concepts, content, and ability to practice after graduation as compared between graduates of integrated curricula and of programs that separate subjects by clinical areas of practice. Another would be the relative advantages of including a community assessment component in graduate nurse clinician programs as opposed to concentrating on further depth in clinical content. A third might be to study the value of clinical research assistantships for doctoral students in the gradual development of their ability to conceptualize clinically relevant research questions and methods.

Research Methods Applied to Community Health Nursing

Six papers were found that contributed primarily to ways of thinking about community health nursing (categorization) or to the ways of studying this practice. In a two-paper series, an approach to categorizing the kinds of practice engaged in by "community nurse practitioners" is described (Archer and Fleshman 1975; Archer 1976). The second paper in this series recategorizes the typology presented in the first paper. As typologies are demanded by the research question involved, or boundaries necessary to define a specific group are needed, categorization schemes such as this one will prove useful.

The remaining four studies in this section report on participant observation as a methodologic approach especially suited to the study of community health nursing (Kratz 1975; Dingwall 1976; Cunningham 1978; Luker 1978). Included in these papers are (a) the philosophic suitability for participant observation of a "naturalistic" method or a "scientistic" method, (b) complete descriptions of the application of the method in community nursing settings, (c) a method of recording observations, (d) responses of the observed, and (e) a description of the categorization of content in specific samples studied.

While many other methods of research are used in community health nursing, no other papers were found that specifically addressed their application to this field. A review of strengths and weaknesses of other methods is needed, as well as a fuller critique of the applicability of methods and research techniques used. Many tools are developed for use by clinicians or to study the practice of clinicians, but no studies have been found reporting the reliability and validity of these instruments. Nurse researchers who can carry out this work are now being prepared in greater numbers, which may result in more methodological studies being reported in the future.

Research Related to Ethics of Community Health Nursing

Three very different topics are involved in the studies of areas of attitudes and values of community health nurses as these relate to the care given to clients. One of these investigations studied attitudes of nurses toward death and dying (Gow and Williams 1977). The data are examined for differences among nurses employed by agencies with different patient types and varying philosophies. The premise tested was if the attitudes of the nurses did not differ, presumably the care given to the dying person and their family would not differ either, regardless of the agency philosophy.

In another study, the values of nurses and their administrators toward care of patients with stroke are examined (Kratz 1976). In this study, the interface between the education of the nurses, their relative autonomy in community health nursing practice, and the role of the administrator are discussed in relation to the care that the patient "deserved." The amount of care "dispensed" to each client is regarded as a function of these factors, with the expectation that the patient and caregiver would work toward the assumption of self-care as soon as possible.

On a very different issue, a survey of attitudes toward professionalism and collective bargaining examines the shifting value system of public health nurses. The relative compatibility of professionalism, militancy, and unionism is assessed among nurses in relation to their demographic characteristics (Bloom et al. 1979).

CONCLUSION

A baseline of research has been developed in the field of community health nursing — slowly for the first half of the century, and more rapidly since support from the federal government became available for graduate education in nursing. Two major reviews in community health nursing research have been conducted, and together with the additional research reported in this chapter, show a broad range of topics that have been studied in this field. The topics cover practice, administration, education, research methods, and ethics.

That this much research has been done is a tribute to the profession. It was conducted during a time when research training was not the emphasis of nursing education, time for research was minimal compared to that available in other fields, and major grants for research in community health nursing were few and far between. The conviction that this practice warrants serious study has led the list of motivating forces for those who have laid the baseline of research during the past century.

Now it is time to increase the value of the research to the profession by providing more rigorous training for future researchers and by structuring practice to facilitate its study. The first task is developing outcome measures that more nearly reflect the client responses we are seeking, and process measures that include the full range and depth of the activities carried out by the nurses. These must be based on conceptual frameworks consistent with the practice under study. Step by step, models will be built and the elements tested until we have a picture from which we can generalize about the critical factors influencing effective practice, whether directed to aggregates, families and groups, or to individuals.

That community health nursing is on the verge of moving rapidly ahead in the study of its own field is demonstrated by the vitality and creativity shown in the studies already accomplished. Considerations and approaches that will move us ahead toward explanatory, rather than the primarily descriptive, levels have been given in the studies reported in this chapter. The researcher in community health nursing will need to go to the original sources for fuller detail on the thinking and processes developed by these earlier researchers upon whose work we must now build.

The building blocks to be used in designing the studies of the future are discussed in Chapter 7. Through such research approaches we can move well beyond the phase of describing the phenomenon of community health nursing interventions and into the development of tested concepts and constructs that can form the underpinnings of our practice. By melding the practical art of community health nursing with the rigors of scientific inquiry, more predictable care with more reliable outcomes will result.

REFERENCES

Abbott EV. Screening for scoliosis: a worthwhile measure. Can J Public Health 1977; 68:22.

Allen WH, and King VM. A study of health visitor attachment to general practitioners in Hertfordshire. Nurs Times 1968; 64:177.

American Nurses Association. Cabinet on Nursing Practice. Memo from steering committee on classification of phenomena for nursing practice. Kansas City, MO. April 1983.

American Nurses Association. Nurse practitioners: a review of the literature 1965–1979. Kansas City, MO. 1980.

Anderson R, and Newman J. Societal and individual determinants of medical care utilization in the United States. Milbank Mem Fund Quart 1973; 51:95.

Archbold PG. Impact of parent caring on middle-aged offspring. J Gerontol Nurs 1980; 6:78.

Archer SE. Community nurse practitioners: another assessment. Nurs Outlook 1976; 24:499.

Archer SE, and Fleshman RP. Community health nursing: a typology of practice. Nurs Outlook 1975; 23:358.

Asbed RA, Schipper MT, and Varga LE. Preschool roundup: costly rodeo or primary prevention? Health Ed 1977; 8:17.

Barber JH, and Wallis JB. Assessment of the elderly in general practice. J Roy Coll Genl Prac 1976; 26:106.

Benson KD, Wade B, and Benson DR. Results of school screening for scoliosis in the San Juan Unified School District, Sacramento, California. J Sch Health 1977; 47:483.

Bergman R. Evaluation of community health nursing. NZ Nurs 1978; 71:23.

Bergman R, and Hellman G. Community nursing services as perceived by posthospitalized patients. Am J Public Health 1969; 59:2168.

Bessman A. Comparison of medical care in nurse clinician and physician clinics in medical school affiliated hospitals. J Chron Dis 1974; 27:115.

Bey M, Taylor B, Edwards LE, and Hakanson EY. Prenatal care for pregnant adolescents in a public high school. J Sch Health 1979; 49:32.

Bishop B. A guide to assessing parenting capabilities. Am J Nurs 1976; 11:1784.

Bloom JR, O'Reilly CA, and Parlette GN. Changing images of professionalism: the case of public health nurses. Am J Public Health 1979; 69:43.

Breslau N. The role of the nurse-practitioner in a pediatric team: patient definitions. Med Care 1977; 15:1014.

Bridges HM. A survey report on the expanding role of the industrial nurse. Occup Health Nurs 1976; 24:22.

Brophy HE. "Project Pursuit," a health defect follow-up activity. J Sch Health 1970; 40:186.

Brown BI. Realistic workloads for community health nurses. Nurs Outlook 1980; 28:233.

Bryan DS, and Cook TS. Redirection of school nursing services in culturally deprived neighborhoods. Am J Public Health 1967; 57:1164.

Bryant GM, Davies KJ, Richards FM, and Voorhees S. A preliminary study of the use of the Denver Developmental Screening Test in a health department. Develop Med Child Neurol 1973; 15:33.

Caldwell LR. Use of the social readjustment rating scale combined with the P.O.R. in a college health service. Nurs Prac 1977; 3:24.

Callan LB, and McCray A. Case studies on remediable health defects. J Sch Health 1942; 42:528.

Cauffman JG, Warburton EA, and Schultz CS. Health care of school children: effective referral patterns. Am J Public Health 1969a; 59:86.

Cauffman JG, Casady LL, Randall HB, Warburton EA, and Schultz CS. The nurse and health care of school children. Nurs Res 1969b; 18:412.

Christensen K, and Lingle JA, Evaluation of effectiveness of team and non-team public health nurses in health outcomes of patients with strokes or fractures. Am J Public Health 1972; 62:483.

Clark J. The role of the health visitor: a study conducted in Berkshire, England. J Am Nurs 1976; 1:25.

Coejic H, and Smith A. The evolution of a school-based mental health program using a nurse as a mental health consultant. J Sch Health 1979; 49:36.

Cox CL. An interaction model of client health behavior: theoretical prescription for nursing. ANS 1982; 5:41.

Cox CL, and Baker MG. Evaluation: the key to accountability in continuing education. J Cont Ed Nurs 1981; 12:11.

Cunningham R. Participant observation: a research technique in public health nursing. Can J Public Health 1978; 69:101.

Currie G, MacNeill RM, Walker JG, Barnie E, and Mudie EW. Medical and social screening of patients aged 70 to 72 by an urban general practice health team. Br Med J 1974; 2:108.

Davis AE, Dinitz S, and Pasamanick B. The prevention of hospitalization in schizophrenia: five years after an experimental program. Am J Orthopsych 1972; 42:375.

Davis F, and Eardley A. Coping with colostomy. Nurs Times 1974; 70:580.

Dennison D, and Fenimore JA. A heart sound screening program for elementary children. J Sch Health 1971; 9:349.

Dingwall R. The social organization of health visitor training. Nurs Times 1976; 72:37.

Edwards LE, Steinman ME, and Hakanson EY. An experimental comprehensive high school clinic. Am J Public Health 1977; 67:765.

Epstein LM, Avni A, Hopp C, and Flug D. Evaluation of a program of aftercare for patients discharged from the hospital. Med Care 1973; 11:320.

Esler A. Attitude change in an industrial hearing conservation program. Occup Health Nurs 1978; 26:15.

Flight RM, and Schussler T. A post-hire evaluation of nurse-conducted preplacement health assessments. J Occup Med 1976; 18:231.

Flynn BC. The effectiveness of nurse clinicians' service delivery. Am J Public Health 1974; 64:604.

Forbes O. The role and functions of the school nurse as perceived by 115 public school teachers from three selected counties. J Sch Health 1967; 37:101.

Ford A, Katz S, Downs T, and Adams M. Results of long-term home nursing: the influence of disability. J Chron Dis 1971; 24:591.

Forman JAS. Nurse attachments to general practice in south-west England. J Roy Coll Genl Prac 1974; 24:579.

Fricke IB. The Illinois study of school nurse practice. J Sch Health 1967; 37:24.

Gerson L, and Hughes O. A comparative study of the economics of home care. Int J Health Serv 1976; 6:543.

Gilman S, Williamson MC, Nader PR, Dale S, and McKevitt R. Task differentiation among elementary, middle, and high school nurses. J Sch Health 1979; 49:313.

Goodman HC, and Perrin EC. Evening telephone call management by nurse practitioners and physicians. Nurs Res 1978; 27:233.

Gow CM, and Williams JI. Nurses' attitudes toward death and dying: a causal interpretation. Soc Sci Med 1977; 11:191.

Greenhill ED. Perceptions of the school nurses' role. J Sch Health 1979; 49:368.

Haerer AF, Wiygul FM Jr, and Parish G. Out-state charity neurology clinics: appraisal and follow-up of a comprehensive neurology project in a thinly populated area. South Med J 1974; 67:587.

Hally MR, Holohan A, Jackson RH, Reedy BLEC, and Walker JH. Pediatric home nursing scheme in Gateshead. Br Med J 1977; 1:762.

Hanchett E, and Forrens PR. A public health home nursing program for outpatients with heart diseases. Public Health Rep 1967; 82:683.

Heath PJ, and Fitton JM. Survey of over-80 age group in a GP population based on urban health centre. Nurs Times 1975; 71:109.

Hengstberger C. Domiciliary follow-up of the patient with acute myocardial infarction and myocardial ischaemia. Med J Aust 1976; 2:204.

Henzell JM. The expanded role of the school health nurse in paediatric screening. Aust Paediatr 1977; 13:44.

Highriter ME. The status of community health nursing research. Nurs Res 1977; 3:183.

Highriter ME. Public health nursing evaluation, education, and professional issues: 1977–1981. In: Werley HH, Fitzpatrick JJ, eds. Ann Rev Nurs Res, Vol. 2. New York: Springer 1984.

Hilbert H. Abstracts of studies in public health nursing. Nurs Res 1959; 8:42.

Holt SJ. The school nurse's "family assessment tool." Am J Nurs 1979; 79:950.

Howard J, Lawrence J, and Rasile K. A survey of public health nurses' knowledge and attitudes about family planning. Am J Public Health 1972, 62:962.

Hughes J, Stockton P, Roberts JA, and Logan RF. Nurses in the community: a manpower study. J Epidemiol Community Health 1979; 33:262.

Humphrey P. Height/weight disproportion in elementary school children. J Sch Health 1979; 49:25.

Hyman C. Accidents in the home to children under two years. Health Visitor 1974; 47:139.

Kaufert J, and Green S. Assessing functional status among elderly patients. Med Care 1979; 17:807.

Klein MC, and Schlageter M. Non-treatment of screened children with intermediate blood lead levels. Pediatrics 1975; 56:298.

Komrower GM, Sardharwalla IB, Fowler B, and Bridge C. The Manchester regional screening programme: a 10-year exercise in patient and family care. Br Med J 1979; 2:635.

Kornder LD, Nursey JN, Pratt-Johnson JA, and Beattle A. Detection of manifest strabismus in young children. 1. A prospective study; 2. A retrospective study. Am J Ophthalmol 1974; 77:207.

Kratz CR. Participant observation in dyadic and triadic situations. Int J Nurs Stud 1975; 12:169.

Kratz CR. Some determinants of care of patients with stroke who were nursed in their own homes. Am J Nurs 1976; 1:89.

LeSueur C, Geiger F, Held B, Gilibert J, and Prystowsky H. Research in the delivery of female health care: manpower development — expanded roles for nursing and the non-professional in family planning. Am J Obstet Gynecol 1972; 112:785.

Lewis CE, Lorimer A, Lindeman C, Palmer BB, and Lewis MA. An evaluation of the impact of school nurse practitioners. J Sch Health 1974; 44:332.

Lewis CE, Lewis MA, Lorimer A, and Palmer BB. Child-initiated care: the rise of school nursing services by children in an "adult-free" system. Pediatrics 1977; 60:499.

Logan AG, Archber C, Milne BJ, Campbell WP, and Haynes RB. Work-site treatment of hypertension by specially trained nurses. Lancet 1979; 2(8153):1175.

Long GV, Whitman C, Johansson MS, Williams CA, and Tuthill RW. Evaluation of a school health program directed to children with history of high absence. Am J Public Health 1975; 65:388.

Lowis EM. An appraisal of the amount of time spent on functions by Los Angeles city school nurses. J Sch Health 1969; 39:254.

Luker KA. Goal attainment: a possible model for assessing the role of the health visitor. Nurs Times 1978; 74:1257.

Lyall WA, Parry RS, and Wright J. Community psychiatry and the public health nurse: evaluation of a training program. Can Psychiat Assoc 1972; 17:S-39.

MacIntyre LJ, and Haywood LJ. Survival factors following myocardial infarction recorded by a nurse. Heart Lung 1975; 4:233.

Managan D, Wood J, Heinichen C, Hoffman M, Hess G, and Gillings D. Older adults: a community survey of health needs. Nurs Res 1974; 23:426.

Manisoff M, Davis LW, Kaminetzky HA, and Payne P. The family planning nurse practitioner: concepts and results of training. Am J Public Health 1976; 66:62.

Mayers MG. A search for assessment criteria. Nurs Outlook 1972; 20:323.

McAtee PA. Nurse practitioners in our public schools? An assessment of their expanded role as compared with school nurses. Clin Pediatr 1974; 13:360.

McCarthy E. Comprehensive home care for earlier hospital discharge. Nurs Outlook 1976; 24:625.

McGrath P, and Laliberte EB. Level of basic venereal disease knowledge among junior and senior high school nurses in Massachusetts. Nurs Res 1974: 23:31.

McNeil HJ, and Holland SS. A comparative study of public health nurse teaching in groups and in home visits. Am J Public Health 1972; 62:1629.

Mechaber J, McNerney H, and Charney E. Analysis of the triage system in a neighborhood health center. J Nurs Adm 1974; 4:29.

Nader PR, Emmel A, and Charney E. The school health service: a new model. Pediatrics 1972; 49:805.

Ortin EL, Laurente CM, and Limson SG. A demonstration of primary care nursing in a community setting — the Heveriza project. The ANPHI Papers 1978; 13:2.

Patterson J. Effectiveness of follow-up of health referrals for school health services under two different administrative patterns. J Sch Health 1969; 39:686.

Perrin EC, and Goodman HC. Telephone management of acute pediatric illnesses. N Engl J Med 1978; 298:130.

Powell C, and Crombie A. The Kilsyth questionnaire: a method of screening elderly people at home. Age Aging 1974; 3:23.

Prescott PA, and Driscoll L. Evaluating nurse practitioner performance. Nurs Prac 1980; 6:28.

Regnery G. Patient care needs — an index for community health staffing. Nurs Adm Quart 1977; 2:79.

Rice DM. An instrument for the recording of student health complaints. J Sch Health 1978; 48:362.

Robertson LH, McDonnell K, and Scott J. Nursing health assessment of preschool children in Perth county. Can J Public Health 1976; 67:300.

Rosenstock I. The health belief model and preventive health behavior. Health Ed Mono 1974: 2:354.

Ruckley CV, Garraway WM, Cuthbertson C, Fenwick N, and Prescott RJ. The community nurse and day surgery. Nurs Times 1980; 76:255.

Rye F, Van Nalta P, and Paegel B. Attitudes of public health nurses and neighborhood health program participants about nurses' working apparel. Health Serv Rep 1973; 88:968.

Sahin ST. The nurse and the early identification of young children at risk. Int J Nurs Stud 1979; 16:141.

Schimmenti C. Military public health nurse program at David Grant USAF Medical Center. Aerospace Med 1973; 44:84.

Schwenger CW, and Sayers LA. A Canadian survey by public health nurses of the health and living conditions of the aged. Am J Public Health 1971a; 61:1189.

Schwenger CW, and Sayers LA. Services to the aged by the Canadian public health nurse in the official health agency. Am J Public Health 1971b; 61:1846.

Shaffer MK, and Pfeiffer IL. Home visit: a gray zone in evaluation. Am J Nurs 1978; 78:239.

Shah PM, Wagh KK, Kulkurni PV, and Shah B. The impact of hospital and domiciliary nutrition rehabilitation on diet of the child and other young children in the family and in neighborhood. Indian Pediatrics 1975, 12:95.

Smiley OR. Public health nurses and teachers in school health programs: a problem in communication. Int J Nurs Stud 1975; 12:211.

Snyder AA, Minnick K, and Anderson DE. Children from broken homes: visits to the school nurse. J Sch Health 1980; 50:189.

Strong PG, and Sandland ET. Subnormality nursing in the community. Nurs Times 1974; 70:354.

Suchman E. Preventive health behavior: a model for research on community health campaigns. J Health Soc Behav 1967; 8:197.

Sullivan JA. Research on nurse practitioners: process behind the outcome? Am J Public Health 1982; 72:8.

Sullivan JA, Grover PL, Lynaugh JE, and Levy A. Video-mediated self-cognition and the Amidon–Flanders Interaction Analysis Model in the training of nurse practitioners' history taking skills. J Nurs Ed 1975; 14:39.

Sullivan JA, and Armignacco F. Effectiveness of a comprehensive health program for the well elderly by community health nurses. Nurs Res 1979; 28:70.

Sultz HA, Henry OM, and Sullivan JA. Nursing Practice: USA. Lexington, MA: Lexington Books, 1979.

Thordarson L, and Costanzo GA. An evaluation of the effectiveness of an educational program for expectant parents. Can J Public Health 1976; 67:117.

Vernon TM, Conner JS, Shaw BS, Lampe JM, and Doster ME. An evaluation of three techniques for improving immunization levels in elementary schools. Am J Public Health 1976; 66:457.

Wagener JM, and Carter G. Patients' evaluations of gynecologic services provided by nurse practitioners. J Am Coll Health Assn 1978; 27:98.

Watts D. District nurses in East Birmingham health district. Nurs Times 1976; 72:157.

Worrall J, and Goldstone LA. A general study of district nursing in Wigan. Nurs Times 1980; 76:21.

Yankauer A, and Sullivan JA. The new health professionals: three examples. Ann Rev Public Health 1982; 3:249.

Yauger RA. Does family-centered care make a difference? Nurs Outlook 1972; 20:320.

TECHNIQUES TO ADVANCE RESEARCH IN COMMUNITY HEALTH NURSING

7

Thomas R. Zastowny

Public health nursing research has come of age and must take on the scientific rigor expected of a discipline accountable for its own practice. Within the current political and economic trends impacting upon the health care system, all professions must justify the content and process of client care in relation to health outcomes of individuals, families, and communities. The challenge in public health nursing research is to develop further clarity and measurability of a practice with such broad scope and such a variety of interventions. For the first time, nurse researchers in enough numbers to make a difference have been prepared to accept this challenge.

As a scientific area of study, community health nursing has two basic functions: (a) to offer an adequate description of those objects or events that are under investigation and (b) to establish theories by which these objects and events may be explained or predicted. In general, the objects and events of importance to community health nurses are families, communities, individual clients, their environment, their health states, and nursing interventions to maintain or promote the same.

As demonstrated in the preceding chapter, community health nursing has focused largely on descriptive research; it has been slower to move to applied experimental and quasi-experimental designs then have other areas of nursing practice. Conducting applied experimental research in the community is difficult at best. Community health nurses face special problems in the design and execution of research in the field. These problems include difficulties in achieving and maintaining experimental control, interfacing with community agencies and organizations involved in the research, the selection of theoretically and clinically relevant factors for study, and the practical problems of implementation and analysis.

Despite these problems, community health nurse researchers need to move in the direction of applied experimental design and more sophisticated analytic approaches than have been demonstrated to date. Through such progress, community health nursing will be better able to develop and test theories and conceptual models that are grounded in rigorous research efforts, as well as to address specific clinical problems.

This chapter addresses the utilization of applied experimental and quasi-experimental research in the field. It focuses on research models; methodological, measurement, and analysis issues; and computer application to research. Presented along with this discussion is an introduction to approaches that have been used in other research field settings and that seem highly applicable to the issues needing investigation in community health nursing.

PRELIMINARY STEPS

Problem Definition

Often the first step in the research process is a straightforward one: to pinpoint problem definition and description. A clear and concise definition of the issue or question under investigation is essential to the research process. Ill-defined problems will only add expense to the investigation and weaken any set of conclusions based on the findings. The care given to precise definitions, objectives, and larger hypotheses early in the research process will influence its overall success or failure. The problem definition should include ideas that provide a good conceptualization of the issue and an operational and quantifiable outcome for measurement.

Estimating Research Effort

One of the most important, but frequently overlooked aspects of the research process is estimating the amount of effort that will need to go into a project under consideration. The first step is making sure that the project is really achievable. Possible choices here are pilot testing, trial runs of procedures, talking to staff likely to be involved in the project, getting other researchers' opinions, and anticipating pitfalls. Next is the development of a plan for the recruitment and organization of the research team. As the work continues there will be other important considerations. Making and managing a budget is an area in which researchers can benefit from the example of the business world. Research funds are often ill managed and exhausted prior to the actual analysis of data. Careful planning and tightfistedness in the beginning are keys to success. Establishing deadlines in the beginning and adhering to them closely will set the right atmosphere for high staff productivity and help ensure that tasks are completed on time. Staff management calls for early estimation of motivation and commitment early and being ready to replace staff if necessary. Backup resources in the consultant community should be identified if staff attrition becomes a problem or internal organizational roadblocks develop. Finally, the allocation of large blocks of time for writing as the project draws to completion is needed to pull together findings and make overall sense of the project.

Pilot Work

Pilot surveys or studies are useful steps in the research process that are particularly critical for survey design. Since the experimenter or researcher may never actually be involved in firsthand data collection, good piloting is essential: the questionnaires involved, for instance in a mail survey, may be the only source of information. Pilot work is directed at "testing" the proposed measurements of the research project and examining assumptions of the project. It allows for incorporating feedback and errors uncovered in methods and other areas during the trial phase. Conceptualization of these studies is as a trial run of the entire research project, using a limited sample size to reveal methodological, substantive, and practical difficulties that might be encountered in the actual study. The initial distributions on the pilot data should be carefully examined and response rates calculated that gauge the percentage of completed return. Often special characteristics of nonresponders can be uncovered, allowing estimation of the sample bias.

EXPERIMENTATION AND RESEARCH STRATEGY

An Experimental Approach

Often in experimental or quasi-experimental research, the process of specifying effects of interventions or treatments can be viewed as a two-stage sequence. In certain experimental approaches the first step, or the first series of studies, is directed at examining the overall effects of treatments or interventions and asks the simple question "Does the treatment make a substantial difference in outcome?" The answer is hopefully found in the findings of the first set of experiments. Whether statistical differences found have clinical relevance is another issue. Their importance relative to the clinical aspects of the experiment remains a judgment left to the researcher and the larger scientific community.

A second, related issue — addressed by the next series of experiments in the same path of research and often calling for more rigorous experimental designs — is the examination of various intervention components comprising the treatment. This stage addresses questions such as "Given a significant treatment effect, what are the most salient components of the intervention that produces that effect?" Other questions can certainly be posed in the context of experimentation that do not neatly fit into the above described approach, but this conceptualization provides one useful way of categorizing research that facilitates thinking about research projects in a systematic and programmatic style.

Theories, Hypotheses, and Objectives

Returning to the task of problem definition, it is particularly important to consider, first, the theories, hypotheses, and objectives in a given research project. Theory provides the broadest background and highest level of conceptual understanding of the project problems and issues. Hypotheses are usually mid-level specific statements that are testable and contain a researcher's expectations about the outcome of an experiment. They "translate" theory into more specific and observable events. Objectives are discreet goals that need to be achieved for the research project to succeed. All of these elements, and especially their interrelationships, need to be specified during the early phases of work. After a conceptual orientation and research framework have been determined, major methodological choices are examined in more detail as they relate to the problem under study.

Essential Properties of Experimentation

Most "good" research shares a number of essential features that involve conceptualization, experimental design and implementation, analysis, final write-up, and dissemination. A beginning requirement is a clear and concise statement of the objectives and conceptualization. A second series of elements relevant to experimentation include a condition (a) that only the intervention is included in the experimental manipulation (that is, that other variables or factors are not also being systematically varied along with the treatment condition by the experimentors), (b) that both the independent (treatment or intervention condition) variables and dependent (outcome or evaluation criterion) variables are well defined and measured, and (c) that a plan or experimental design chosen, which specifies the allocation of subjects to treatments, is adequate and appropriate to the questions under consideration (Nunnally 1978). A third criterion is that valid and reliable data have been collected during the experiment. Fourth is the appropriateness of the statistics applied to the data. Finally, good research ends with findings specified as to their generalizability and limitations. Guidelines for replication may also be added.

Existing scientific guidelines lay out a fairly demanding and rigorous set of principles to achieve, especially when research is undertaken in community health field settings. For an excellent review of methodologic issues in clinical research that fleshes out many of the above principles, see the special issue of the *Journal of Consulting and Clinical Psychology* (1978). Attention to such standards will help ensure a high-quality product and instill faith in the research findings.

Types of Experimental and Quasi-experimental Designs

Much has already been written to assist the researcher in the choice of experimental designs (Campbell and Stanley 1963; Campbell 1969; Paul 1969; Hersen and Barlow 1976). The following section is limited to a discussion of some general issues to consider when selecting designs and some of the advantages and disadvantages of various approaches.

True experimental designs include randomization of subjects to treatment conditions and assure the researcher of a "fair to high" amount of control over potentially confounding variables. Quasi-experimental designs, in contrast, are marked by use of naturally occurring or unrandomized subject groupings and, generally, give less control over important confounding influences. Other distinctions such as "within," "between," and "single case" subject classifications are useful and are also discussed. Twelve of the more common experimental designs are illustrated in Table 7.1 which is taken from Campbell and Stanley (1963) and Mahoney (1978). In the table, a "0" refers to an assessment and an "X" refers to a treatment.

Subject designs that focus on variation of individuals within a single group are often used to evaluate individual changes where treatments are characterized by large individual subject variation. This design is also used in study areas where reversal of the experimental effects is possible (Wilson 1978). Problems encountered with this approach include comparing the large variability and difficulties in generalizing the findings beyond the present study (Hersen and Barlow 1976).

Between-subject designs are more appropriate for relative efficacy experiments such as those that attempt to isolate salient treatment factors in treatment packages, or for the purposes of comparing different intervention groups. Problems with this approach include an averaging of results because the results are often reported by group means, and minimization of real between-subject differences when variability is largely allocated to error variance. In addition, there may be ethical objections to withholding treatment from subjects or patients who could benefit from treatment (controls). Replication studies are equally difficult using either classification system.

Single-subject designs represent another experimental approach and are particularly effective when all subjects receive all treatment conditions; hence, subjects serve as their own controls. This experimental approach represents an extensive and intensive study of the individual. On the positive side, single-subject methodology provides more control over within-subject variability and research cost and often yields very detailed longitudinal data (Shontz 1976). On the other hand, statistical analysis and generalization are more complicated in these models.

A compelling approach with an emphasis on flexibility is the use of experimental designs in combinations and sequence (Bergin and Strupp 1972). Single-subject designs can be used to isolate important treatment or intervention factors. Replications can then be undertaken in group settings with between-group comparisons. Once treatments have been isolated and refined, a series of small studies can be used for the next stage of evaluation. Finally, more complicated explorations with larger multivariate studies can be initiated, especially including replications with different populations at different sites.

Table 7.1 The 12 Most Common Experimental Designs

Design	Symbol	Description	Comments
		Within subject	
1. Posttest only	X0	A person or group experiences a manipulation (X) (e.g., therapy), and the dependent variable is then measured (0).	Extremely weak and uninformative design; no strong conclusions can be drawn.
2. Pretest–posttest	0X0	The dependent variable is measured (0) before and after the experimental manipulation (X).	Weak design; it may be concluded that there was (or was not) a change in the dependent variable, but one cannot determine whether this change would have occurred anyway (without the experimental manipulation).
3. Reversal	0X0X0	Two separate manipulations of the independent variable are each preceded and followed by measurement of the dependent variable.	More adequate design in that it can replicate the observed effect of an experimental manipulation; conclusions are limited to the subject or group in question, however, and this design does not rule out the possible influence of factors other than the independent variable; reversal may pose practical and ethical problems in some situations.

4.	Equivalent time samples	0X0X0X0X0X	An extension of the reversal design in which an independent variable is sequentially presented and removed (or otherwise manipulated) with alternating measurements of the dependent variable.	Moderately adequate design in the sense of multiple replication and possible control of some time-related factors; limitations include the possibility that the effects of a manipulation may change due to its repeated presentation and withdrawal.
5.	Multiple baseline	0X000 00X00 000X0	The timing of an experimental manipulation is systematically varied across different behaviors or situations.	Moderately adequate design in that it includes replication and partial control of time-related factors; limitations vary with the specific procedures.
6.	Time series	000X000	The stability of a dependent variable is measured; deviations from that stability after an experimental manipulation are used to infer causal relationship.	Somewhat controversial in terms of adequacy; limitations include failure to rule out factors that changed simultaneously with the experimental manipulation and failure to replicate.
7.	Changing criterion	$0X_1 0X_2 0X_3$	Similar in some respects to equivalent time samples design, except that the value of the independent variable is systematically altered; if changes in the dependent variable reliably covary with these manipulations, a causal relationship is inferred.	Moderately adequate design that shares many of the strengths and weaknesses of the equivalent time samples design; in addition, this may be problematic with some patterns of criterion change.

From Mahoney M. Experimental methods and outcome evaluation. In: Special issues: methodology in clinical research. Journal of Consulting and Clinical Psychology 1978; 46(4):666–667.

Certainly not all community health nurse researchers will want to take all the projects they work on to the most comprehensive and rigorous level of evaluation and analysis. Keeping in mind the study purpose, the available resources, the power of the sample size, and the experimental approach will allow the researcher to choose the best evaluation perspective for any experiment.

Research Models

Research can be undertaken for a variety of reasons: unexplained experiences in everyday life, organizational problems needing solutions, unanswered questions or unresolved issues from previous research, to name a few. The original stimulus for the research and how it is supported (a National Institutes of Health (NIH) grant or a local funding source) and the characteristics of the research and service teams (e.g., all R.N. Ph.D.s, a mix of M.D.s, Ph.D.s, R.N.s, and M.S.W.s) will also shape the research process. For an interesting sample of how the mix in health teams affects process and outcome, see a thoughtful study by Feiger and Schmitt (1979). For example, applied research undertaken in response to real world crises usually seeks to define and solve pragmatic problems (e.g., does travel distance to health care providers serve as a barrier to health care for the economically disadvantaged?). Basic research, often supported by government grants, addresses theoretically interesting and more elemental questions the practical and clinical relevance of which varies (e.g., what are the disease processes underlying cancer development?).

There are also conceptual differences of many kinds. The first, as implied above, is the nature of the problem (basic research versus applied). The second is the approach to methodology (see Table 7.1). The third is related to the experimental environment and focuses on the differences between laboratory and field settings. An important point to note is that any combination of the described dimensions can exist. While no "ideal types" exist in the world of community health nursing research, analysis of a study according to these dimensions can give the researcher valuable information for its planning, execution, and analysis.

Another critical aspect of the research process is the formation of the research team. Any researcher about to undertake an investigation is faced with a decision between working independently or in some sort of collaborative research arrangement. Continued experience in research endeavors permits the conceptualization of certain types of research organizations, such as those shown in Figure 7.1. Model 1 is a hierarchic structure, Model 2 is collaborative, Model 3 is a hybrid conceptualization, and Model 4 indicates a researcher working independently. To facilitate our discussion, let X = principal investigator; Y = associate investigator; and Z = support staff.

As one reviews the various models, several similarities and differences emerge. First, for all the models except the hybrid, the power lines are largely

Model 1

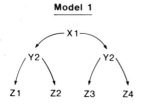

Model 2

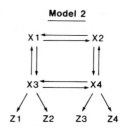

Model 3

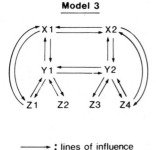

Model 4

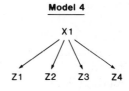

——→ : lines of influence

⇉ : reciprocal influence

Figure 7.1.   Research models

hierarchical; that is, decisions start at the top and are handed down. This process consolidates power in the hands of the principal investigators. All models use some support staff. Even an independent investigator will be likely to rely on technical and other manpower supports to accomplish a research project, especially in field studies.

The differences in the models are perhaps more striking and serve to assist the researcher in matching research team organization with the stated research goals. In Model 3, for example, organization goals and strategies can be influenced even by support staff. Model 2 also benefits from reciprocal influence and decision making, but only among upper staff levels. Such organizational staff might be appropriate to use where creativity and multidimensional/multilevel perspectives are required. Models 1 and 4 are more task oriented and efficient designs, once plans and research decisions are established.

More complicated time- and stage-dependent organizational structures can be conceptualized whereby a research team might adopt Model 3 in the early phases of a project and move to a structure more like Model 1 or 4 during the later phases of the project. Important to note is that the organizational structure and research team characteristics can impact greatly on the conceptualization, implementation, and analysis phases of the research. Investigators who can succeed in matching research team structure to the tasks at hand will administer projects more efficiently and productively.

IMPLEMENTATION

With regard to field study, the conceptualization and determination of the research methodology is only part of the process. What remains is the implementation of the research project. Implementation on a simple level means getting the job accomplished, setting up the measurement system, collecting the data, engaging in field work, and anything else that becomes necessary to complete the project.

A first step that must be accomplished prior to the research actually beginning is gaining access to the specified data source or sample, and at the same time earning acceptance in the organization where the work will take place. At this point or before, the researcher will need to present the research plan and methodology to the organization in order to gain its approval. Entry negotiations are often a crucial and necessary aspect of applied research. The relationship established early on can lead to productive contacts or set up the research project for failure.

A second, related aspect of organization and community negotiations helpful when conducting naturalistic (field) studies focuses on individual and organizational goals. Any organization will have its own sets of goals, objectives, and ongoing projects. One useful strategy is for the researcher to become aware of those goals and search for methods to include them, perhaps in indirect ways, in the course of the research project. One sure way to disaster is to attempt to implement a research project with specific objectives that are in opposition to the goals of the organization with whom the work is being initiated. Detailed analysis of organizational goals and structure, of time demands of the anticipated research project on existing staff, of potential benefits of the research to the organization, and of the political impact of the project will be worthwhile and prevent unneeded delays and other logistical problems.

Data: General Considerations

Measurement

Two basic issues are central to all research projects: reliability and validity. Reliability refers to the extent to which the same measure or recording yields the same or nearly the same results on multiple applications. In other words, the measurement has to maintain consistency with a minimum of random error. Validity, in contrast, refers to the extent to which a measure actually captures what it intends to measure. This concept can be formulated as a question: "Is this the right measure, theoretically, for the task at hand?"

Clearly, both properties are essential for sound research. By and large, if researchers use existing instrumentation already developed, reliability and validity problems should be already worked out, with estimates of the properties usually available in the literature; at that point, only a minimum of attention and effort is needed to adapt these measures to the present research. When testing new measures, generally much more effort is required to establish reliability and validity. A wise policy in research is to complement newly developed tools with other more established measures with known reliability and validity. The new and old measures can then be used in tandem on the sample, thus providing some preliminary data on the psychometric properties of the new measures. A fuller discussion of these procedures can be found elsewhere (Nunnally 1978; Rao 1967).

Selection

One of the first steps in the implementation phase, one that helps assure a high-quality and purposeful investigation, is the care and effort attached to the collection and preparation of data. Data form the heart of the research project; and choosing what data to collect is probably the first decision encountered in implementation. The answer to this question is, of course, largely a function of the nature and essence of the research question. Other more practical considerations, such as time and money resources, availability and ease of data collection, reliability and validity issues, will also impact on this choice.

A general rule is to collect enough data and in detailed enough form to answer adequately the research questions under consideration. Another rule is to collect data in the most detailed form that is possible given the structure of the project. Despite these general rules, proper data collection is not easy. Too much data, especially with regard to the number of variables, can yield an unwieldy amount of information (data matrix) that is uneconomical and wasteful. As variables are added (and sample size remains constant), precious power to detect relative differences drops, and the probability of finding spurious relationships increases. Too large a sample size squanders resources with few gains; one rapidly approaches a point of diminishing return. On the other hand, too few variables measured, or too few subjects assessed, may leave the researcher without having captured an important covariate or factor essential for an acceptance or rejection of the null hypotheses.

Helpful considerations for determining sample size and number of variables to be measured are

1. Examine the past and present literature to arrive at "expected" numerical values of the relationships under study. This converts, in part, to the question of whether the researcher is looking for large effects, midrange effects, or relatively small effects (Cohen 1962).
2. Be aware of power calculations and estimated sampling procedures that ensure a minimal ability to detect expected effects (Cohen 1962, 1968).

3. Consider the proposed analysis and determine, by anticipation or by computer simulation, the variable/sample size/power ratios. Also consider the number of statistical tests to be performed in relation to the total number possible (Cohen 1962; Hummel and Sligo 1971; Harris 1975), and the appropriateness of the statistical models.

Quality Control

From time to time, in any research project, it is wise to conduct periodic reliability checks on the data collection. Without continued fine tuning initial acceptable reliability may diminish over time. Included in this recommendation are not only strict mathematical interpretations of reliability but also regular general assessments of research procedures over time. Researchers should spend time with the people observing the phenomena under study and speak with adjunct data sources to check for consistency — even with keypunchers or other support personnel in an effort to obtain the most comprehensive view of the entire project as possible. If data collection goes awry, as it is apt to do at times, ongoing monitoring is one of the best safeguards for a quick resolution of problems and restoration of a quality product.

Available Data

The way in which an investigator obtains the data needed to examine a research question ranges from the collection of new data (primary analysis) to the analysis of already existing data files (secondary analysis). Combinations of the two approaches are also possible and increasing in use. Some advantages of primary collections are (a) reliability and validity can be better estimated; (b) data most relevant to the research question can be collected, (c) measurements of choice can be used, (d) sample size can be directly determined, and (e) data processing costs are usually lower. Advantages of secondary analysis include (a) cost resource savings of direct data collection, (b) additional interesting variables available in established data files, (c) large sample sizes, (d) longitudinal data, which are often available, and (e) time savings for data coding and preliminary review of variables' distributions. Issues for resolving the choice of data question include time and resources at hand, the quality of the secondary files available for analysis, and the sample size and measurement precision required to examine the research hypotheses. One of the more difficult challenges for secondary analysis is the tailoring of appropriate designs to fit existing data files. For primary analysis, the difficulties lie in conducting tight, well-formulated studies that hold good promise for replication.

Coding

Before and/or after data are collected, data coding strategies must be explored. The investigator may have used a questionnaire, an observational schema, or a form to record information from existing records; but in each case, use of a computer mandates arranging information for counting. Data coding is an important but often overlooked part of the research process. If by not capturing the variables of interest, poor coding results in their loss; this compromises analysis, which can only be as good as the data input. The following discussion suggests some ways to organize data into a form that will permit computer analysis.

In some investigations, the factors to be studied are identified clearly and built into the data collection process in such a way that they can be tabulated with other factors easily. For example, if an investigator wants to note whether a teacher-nurse conference was held, a space is included on the data collection form for checking "yes" or "no" to this variable. Suppose later in the study it is of interest to know whether more student problems were discovered through teacher-nurse conferences, through physical examinations, or through a combination of the two. Each of the two occurrences would have to be coded so that the computer could be programmed to calculate how many children had physicals only, how many had been the subject of a teacher-nurse conference only, how many had both, and how many had neither.

When coding information, the investigator needs to consider the general purpose of codes and kinds of codes that can be used. Below is a listing of several single-coding schemes. Other schemes are available and often research will generate new codes and coding schemes as the set of research instruments becomes finalized.

1. *Simple codes*: Simple codes are any instance of attaching numbers to qualified states. For example, *race* where 1 = white, 2 = black, 3 = Hispanic.

2. *Geometric codes*: These are very useful where combinations of items can occur. For example, let 0 = no treatment, 1 = group health education program, 2 = home visit; then by definition 3 = health education program and home visit. A two-field (00) digit scheme could also be used; for instance, a 12 could indicate health education and home visit.

3. *Dummy codes*: These are simple codes, usually binary (0, 1), in which the presence (yes = 1) or absence (no = 0) of something (drug treatment, married) is coded, although other numeric notation can be used.

4. *Combination codes*: These codes lump together two or more variables such as race and sex: 1 = white male, 2 = white female, 3 = black male, 4 = black female; this can be a valuable space saver. Should the researcher want to examine the independent effects of either factor (in this case, race or sex) in a detailed analysis, however, new variables that represent the factor of interest (race or sex alone) would need to be computed.

Combination codes may be very useful when outcomes are to be coded. For example, a student may have had a problem identified in the teacher-nurse conference that the nurse investigated and resolved. Other problems may have taken longer to investigate or follow through on and are not resolved. Also, some problems may have been discovered through physical assessment methods with the same two outcome possibilities: resolution and no resolution. Combination codes can supply the researcher with multiple choices for coding information on where a problem was discovered and whether it has been resolved.

Use of Computers

Introduction to Computers
Before data management and statistical analysis are discussed, a brief introduction to computers is in order. Increasingly, the computer has become one of the major tools of quantitative, and sometimes qualitative research. Use of the computer gives the researcher access to many specific languages and exact mathematical processing functions. Besides simple functions (addition, subtraction), sets of commands organized in a logical sequence called programs (or "software") can be written to accomplish a great many tasks in increasingly shorter periods of time.

Most of the time computer programmers, formally trained in special languages or generally in computer science, do most of the programming. However, more and more scientists and practitioners are using prepackaged programs to gain independent access to systems (e.g., Statistical Package for Social Sciences [SPSS]) (Nie et al. 1975). Considerable efforts have been invested in devising computer languages that are close to spoken and written language systems. Usually these higher-level languages get "converted" by computers to more powerful, but more complicated, symbol systems (machine languages) that can be utilized by the computer.

Communication with computer systems can be accomplished in a variety of ways. Input/output devices include cards, tape, keyboards, light sensitive pens, printers, plotters, and cathode ray terminals. Feedback from the system often takes the form of printed output of specified programs.

General advantages of computer use include its speed, built-in access to prewritten algorithms, and dependability. Specific functions that also greatly facilitate research are the computer's data handling and number manipulation abilities. Data handling tasks may on one hand involve a great deal of reading and writing with a minimum of calculations. Matching newly reported tuberculosis cases to a local health department's general cumulative tuberculosis registry to check for history of previous contacts is an example of a simple, but otherwise time-consuming, data processing task. On the other hand, solving a series of simultaneous equations for the development of a causal model to predict depression among the elderly requires a repeated and complicated set of calculations. These characteristics serve to determine the type of job and, often, the associated cost of the computer time used.

Storage Devices
Cards are usually the first storage method the researcher will encounter, unless the research is being conducted on prepared data sources. Cards are usually sufficient for initial input of data, but for continued access, other forms of

storage are more efficient. Cards are largely out of date at present and most data storage goes directly to disk. Many existing data files, for example, exist on magnetic disk or tape.

Disk storage provides a way of storing relatively small amounts of data in a form that can be conveniently and rapidly retrieved. Disk storage advantages include ease of availability and access, and overall flexibility with regard to changing organization, format, and data elements of the file. Disadvantages include cost, particularly as the data file increases in size.

Magnetic tape, probably the most universal technique of computer storage, is also the most economical in terms of cost per character of information stored. Data on magnetic tape are recorded in chunks called blocks. The size of the blocks may vary and the amount of tape a block uses is proportional to its length. Tapes can be read or written on any number of times and give the researcher great flexibility with regard to storage. Often a minimal charge is associated with the mounting of the tape before it can be accessed. Tape storage is an attractive alternative when the data are seldom accessed and the data matrix is large and hence expensive to retain on disk.

Probably the most efficient use of these storage methods comes with mixing methods as the situation demands while considering both the short- and long-term benefits of each method.

Preparations for Analysis (the Data Matrix)
Data that have been carefully coded, keypunched, and varified are put into a form that is organized and relatively fixed. Usually this form is a symmetrical matrix, with variables making up the columns of the matrix and with the rows corresponding to subjects.

Complete data matrices, where all subjects have valid responses on all variables, are the easiest to work with. With incomplete matrices, the researcher must watch for missing data in the column (variables) or rows (subjects) and take appropriate action. Once the data are in this form, analysis can be initiated. Copies of the data matrix should be printed at various stages of the project. Errors can then be tracked down and corrected and the researcher can get a clear visual record of the organization of the data.

In summary, a number of coding, data management strategies, and common-sense notions useful when working with computers are worth reviewing:

1. Every subject should have a unique ID number or identifier.
2. Keep as many codes as possible in numeric (number) form, rather than alphanumeric (letters with numbers) or alpha (letters).
3. If processing multiple records per case, it is good practice to include a record or code of the position of the individual record in that specific sequence (sequence in the entire data file can also be added).
4. Always have at least two copies of the data matrix on hand (one for ongoing use, another for backup in case of computer or human-generated error that results in data loss).

5. Always label codes clearly (you might remember while the project is being analyzed which group got which treatment, but as time passes these details are likely to fade from memory).
6. Try to complete analyses well ahead of deadlines, as computers malfunction from time to time, and their "down" time is often quite unpredictable.

Choice of Computer Packages (Languages)

With the mushrooming of the micro- and mini-computer technology together with the standard mainframe computer capabilities, there is an extraordinarily wide variety of hardware, accompanied by prepackaged computer analysis languages and prewritten software packages, available today. The researcher is in an ideal position to evaluate the analysis needs of his or her project and to choose a language or package accordingly. Information that will assist the researcher in choice of computer language and packages is outlined below in a question format.

- What is the level of support for the language or package under consideration? Higher support is usually considered better. That means that there are more staff programmers who are facile in the language for programming assistance; more effort is directed at keeping the language "bug free"; and updates to the language, in terms of new subroutines and functions, are more promptly accomplished.
- Will the analysis demand more "batch" (usually card input) or interactive processing? Use of micro- and mini-computers and/or batch processing by the mainframe is convenient when the data matrix is small and relatively complete. Interactive processing is better when more flexibility is required. Recent technology has permitted the development of software programs that allow several of the mini- and micro-computers to interact with the mainframe. Advances have allowed efficient combinations of batch and interactive processing. In addition, the interactive languages and the smaller computers also permit remote job entry. These possibilities should be investigated before the data are coded and ready for processing.
- What is the projected data management and analysis sequence? Several languages and packages can be used at various stages of the project. This issue is given further elaboration in the section that follows.

Management Sequences and Hierarchies

Within any research project, a certain natural processing sequence takes place with regard to the preparation of data for analysis. The sequence is usually a minor variation of what follows: (a) data collection, keypunching, and verification, (b) data organization, cleaning, and checking, (c) further validity checks and preliminary analysis, (d) hypothesis testing, (e) exploratory data analysis, and (f) permanent revision and storage. Associated with each phase are computer languages or software that are more or less appropriate to use, depending on the tasks required during any one particular phase. Computer languages, like other processes, operate most efficiently within a certain range of functions. This range is largely governed by their design and purpose. Using languages for tasks for which they are not designed creates nonoptimal programming and built-in extra overhead. While many of the languages have capabilities outside their delineated functions, considerable savings can be realized by mixing languages according to management needs. Some down time will undoubtedly be spent switching from language to language, or system to system, as the project demands. However, the added power gained for analysis and the cost saving realized are well worth the trade-offs. Many packages are now able to read and write files from different packages. This feature should further significantly cut conversion time.

ANALYSIS

This section is not meant to be a comprehensive guide to the assumptions and use of the various statistical approaches available today. Other sources can satisfy that need. Rather, it is a presentation of first-step considerations for analysis and a sampling of useful analytic strategies abstracted from several health services' research projects.

Hypotheses Revisited

As soon as strategies for analysis are being decided upon, a researcher will inevitably be led back to the experimental design and the hypothesis under consideration. Analytic strategies should flow naturally from the set of research objectives and the design organization of the project. Therefore, the care and effort given in the early phases of the project to the delineation of ideas for testing is crucial and will be well worthwhile at this phase. If the hypotheses are not in order by this time or if objectives are unclear or not specific enough, reformulation, re-evaluation, and perhaps redefinition and clarification of these issues must take place and be resolved before further progress can be made. Again, reformulation at this phase may be too late; early and concise definition of hypotheses for study and testing is strongly advised.

Preliminary Analysis Issues

It is crucial to consider data analysis issues early in the experiment. How the data are to be analyzed depends on the research objectives and hypothesis under consideration. A practical first step involves getting a "hands-on" idea of the distribution of the data. Close examination of each variable in the study may test preliminary hypotheses and yield valuable information on which to base later choices of more advanced analysis techniques. Analysis of basic distribution involves obtaining a number of basic descriptive statistics, such as the mean, mode, median, standard deviation, range, kurtosis, cumulative distribution, percentiles, and the like. Graphic plots can also be helpful. Without this crucial first step of getting a "feel" for the data, potential errors in scoring can be left uncorrected. The researcher would also fail to acquire a clear understanding of each variable's variation and distributional characteristics. As a result, the finer and more subtle interpretations that accompany more advanced techniques are apt to also be misunderstood or bypassed altogether.

Bivariate and Multivariate Approaches

As advances are made in statistics and quantitative methods, especially with regard to multivariate methods, there is an ever-widening set of analytical procedures available to the researcher (Cooley and Lohnes 1971; Finn 1974; Bock 1975; Cohen and Cohen 1975; Harris 1975). This variety presents enormous and sometimes overwhelming possibilities for analysis. At the same time the danger increases of using many of the procedures that have evolved inappropriately. Another ever-present pitfall, of concern especially if a researcher is quantitatively minded, is of statistical overkill (using too many and too high-powered techniques to answer relatively simple sets of questions).

Once a researcher is satisfied with his or her knowledge regarding the underlying distributions of the data, straightforward relationships between variables, often described by bivariate statistics, can be considered. These may be correlations, contingency tables, means broken down by subcategories of subjects, scatter plots, or other techniques. These analyses may answer the central questions of the study or may reveal factors and potential interactive effects that need to be included in later analysis. Many research questions can be addressed with these analyses.

If the design is more complicated or the effects of testing involve several factors, multivariate techniques may be considered (Jones 1966; Harris 1975; Timm 1975; Olson 1978). Only a few years ago, true multivariate procedures were fairly rare in this line of research. Today, however, they are increasingly being applied to diverse community health research efforts. As the term implies, multivariate procedures examine the interrelations among more than two factors at the same time as well as their effects. These procedures allow for multiple dependent variables, multiple independent variables, or a combination of both. With these procedures, the researcher can address more complicated sets of questions than would be possible with bivariate approaches. Using multiple regression techniques to evaluate the differences in perception of the school nurse's role in Greenhill's study (1979), for example, helped to establish the relative variance among the perceptions within the various professional groups and between each group and the nurses.

Besides augmenting the comprehensiveness of the questions under study, multivariate analysis has the capability of partially removing the effects of covariates or controlling factors before the central study hypotheses are addressed. Another frequent use of these procedures is statistically equalizing study groups on key antecedent measures that were left unmatched by the experimental design.

An additional important feature of multivariate procedures is that they often have built-in safeguards against reporting spurious results. Some overall significance testing is usually provided or can be calculated on the basis of the number of hypotheses tested or number of dependent variables examined. For recommendations on choosing a test statistic in multivariate analysis of variance and as an introduction to this literature, see the article by C.L. Olson (1978).

Additional Research Strategies

Some of the most common workhorses of health service research include techniques such as factor analysis, cluster analysis, multidimentional scaling, discriminant analysis, analysis of variance and covariance, regressional and correlational analysis, path analysis, and stochastic/probability analysis. These techniques, some of their common applications, specific health services research applications, and their common assumptions and additional reference sources are presented in Table 7.2.

Consideration of earlier sections of this chapter will certainly assist the researcher in making some decisions about analytic approaches. Once having worked through these issues, however, more detail is needed to continue into the analytic phase. One approach found helpful in the past is organizing the set of research questions under consideration into a hierarchy. The purpose of this kind of hierarchy is twofold. First, it organizes the research analytical effort into a sequential set of tasks; second, it separates major from minor research questions. While these judgments should have already been made, the sequential organization, at this stage, reinforces and parallels the design and statistical reasoning determined from the earlier phases of the project. Another advantage is that the analysis tasks that are delineated under the hierarchy can be subdivided and shared among research support staff, including those perhaps not cognizant of the entire analytic thrust of the project.

A hierarchy often used in health services research distinguishes between sociodemographic factors and other variables of interest as to effects on important health considerations. Because the sociodemographic factors are usually unchangeable and represent, in some sense, what a patient brings to a situation, their effects are often examined first in isolation on the dependent variables. Certainly they can, and often are, the subject of major theoretical interest themselves.

Table 7.2. Common Techniques Used in Health Services Research

Technique	Common Applications and Issues	Sources	Comments
1. Factor analysis	Multivariate normal distribution; Linear relationship; Data reduction; Exploration of underlying structure; Hypothesis testing	Cattell 1952; Comrey 1973, 1978; Gorsuch 1974; Harman 1967; Horst 1965; Kruskal and Shepard 1972; Mulaik 1972	This procedure is primarily used in a descriptive manner. Several rotational and extraction methods are available. Usually several analyses, using different parameters, (rotation, number of factors) yield the widest perspective to view the data.
2. Cluster & typological analysis	Identifying natural clusters or groupings of objects; Developing conceptual schemes for classification; Search for data structure. Random sampling, reliability and validity, and level of measurement may be issues depending on the specific kind of analysis undertaken. Item to dimension ratio should be appropriate; Many models available for representation of individual differences,	Anderberg 1973; Bailey and Tryon 1960; Everitt 1974; Hartigan 1975; Ball and Hall 1967; Bonner 1964; Fisher 1958; Fleiss and Rubin 1969; Gower 1967; Johnson and Wall 1969; Johnson 1967; Shepard, Romney and Nerlowe 1972. Wolfe 1970; Cattell 1949; Overall 1964; Goldstein and Linden 1969	A statistical routine useful for typing and development of taxonomic groupings. Often described as a procedure that identifies "natural groups."

3.	Multidimensional scaling	Some models are more or less restrictive according to number of missing values, level of measurement, continuous and discrete distributions, and asymmetric tendencies; Goodness of fit ("stress" values); Random versus fixed start positions; metric and nonmetric options.	Green and Carmone (1970); Kruskal 1964; Shepard 1972	One of the most sensitive multivariate scaling pathology currently available. The field of psychometrics to deal with problems of measurement.
4.	Discriminant analysis	Multivariate normal distribution; (sometimes critical) population covariances in groups be equal; Examines significant differences among two or more groups of individuals; Attempts to simplify these differences into a smaller number of factors; predicts individual classification using derived factors.	Bock 1975; Cooley and Lohnes 1971; Cacoullos 1973; Dixon 1973; Edwards 1968; Harris 1975; Lachenbruch 1975; Kirk 1969; Overall and Klett 1972; Rao 1967; Timm 1975; Van de Geer 1971.	Discriminant analysis is a system of multivariate statistical techniques that examine and explain group differences, and provide a predictive classification scheme. Significant tests are robust against minor violations.

Table 7.2.   (Continued)

Technique	Common Applications and Issues	Sources	Comments
5. Analysis of variance and covariance	Normally distributed error variance; Homogeneity of error variance; Independent error components; Addition of components. Estimates differences between the means of populations; Variations include use of covariates, adjustments for nonorthogonal designs, and specification of "independent effects" ordering.	Anderson 1958; Bartlett 1947; Bishop, Fienberg, and Holland 1975; Bock 1975; Cochran and Cox 1957; Finn 1974; Hotelling 1936; Jones 1966; Rao 1952; Wilkinson 1975; Woodward and Overall 1975.	Much of the research in the health services area employs the ANOVA models, or alternatively, regression procedures, described below. Covariance problems are somewhat more complicated. In such analysis the relationship between the covariate and both the independent and dependent variable should be studied before the procedures are used.
6. Multiple regression and correlation	Fixed linear regression model; Residuals from the mean of the predicted value for each independent value are normally distributed (heteroscedastic effects); Identify and clarify the relationships among one dependent or criterion variable and predictor variables. Correlations,	Darlington 1968; Draper and Smith 1966; Kerlinger and Pedhazur 1973; Cohen and Cohen 1975.	Although computation considerations once required researchers to use linear models, computer developments have made access to nonlinear models easier. It is important that the choice of model (linear or nonlinear) be a function of how well the model captures the intrinsic

			qualities of the phenomena under study and the theoretical meaning of the dependent function.
	besides estimating the degree of relationship between independent factors, estimate impact of the predictors on the criterion in several ways (zero-order, squared product moment, squared semi-partial, and squared partial correlation).		Path analysis yields an excellent "picture" of the relationships among variables, especially the indirect and direct pathways of effects. More difficult to find are procedures to estimate the overall fit of the model to the data. The two available statistics (R^2 and multiple R values) and degree of fit between actual and predicted correlations should be used in tandem. Other more systematic procedures are being developed and already in use (see Lisrel).
7. Path analysis	Variables can be temporally ordered and measured on an interval scale; Relationships are primarily linear and additive; Correct specification of the model is possible; Asymmetrical relationships exist. Used for testing and developing theoretical models. Li (1975) described path analysis as a plausible interpretation of the relationships among variables that are compatible with the observed data.	Blalock 1964; Cohen 1968; Duncan 1966, 1975; Heise 1968; Land 1969; Li 1975; Wright 1921, 1934, 1960; Goodman 1973.	

An example of this approach can be seen in the analysis in Table 7.3. In a satisfaction study, Roghmann et al. (1979) examined the relationship between satisfaction with medical care and health care utilization among a low-income population. The analysis is useful to review here, since it illustrates an example of the hierarchical approach using a set of sociodemographics as covariates or controlling factors. In this analysis, hierarchical regressions (where the order of entrance of variables into the equation is predetermined by the researcher) were used to predict utilization on the basis of demographic and satisfaction variables, and in parallel fashion, to predict satisfaction from the demographic and utilization variables. These analyses, it was reasoned, would yield important information on the relative efficacy in predicting utilization from satisfaction, and satisfaction from utilization. Both analyses controlled for sociodemographics.

The findings suggested that utilization could be predicted within a reasonable range; however, satisfaction was generally more difficult to predict (see Roghmann et al. 1979; and Zastowny et al. 1983 for a more elaborate theoretical discussion of these findings).

Though well formulated, the analysis undertaken in this study is not the only appropriate one. Another analytic strategy here would be to reverse the order of entry of predictor variables into the equations and examine the differences in explained variance and regression coefficients. In this case, for predicting utilization, satisfaction could be entered first, followed by the sociodemographic block. These solutions would then be compared and contrasted to the earlier analysis.

A similar analysis in another health services evaluation study can be studied in Table 7.4. Making good use of a longitudinal perspective, Chamberlin et al (1980) examine a variety of factors impacting on mothers' use of positive contact on child's developmental status at a specifically designated point in time. A combination of hierarchical and simultaneous regressions were performed, taking into account the time ordering of the measures. From these analyses, a preliminary causal model was developed that illustrates the paths of influence of important factors impacting on the child's level of general development at 18 months of age. Sometimes, given a case where the assumptions of a more formal model can be satisfied and additional hypotheses can be tested, as in this example, one series of analyses can naturally set the stage and lead to the next. This study used a variety of statistical techniques that form a coherent and logical sequence.

Community Health Techniques

Since a number of techniques have been mentioned here that have not yet been directly addressed, a few brief comments about each approach may be useful. These procedures include survey designs, health diaries, mixed ex-

Table 7.3. Regression Analysis: Prediction of Utilization and Satisfaction Controlling for Socioeconomic Variables

| | Utilization | | Satisfaction | | | |
| | | | General | | Specific | |
	Clinics	Doctors	Positive	Negative	Positive	Negative
Proportion of variance explained						
Step 1: Black	0.086	0.072	0.004	0.011	0.000	0.001
Education	0.040	0.080	0.048	0.000	0.003	0.001
Family size	0.028	0.094	0.008	0.000	0.003	0.020
Age	0.009	0.005	0.000	0.000	0.000	0.002
Poor health	0.001	0.023	0.000	0.001	0.013	0.005
Step 2: Clinic visits	—	—	0.003	0.000	0.009	0.001
Satisfaction	0.016	0.007	—	—	—	—
Total R^2	0.179	0.274	0.062	0.012	0.030	0.030
Standardized regression coefficients						
Black	+0.219*	−0.242*	+0.000	−0.105*	−0.004	+0.032
Education	−0.201*	+0.129*	−0.203*	+0.005	−0.066	−0.002
Family size	+0.184*	+0.106*	+0.080	+0.005	+0.072	+0.142*
Age	−0.098	+0.081	−0.000	+0.008	+0.012	+0.042
Poor health	−0.006	−0.157*	−0.006	+0.032	+0.112*	+0.066
Clinic visits	—	—	+0.056	−0.001	−0.106*	−0.034
General positive	+0.108*	−0.017	—	—	—	—
General negative	0.000	−0.069	—	—	—	—
Specific positive	−0.118*	−0.034	—	—	—	—
Specific negative	−0.027	+0.061	—	—	—	—

* Coefficients above +.10 or below −.10 are significant at $p \leq .01$.

Reprinted by permission from Roghmann K, et al. Satisfaction with medical care. Medical Care 1979; 17(5):474.

Table 7.4. Summary of Regression Equation for Variables Predicting Mother's Use of Positive Contact at Time 1 (N = 494)

Independent Variables	Simple r	Multiple R	R square	RSQ change	Standardized beta weights	F value
Variables in operation at birth of child (Time 0)						
Mother years of education	0.17	0.17	0.03	0.03	0.02	0.20
Mother's knowledge of development (Time 0)	0.17	0.20	0.04	0.01	0.09	3.04*
Mother's religious orientation (Catholic, Other)	−0.10	0.21	0.04	0.01	−0.05	1.34
Father's job classification	−0.16	0.22	0.05	0.00	−0.06	1.34
Mother took child birth classes	−0.04	0.23	0.05	0.00	−0.05	1.63
Child sex (female)	0.06	0.23	0.05	0.00	0.05	1.44
Mother's prior experience with children	0.01	0.24	0.06	0.00	0.03	0.40
Physician teaching input (Time 0)						
Average teaching score per practice (Time 0)	0.13	0.26	0.06	0.01	0.07	2.55*
Mother and child characteristics (Time 1)						
Mother's perception of child's overall functioning	0.19	0.31	0.10	0.03	0.16	13.96*
Child's behavior: friendly–outgoing	0.20	0.34	0.12	0.02	0.14	10.34*
Mother's perception of being helped by MD or nurse	0.13	0.36	0.13	0.01	0.13	8.83*
Child's behavior: aggressive–resistant	0.11	0.37	0.14	0.01	−0.09	4.82*
Mother's gain in knowledge over 1 year	0.11	0.38	0.14	0.01	0.08	3.10*

* $p < .01$; overall F value for complete equation: $F = 6.20$, $df = (13.480)$; $p < .01$

Reprinted by permission from Chamberlin RW, et al. An evaluation of efforts to educate mothers about child development in pediatric office practices. American Journal of Public Health 1979; 69(9):883.

perimental designs, meta-analysis procedures, and multitrait, multimethod paradigms.

Survey Designs

The development of reliable and valid survey instruments is a separate area of research in a wide variety of health-related disciplines. Crucial concepts with regard to survey use include initial piloting of the survey, sampling strategies, response analysis, and final references made with survey data.

Health Diaries

A health diary is a prospective procedure used in order to obtain patients' reports of morbidity (illness and injury), disability, and health actions. In recent years, there has been a return to health diaries in order to get a fuller picture of health and illness. Advantages of this methodology have been described in a useful review article by Verbrugge (1980) and include reduction of recall error, yield of individual level data for analysis of dynamics and time sequences, and excellent data quality.

Additional Methodological Advances

Several additional methodological advances are worth reviewing. These include use of mixed experimental designs, e.g., single-subject embedded in between-group, the use of meta-analysis procedures, and increasing use of procedures such as the multitrait, multimethod (MTMM) paradigms for methodological and treatment research (including evaluation procedures for MTMM matrices).

The use of mixed experimental designs in applied research is increasing. Generally, this strategy offers several advantages: (a) it allows the researcher to get closer to the data and permits a more complete picture of the relationships to emerge, especially in cases such as clinical trials or treatment interventions; (b) it allows for a replication effect to emerge in the same study; for example, in the case of single subject embedded in a between-group comparison, the single-subject effect could replicate or not replicate the group effect; and (c) it allows the individual variability to be taken into full account in the final comparisons.

Meta-analysis procedures combine the results of independent studies for the purpose of integrating findings. They allow researchers to better understand and interpret the research that has already been conducted. The analyses are geared toward removing subjective error from conclusions, e.g., given all the studies on preoperative surgery preparations, are experimental subjects better than controls in postsurgical adjustment? More simply, is there a treatment effect? Analyses are also helpful in estimating the magnitude of the treatment effect. Some researchers argue that the confusion and contradictions in research may not be a function of the results uncovered but more a matter of how the results are synthesized. For those interested, see Cooper (1979) for a suggested, generally applicable meta-analysis evaluation package. See also Devine and Cook's meta-analysis of the effects of psychoeducational interventions on the length of hospital stay (1983). For another method to integrate descriptive and experimental field studies, see the work of Bijou, Peterson, and Aylt (1968).

Originally, multitrait, multimethod paradigms were primarily used, albeit rarely, in the test and measurement areas. From this beginning, later work has made use of similar procedures to assess treatment and intervention efficacy. Depending on what variables fill the rows and columns of the MTMM matrix, a variety of questions can be tested that would otherwise have escaped the researcher's grasp. Known evaluation procedures are difficult. A detailed review and critique of such analyses is available in *Multivariate Behavioral Research* (1977)*12*: 447–478.

COMMON PROBLEMS

Research is plagued by a set of common problems and errors. Knowledge of these pitfalls can be painlessly distilled, so that others may profit without having to pay a high price in terms of ill-spent time or resources. Below is a partial list of such problems, clustered by type. The references give sources where the problematic topics and potential solutions are further elaborated.

A.   Theoretical

1.   Lack of clarity in research objectives (off to a shaky beginning)
2.   Null hypotheses unspecified (crucial, especially with regard to the statistical test employed)
3.   Choice of wrong variables to study or variables taken from weak theoretical frameworks
4.   Lack of connection between the study planned and the prior work reported in the literature

B.   Methodological

1.   Sample size too small, especially for replication studies (Tuersky and Kahnemen 1971)
2.   Nonrepresentation design
3.   Multivariate approach not often taken (very important where covariates are included in the design)
4.   Lack of appropriate control groups (complicated considerations included here, such as experimental set, control for contact with experimenters, etc.)
5.   Lack of follow-up data (especially crucial where intervention effects may take a long time to be realized)
6.   Lack of proper pre-post interval for repeated measure designs
7.   Inappropriate statistics employed (the backbone of the results)

8. Inappropriate experimental design for the set of research questions (sometimes complicated designs needed for complicated questions)
9. Lack of adequate reliability and validity of measurement

C. Practical

1. Consultation services sought too late (problems detected too late may be irremediable)
2. Underestimates for analysis and computer time (frustration of being one or two computer analyses away from completion and running out of funds)
3. Nonoptimal computer languages used for data-handling tasks
4. Working with "unclean" or unchecked data (because of lack of attention to details in the beginning). Examining the early distributions also useful.

REFERENCES

Anderberg MR. Cluster analysis for application. New York: Academic Press, 1973.

Anderson TW. An introduction to multivariate analysis. New York: Wiley, 1958.

Bailey D, and Tryon BC. BC-TRY program. Portland, OR: Tryon-Bailey Associates, 1960.

Ball GH, and Hall DJ. A clustering technique for summarizing multivariate data. Behav Sci 1967; 12:153–155.

Bartlett MS. Multivariate analysis. J Roy Stat Soc 1947; 9:176–197.

Bergin AE, and Strupp HH. New directions in psychotherapy research. J Abnorm Psychol 1972; 76:13.

Bijou SW, Peterson RF, and Ault MH. A method to integrate descriptive and experimental field studies at the level of data and empirical concepts. J Appl Behav Anal 1968; 1:175.

Bishop YM, Fienberg SE, and Holland PW. Discrete multivariate analysis: theory and practice. Cambridge, MA.: MIT Press, 1975.

Blalock HM. Causal inferences in nonexperimental research. Chapel Hill: University of North Carolina Press, 1964.

Bock RD. Multivariate Stat Methods Behav Res Dev 1964; 8:22–33.

Bock RD. Multivariate statistical methods in behavioral research. New York: McGraw-Hill, 1975.

Bonner RE. On some clustering techniques. IBM J Res Dev 1964; 8:22–33.

Cacoullos T, ed. Discriminant analysis and its applications. New York: Academic Press, 1973.

Campbell DT. Reforms as experiments. Am Psychol 1969; 24:409.

Campbell DT, and Stanley JC. Experimental and quasi-experimental designs for research. Chicago: Rand-McNally, 1963.

Cattell RB. r_p and other coefficients of similarity. Psychometrika 1949; 279–298.

Cattell RB. Factor analysis. New York: Harper, 1952.

Chamberlin RW, Szumowski EK, and Zastowny TR. An evaluation of efforts to educate mothers about child development in pediatric office practices. Am J Public Health 1979; 69:875.

Cochran WG, and Cox GM. Experimental designs. 2nd ed. New York: Wiley, 1957.

Cohen J. The statistical power of abnormal social psychology: a review. J Abnorm Soc Psychol 1962; 65:145.

Cohen J. Multiple regression as a general data-analytic system. Psychol Bull 1968; 70:426.

Cohen J, and Cohen P. Applied multiple regression/correlation analysis for the behavioral sciences. New York: Wiley, 1975.

Comrey AL. A first course in factor analysis. New York: Academic, 1973.

Comrey AL. Common methodological problems in factor analytic studies. J Consult Clin Psychol 1978; 46:648–659.

Cooley WW, and Lohnes PR. Multivariate data analysis. New York: Wiley, 1971.

Cooper HM. Statistically combining independent studies: a meta analysis of sex differences in conformity research. J Person Soc Psychol 1979; 37:131.

Darlington RB. Multiple regression in psychological research and practice. Psychol Bull 1968; 69:161–182.

Devine EC, and Cook TD. A meta-analytic analysis of psychoeducational interventions on length of post-surgical hospital stay. Nurs Res 1983; 32:267–274.

Dixon WJ, ed. Biomedical computer programs (BMD). Berkeley, University of California Press, 1973.

Draper NR, and Smith H. Applied regression analysis. New York: Wiley, 1966.

Duncan OD. Path analysis: sociological examples. Am J Soc 1966; 72:1–16.

Duncan OD. Introduction to structural equation models. New York: Academic Press, 1975.

Edwards AL. Experimental design in psychological research. 3rd ed. New York: Holt, Rinehart, and Winston, 1968.

Everitt B. Cluster analysis. London: Heinemann Educational Books, 1974.

Feiger SM, and Schmitt MH. Collegiality in interdisciplinary health teams: its measurement and its effects. Soc Sci Med 1979; 13A:217.

Finn JD. Multivariance: univariate and multivariate analysis of variance, covariance and regression. Chicago: National Educational Resources, 1974.

Fisher WD. On grouping for maximum homogeneity. Am Stat Assn 1958; 53:789–798.

Fleiss JL, and Rubin J. On the methods and theory of clustering. Multivariate Behav Res 1969; 4:235–250.

Goldstein SG, and Linden JD. A comparison of multivariate grouping techniques commonly used with profile data. Multivariate Behav Res 1969; 4:104–114.

Goodman LA. The analysis of multidimensional contingency tables when some variables are posterior to others: a modified path analysis approach. Biometrika 1978; 60:179–192.

Gorsuch RL. Factor analysis. Philadelphia: Saunders, 1974.

Gower JC. A comparison of some methods of cluster analysis. Biometrics 1967; 23:623–637.

Green PE, and Carmone FJ. Applied multidimensional scaling and related techniques in marketing analysis. Boston: Allyn and Bacon, 1970.

Greenhill ED. Perceptions of the school nurses' role. J Sch Health 1979; 49:368.

Harman HH. Modern factor analysis. Chicago: University of Chicago Press, 1967.

Harris RJ. A primer of multivariate statistics. New York: Academic Press, 1975.

Hartigan JA. Clustering algorithms. New York: Wiley, 1975.

Heise DR. Problems in path analysis and causal inference. In: Borgatta EF, ed. Sociological methodology. San Francisco: Jossey-Bass, 1969.

Hersen M, and Barlow DH. Single case experimental designs. New York: Pergamon Press, 1976.

Horst P. Factor analysis of data matrices. New York: Holt, 1965.

Hotelling H. Relations between two sets of variates. Biometrika 1936; 28:321–377.

Hummel TJ, and Sligo JR. Empirical comparison of univariate and multivariate analysis of variance procedures. Psychol Bull 1971; 76:49.

Johnson RL, and Wall DD. Cluster analysis of sematic differential data. Ed Psychol Measurement 1969; 29:796–780.

Johnson SC. Hierarchical clustering schemes. Psychometrika 1967; 32:241–254.

Jones LV. Analysis of variance in its multivariate developments. In: Cattell RB, ed. Handbook of multivariate experimental psychology. Chicago: Rand-McNally, 1966.

Kerlinger FN, and Pedhazer EJ. Multiple regression in behavioral research. New York: Holt, Rinehart, and Winston, 1973.

Kirk RE. Experimental design: procedures for the behavioral sciences. Belmont, CA: Brooks/Cole, 1969.

Kruskal JB. Multidimensional scaling by optimizing goodness of fit to a non-metric hypothesis. Psychometrika 1964; 19:1–10.

Lachenbruch PA. Discriminant analysis. New York: Hafner, 1975.

Land KC. Principles of path analysis. In: Borgatta EF, ed. Sociological methodology. San Francisco: Jossey-Bass, 1969.

Li CC. Path analysis—a primer. Pacific Grove, CA.: Boxwood Press, 1975.

Mahoney MJ. Experimental methods and outcome evaluation. J Consult Clin Psychol 1978; 46:660.

Mulaik SA. The foundations of factor analysis. New York: McGraw-Hill, 1972.

Nie NH, Hull CH, Jenkins JG, Steinbrenner K, and Bent D. SPSS: Statistical Package for the Social Sciences. 2nd ed. New York: McGraw-Hill, 1975.

Nunnally JC. An overview of psychological measurement. In: Wolman B, ed. Clinical diagnosis of mental disorders: a handbook. New York: Plenum Press, 1978.

Olson CL. On choosing a test statistic in multivariate analysis of variance. Psychol Bull 1978; 83:579.

Overall JE. Note on multivariate methods for profile analysis. Psychol Bull 1964; 61:195–198.

Overall JE, and Klett CJ. Applied multivariate analysis. New York: McGraw-Hill, 1972.

Paul GL. Behavior modification research: design and tactics. In: Franks CM, ed. Behavior therapy: appraisal and status. New York: McGraw-Hill, 1969.

Rao CR. Advanced statistical methods in biometric research. New York: Wiley, 1967.

Roghmann KJ, Hengst A, and Zastowny TR. Satisfaction with medical care: its measurement and relation to utilization. Med Care 1979; 17:461.

Shepard RN. Introduction. In: Shepard RN et al., eds. Multidimensional scaling, Vol. I. New York: Seminar Press, 1972.

Shepard RN, Romney AK, and Nerlove SB. Multidimensional scaling. Vol. I, Theory. New York: Seminar Press, 1972.

Shontz FC. Single-organism designs. In: Bentler PM, Lettieri DJ, Austin GA, eds. Data analysis strategies and designs for substance abuse research (Research Issue 13). MD: National Institute on Drug Abuse, 1976.

Timm NH. Multivariate analysis with applications in education and psychology. Belmont, CA: Brooks/Cole, 1975.

Tversky A, and Kahneman D. Belief in the law of small numbers. Psychol Bull 1971; 76:105.

Van de Geer JP. Introduction to multivariate analysis for the social sciences. San Francisco: Freeman, 1971.

Verbrugge L. Health diaries. Med Care 1980; 18:73.

Wilkinson L. Response variable hypothesis in the multivariate analysis of variance. Psychol Bull 1975; 82:408–412.

Wilson GT. Methodological considerations in treatment outcome research on obesity. J Consult Clin Psychol 1978; 46:687.

Woodward JA, and Overall JE. Multivariate analysis of variance by multiple regression methods. Psychol Bull 1975; 82:21–32.

Wright S. Correlation and causation. J Agric Res 1921; 20:557–585.

Wright S. The method of path coefficients. Ann Math Stat 1934; 5:161–215.

Wright S. The treatment of reciprocal interaction, with and without lag, in path analysis. Biometrics 1960; 16:423–445.

Zastowny TR, Roghmann KJ, and Hengst A. Satisfaction with medical care: replications and theoretical reevaluation. Med Care 1983; 21:294.

PROGRAM EVALUATION IN COMMUNITY HEALTH NURSING

8

Christy Z. Dachelet

The community health nursing process applied to the community, family, or individual as client involves six components: (a) an identification or diagnosis of health and social needs, (b) goal setting based on the needs identified, (c) a consideration of alternative interventions or programs to alleviate or diminish the identified need; (d) a decision as to which intervention or program is the most desirable based on assorted considerations such as feasibility, political expediencies, and resources, (e) the planning, design, and implementation of the intervention, and (f) a judgment as to the "value" of the intervention finally instituted. Performance of each of these role components in and of itself requires special skills and know-how. The professional community health nurse must blend talents and skills gleaned from formal education and practical experience to meet the challenge of these multiple dimensions.

This chapter focuses on the later component of the community health nursing process — namely, evaluation. While it is equal in importance to the other components of the nursing process, it is too often given less than adequate attention. The first reason for such treatment is that providers' priorities tend, quite naturally, to favor direct service to clients. Evaluation is, however wrongly, often viewed as of only tangential relevance to the clients' or communities' needs. Second, the community health nurse often feels inadequate to the challenge of evaluation. The special skills required for performance in this component of the nursing role often are not acquired in the course of the community health nurse's basic preparation. Yet a third reason is the threat perceived to be associated with evaluation: it conjures up visions of exposed inadequacies and ineffectiveness. Finally, while lip service is consistently paid to the importance of thorough, rigorous evaluation, in reality there is precious little time or funds allocated to this function.

Listing these factors is not meant to imply that evaluation does not in fact occur; it does. Evaluation is natural; it is second nature for responsible community health nurses to question the effectiveness, efficiency, and appropriateness of their efforts, as well as clients' satisfaction with their service. Each community health nurse daily makes impromptu judgments about the relative worth or value of services performed. What too often is lacking, however, is a systematic, organized scientific approach to substantiating and documenting the value realized from the program or intervention implemented.

The time has come when intuitive or seat-of-the-pants evaluations are no longer sufficient. Competing demands for limited resources throughout the health care system require each professional to substantiate his or her claim for support. Choices will be made among competing programs, or competing services. Through the conduct of evaluations, information will be available to ensure that the best choices are made.

Definition of Program Evaluation

Attkisson et al. (1978) provides a comprehensive working definition of program evaluation. It is a process

1. of making reasonable judgments about program effort, effectiveness, efficiency, and adequacy.
2. based on systematic data collection and analysis.
3. designed for use in program management, external accountability, and future planning.
4. focused especially on accessibility, acceptability, awareness, availability, comprehensiveness, continuity, integration, and cost of services.

These criteria characterize program evaluation and introduce many of the terms and concepts to be discussed in this chapter. This working definition is still incomplete, however; it needs to be augmented with the following companion definition emphasizing the difficulties in evaluation.

Once again, evaluation is

1. a value-laden, subjective, frequently misunderstood process.
2. based too often on inadequate, imprecise data gathered with instruments of questionable reliability or validity.
3. designed for use in justifying the status quo or appeasing a grant requirement or stipulation.
4. conducted in an emotionally charged environment of political expediency and unspoken threat.

Together these definitions set the stage for this chapter.

Purpose and Scope of the Chapter

The purpose of this chapter is threefold:

1. To establish program evaluation within the context and responsibility of the community health nurse role.

2. To introduce the community health nurse to the evaluation literature and to the generally recognized frameworks for considering evaluation as described in this literature.
3. To offer a practical guide to the community health nurse undertaking a program evaluation.

Evaluation is a growing, challenging field — a field whose relevance and importance increases as more critical eyes are focused on a costly, imperfect health care system. Evaluation will become an increasingly important dimension of the community health nursing role and an imperative responsibility of the professional community health nurse. This chapter is intended to introduce the community health nurse to the terminology, concepts, and basic tenets of the field of evaluation. It will provide the context for further study in this field, and it will offer a practical guide to the community health nurse undertaking an evaluation.

Activities Subject to Evaluation

Evaluation is a broad term with an indefinite scope and focus. In the field of health care services there are essentially three types of activities that might be evaluated: (a) agency management and operations, (b) provider performance, and (c) specific programs or interventions.

Agency Management and Operations

Overall agency management and operations is one type of activity that might be evaluated. Such an evaluation is broad in scope and focus, involving an overall assessment of the viability, fiscal stability, and structural soundness of an agency. An evaluation of an agency requires examination of such diverse elements as the mechanisms for goal and policy setting; the relevance of broad goals to the community served; the composition and representativeness of the governing body; the responsiveness of the management to the community, governing body, and staff; the benefits and responsibilities derived from interagency affiliation; the consistency of the staffing pattern to the organization's goals; the sources of income and the soundness of the allocation of these resources; the constraints put on endowments; the condition of physical properties; the adequacy of information systems; and the consistency between organization goals and program objectives. An agency evaluation is most often undertaken by a committee or a board of directors, an outside consultant, or sometimes by an agency director or administrator. By attempting to judge the overall well-being of the organization, attention is focused on how successfully the governing, management, and service components combine to result in a smooth-running, effective, efficient body. While an agency may accomplish its service goals through several program components, an agency evaluation usually forgoes in-depth evaluation of specific problems. Rather, the agency evaluation attempts to assess how the several programs *combine* to accomplish the goals of the organization as a whole.

Provider Performance
A second type of activity that is often subject to evaluation in the health services field is provider performance. Evaluation of provider performance is frequently referred to as quality assurance or quality of care evaluation. Essentially, quality assurance evaluation involves peer review or a comparison of the calibre of professional services provided to specific standards or criteria agreed upon by clinical peers as indicative of the optimal or most appropriate treatment for a given illness or behavioral condition. The objective of this type of evaluation is to identify possible errors in provider judgments and to correct deficiencies uncovered, all to ensure that the client receives the highest standard of care possible. Methods used in quality assurance evaluation include record audits, length of stay reviews, drug use profiles, utilization reviews, and level of care reviews. Donabedian's classical model (1966) for evaluating quality of care offers a framework for understanding this type of evaluation activity.

Specific Programs or Interventions
A third type of activity subject to evaluation is a specific program or intervention. It is this type of evaluation that receives the most emphasis in the remainder of this chapter. A program has three components: goals or objectives, activities or functions, and resources. The definition of a program offered by Deniston and Rosenstock (1970) reflects these components: "An organized response to eliminate or reduce one or more problems where the response includes one or more objectives, performance of one or more activities, and expenditures of resources." Program evaluations can have simple or multiple foci, covering one or more of the following aspects: effectiveness, efficiency, adequacy, accessibility, acceptability, and/or availability.

There is obvious overlap among these three types of evaluations. A total agency evaluation would be somewhat sterile if not even a limited amount of attention were given to assessment of the quality of services provided by the agency or to accomplishment of the goals of specific programs conducted by the agency. Similarly, quality assurance evaluation would be incomplete without attention to whether the type of services being provided was in fact relevant to the defined need. And program evaluation would be less than complete if some consideration were not given to the organizational context within which the program operated or to the quality of the specific services provided via the program.

Woy et al. (1978) provides a thoughtful examination of the interrelationship between quality assurance and program evaluation. A comparison and contrast of these two evaluative activities is made along the dimensions of legislative sanctions, degree of reliance on peer and administrative review, level of analysis, basic objectives, and principal methods. While the authors conclude that the distinctions between these two evaluation activities are becoming less sharp and more complementary as evaluation efforts intensify, the differences that they outline provide a succinct comparison, useful to those conducting evaluations.

Program or intervention evaluation is worthy of emphasis here because of its particular applicability and relevance to the community health nurse in practice. The community health nurse in clinical practice is frequently faced with assessing the "value" or "goodness" or "worth" of an intervention or program instituted on behalf of a client. Many of the terms, concepts, and methodologies introduced in the discussion of program evaluation are equally applicable to agency or quality assurance evaluation. While the examples and specific methodologic approaches discussed in this chapter are for program or intervention evaluation, the parallel to the other activities subject to evaluation will often be apparent.

EVALUATION WITHIN THE CONTEXT AND RESPONSIBILITY OF THE COMMUNITY HEALTH NURSE ROLE

It is perhaps unnecessary to belabor the point that program evaluation falls within the responsibility of the community health nurse role. For reasons already cited, program evaluation is today more a necessity than a frill. As health care dollars become more scarce and consumer expectations become more abundant, those programs and providers shown to be effective and efficient will have an advantage in the competition for limited resources.

For the community health nurse, program evaluation must be acknowledged as a personal and professional responsibility. Keeler (1972) stressed this requirement of the role, concluding:

. . . We need to accept responsibility for program evaluation not just in response to the requirements of others but also because full maturity of our kinds of services and our future role in the health care system depend on our assumption of this responsibility. We must undertake to evaluate the program in terms of what the effort is producing.

Successes and failures of specific interventions, approaches, programs, and techniques must be convincingly determined. Only in this way will the community health nurse be able to document where, how, and under what conditions specific interventions or programs make a difference.

Program evaluation has been associated with another acknowledged responsibility of the professional nursing role — practice research. The typology for nursing research presented by Abdellah and Levine (1979) is reproduced in Figure 8.1. This typology places program evaluation within the category of explanatory research. Program evaluation aims to discover why a phenomenon occurred. In its most successful application a program evaluation establishes a causal relationship between program effort and client outcome.

I. Research Aims
   A. Methodological Research
      1. To develop research methodology
      2. To develop tools for nursing administration or education
      3. To develop theories and models
   B. Descriptive Research
      1. To discover new facts
      2. To gather exploratory data as a prelude for further research
   C. Explanatory Research
      1. To discover causal relationships
      2. To make predictions
      3. To evaluate a program, method, procedure, product, system, individual or group behavior
II. Research Design
   A. Experimental design
   B. Partially experimental design
   C. Nonexperimental design
III. Research Content
   A. Nursing practice
   B. Nursing education
   C. Nursing administration

Figure 8.1.   A typology of research in nursing. (From Abdellah FG and Levine E. Better patient care through nursing research, 2nd ed. London: MacMillan, 1979; p. 467.)

Examples of evaluation studies relevant to community health nursing can be found in the nursing literature. Highriter (1977) reviews the community health nursing research literature for the years 1972 to 1976. Her categorization of 115 studies according to their main purpose is a useful measuring stick by which to place evaluation studies within the context of the body of community health nursing research. She identifies six categories of studies, which are listed in order of decreasing frequency of occurrence (see Fig. 8.2). Service evaluation studies provide the largest group of studies (44 in number, or nearly 40 percent); and they are grouped into three subcategories: evaluation of total service programs, including screening programs; evaluation of performance of specific techniques and nursing activities; and evaluation of performance in a role.

Program evaluation and research are both within the context and responsibility of the community health nurse role. A consideration of the relationship between these two endeavors deserves a short digression. The recurrent question is: Is evaluation research? Not unexpectedly, contrasting positions on this issue are frequently based on definitional distinctions. Suchman (1967) offers the most thoughtful and comprehensive discussion of the relationship between evaluation and research. Of particular usefulness is the distinction he makes between evaluation and evaluation research:

1. Service evaluation studies
   a. evaluation of total service programs
   b. evaluation of performance of specific techniques and nursing activities
   c. evaluation of performance in a role
2. Client need assessment studies
3. Service description studies
4. Community health nursing education studies
5. Attitude studies
6. Study reviews and methodology studies

Figure 8.2. Categories of studies reported in the community health nursing research literature) (Reprinted by permission from Highriter ME. The status of community health nursing research. Nursing Research 1977; 26:183–192. Copyright, 1977. The American Journal of Nursing Company.)

. . . we will make a distinction between "evaluation" and "evaluative research." The former will be used in a general way as referring to the social process of making judgments of worth. This process is basic to almost all forms of social behavior, whether that of a single individual or a complex organization. While it implies some logical or rational basis for making such judgments, it does not require any systematic procedures for marshaling and presenting objective evidence to support the judgment. Thus, we retain the term "evaluation" in its more common usage as referring to the general process of assessment or appraisal of value.

"Evaluative research", on the other hand, will be restricted to the utilization of scientific research methods and techniques for the purpose of making an evaluation. In this sense, "evaluative research" becomes an adjective specifying a type of research. The major emphasis is upon the noun "research", and evaluative research refers to those procedures for collecting and analyzing data which increase the possibility for "proving" rather than "asserting" the tremendous social significance of the latter, but only to propose the application of empirical research techniques, insofar as they have been developed in the social sciences today, to the process of evaluation.

Suchman develops the position that evaluation becomes evaluative research when there is adherence to the canons of proof and laws of inference central to the logic of the scientific method. The more closely an evaluation effort strives to achieve validation, explanation, and prediction — elements central to the scientific method — the more nearly it approaches research. Evaluative research itself "is a specific form of applied research whose primary goal is not the discovery of knowledge, but rather a testing of the application of knowledge." Suchman maintains that the scientific method is as applicable to applied research as it is to basic research.

Overton and Stinson (1977) addressed the issue of the relationship between evaluation and research. They too, maintain that the major factor that differentiates evaluation research from other research is the objective or purpose of the study, not the design or execution of the study.

Both research and evaluation are legitimate, indeed mandatory, elements of the role of the community health nurse. Their relationship is often comple-

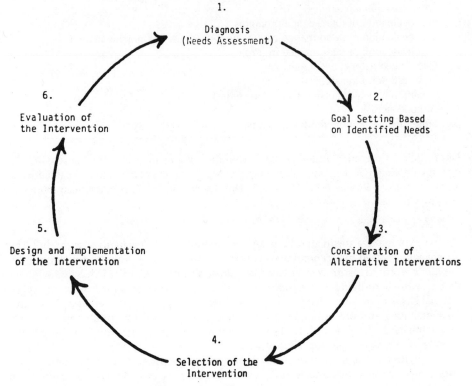

Figure 8.3.   The nursing process

mentary; often they are even identical aspects of that role. Evaluation studies offer the community health nurse both challenges and rewards. Evaluation challenges the community health nurse to apply a variety of competencies acquired from the field of epidemiology, administration, research methods, and political science. The community health nurse who meets the challenge of evaluative research is rewarded with an answer to the critical question: Does this program make a difference?

EVALUATION WITHIN THE CONTEXT OF THE NURSING PROCESS

The components of the nursing process as identified in the opening paragraph of this chapter are most accurately depicted as cyclical phenomena. (See Fig. 8.3) While this figure depicts evaluation as a discreet step or element in the nursing process, in fact it assumes and requires the occurrence of every other component identified in the cycle. That is, evaluation does not occur in a vacuum. It presupposes that a need was identified; that a goal was set, the accomplishment of which would alleviate or lessen the need; that alternative

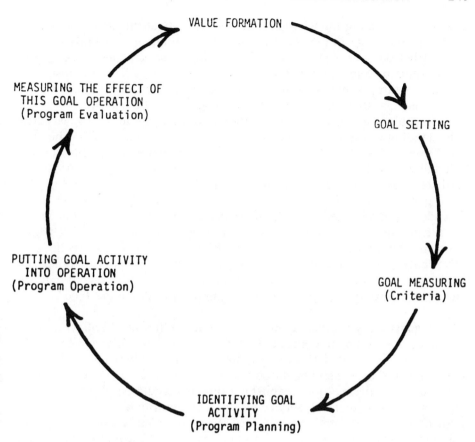

Figure 8.4.   The evaluation process

interventions for accomplishing the goal were reviewed; and that an intervention was selected, designed, and implemented. It is also less than accurate to maintain that the nursing process occurs in such discrete sequential steps as this figure implies. Rather, various activities occur simultaneously. Ideally cyclical, the process allows for the continued operation of various feedback loops.

There is a close interrelationship between the evaluation process and the nursing process. The parallels between these two processes are well illustrated by comparing the nursing process depicted in Figure 8.3 with the evaluation process depicted in Figure 8.4. Suchman specifies six components in the evaluation process: value formation, goal setting, goal measuring, identifying goal activity, putting goal activity into operation, and assessing the effect of this goal operation.

A comparison of these figures underscores the conceptual similarity of the nursing and evaluation process. Whether this cyclic process is labeled the nursing process or the evaluation process largely depends on the perspective of the person describing the events. A nurse going about the activities of planning, implementing, and evaluating as part of the nursing role takes part in what is labeled the nursing process. Conducting these activities in the context of the evaluator role suggests the label *evaluation process*. It is interesting to note that health planners identify a nearly identical cycle of activities, which, not surprisingly, they label the *health planning process* (Blum 1974).

A prerequisite for successful application of the evaluation process is a clear understanding of the components of that process (Suchman 1967). The evaluation process begins with some value orientation that assumes the worth or desirability of a certain state or condition of being; for example, it is "good" that babies are born free of birth defects. Through both implicit and explicit values goals are set. Given this inextricable link, knowledge of a value would allow identification of the goal. Or, alternatively, knowledge of the goal would facilitate identification of the value orientation precipitating that goal. The goal statement "To work toward less than (a specified percent) of babies being born with a birth defect" directly implies the value specified above. The specific goals that are set are likely to originate from, or at least be consistent with the conceptual framework developed by the community health nurse. (See Chapter 3.)

Once goals are set, a means must be identified that would allow a determination or measurement of the attainment of the goal. In the present example, a way would be needed to discover the number of babies born with birth defects. Birth records might be the source of such information. Next a program or intervention specific to accomplishing the goal would be planned. For example, a genetic counseling service or a prenatal nutrition program might be planned and implemented. Finally, goal-measuring criteria would be applied to the outcome of the program and a judgment as to the extent of the success would be made based on the pre-established goals. (See the final section of this chapter for a description of the mechanics of accomplishing these steps.)

FRAMEWORKS FOR APPROACHING THE EVALUATION LITERATURE

Not unlike other disciplines, the field of evaluation has an established body of literature. And, again not unlike other disciplines, this literature has its own jargon, its particular way of talking about what is going on in the field. As the community health nurse ventures into the field of evaluation, he or she encounters familiar words that are used in a precise or specialized context. For example, words such as effectiveness, appropriateness, and effort have a particular meaning when used in the context of evaluation literature. This section introduces the community health nurse to the terminology and basic concepts of the evaluation field. At the same time it introduces the names and ideas of the prominent scholars in evaluation — names and ideas that the community health nurse will encounter in the course of reading in the field. Admittedly, the survey does not present models in great detail; the reader is encouraged to examine these models more closely by referring to the original sources.

The Donabedian Paradigm

While the emphasis of this chapter is program evaluation, a model originally introduced in the context of quality assurance evaluation deserves mention. Donabedian (1966) originated a paradigm of "structure," "process," and "outcome" in relation to the evaluation of quality of care. More specifically, he introduced this now classical tripartite model in relation to the evaluation of the quality of medical care. Its relevance and direct applicability to the evaluation of the quality of nursing care has been recognized. (Donabedian 1969; Block 1975). This conceptual model is described here because of its ready adaptability and application to program evaluation. Through it, programs or interventions can be evaluated in terms of their structure, process, and/or outcome.

Structure
The structural aspect of the evaluation paradigm focuses attention on the organizational and administrative structure of a program. The evaluator examines such elements of the program as the organization chart, the size and credentials of the staff, the adequacy of the physical facility and equipment, the fiscal resources, and the intra- and/or interagency affiliations. This type of evaluation has been variously referred to as pre-evaluation or quasi-evaluation (Greenberg 1968). Its underlying assumption is that a program that is well organized, competently staffed, adequately funded, and well equipped will necessarily produce good outcomes. A structural evaluation has the advantage of fairly concrete and assessible information. Its significant limitation is the often poorly established cause-effect line between structure and outcome.

Process
Process evaluation essentially relies on counts of program activities, or on what the program does. It assumes that if a certain amount of effort is expended, certain results will be achieved. Its requiring a consensus on what amount of effort represents "good" performance in the context of the specific program area means that accepted standards of performance, either empirical or normative, must be available. For example, to evaluate a home visit program for stroke victims in terms of process involves knowing how many posthospitalization home visits clinical peers judged appropriate for these patients. Evaluation studies relying on process criteria are quite readily identified by the type of data sources used and the type of data reported. Process-related data are culled from clinical records, activity logs, appointment logs, laboratory reports, and billing records. Reports of evaluation studies focusing on process frequently cite such data as number of visits made, group sessions conducted, well-baby physicals completed, and parents counseled. As with structure-

focused studies, an advantage of process studies is fairly accessible "countable" data. The same limitation also exists: the ambiguous and tenuous link between "good" process and "good" outcome that is assumed. Structure and process evaluations have been quite aptly referred to as presumptive in nature (Stanley 1964).

Outcome
Donabedian's third approach to evaluation is that based on outcome. Program evaluation in terms of outcome assesses or measures end-results in terms of the health status of the individuals or group to whom the program was applied. Outcome studies are generally recognized as the essential element of evaluative research. The goals of programs in the health field are nearly always stated in terms of improving the health status of the recipients of the program's services. Because outcome studies provide direct data on the extent to which these goals are achieved, they have obvious appeal. However, outcome studies are difficult to design and carry out: frequently reliable, valid measures of outcome in terms of health status are nonexistent. Outcome studies require rigorous design and considerable fiscal resources and time.

Other Models

Of particular interest to the community health nurse is an extension of this paradigm suggested by Attkisson et al. (1978) in relation to human service program evaluation. In their discussion of the future directions for program evaluation, Attkisson et al. extend Donabedian's structure-process-outcome paradigm to include evaluation of the *community impact* of programs. They advocate that programs begin to be evaluated within the context of the larger community service network of which they are a part. They lament the lack of integration of human services at the community level and the crises this separation has precipitated. Developing a method of measuring the degree of human services integration in a community is one goal these researchers set for future work in the field.

Describing structure, process, and outcome as discreet approaches to evaluation might lead to the unfortunate conclusion that these approaches are in practice applied singly. In fact, only a combination of the three approaches assures adequate program evaluation. Ideally an evaluation includes assessment of structure, process, and outcome and establishes a cause-effect relationship between the structure of a program, the processes implemented, and the outcome realized.

Two models for organizational analysis described in evaluation literature will acquaint the community health nurse with the terminology likely to be encountered in the literature. A critique of these two approaches to organizational analysis — the goal attainment model and the systems model — can be found in Etzioni (1969). In the goal attainment model the criterion for assessment of effectiveness is derived directly from the stated goals of the organization. Etzioni elaborates on the shortcomings of the goal attainment model for evaluating complex social organization and advocates instead that the systems model be applied in these evaluations. The systems model recognizes the organization as a multifunctional unit that performs not only goal attainment activities but also maintenance and custodial activities. Application of the systems model to the evaluation of an agency or organization requires looking at more than whether the organization is performing its goal activities; it requires an assessment of how appropriately resources are allocated among program service and administrative functions of the organization.

While Etzioni's critique of these two models for organization evaluation deserves note, the reader is advised against transference of his conclusions to the activity of program evaluation. In fact, the goal attainment model is often the more satisfactory model to apply to the evaluation of specific interventions or programs. Program evaluation is a more circumsubscribed effort than total agency evaluation. While it must be granted that a program's success is influenced by the organization structure of which it is a part, the purpose of program evaluation is to assess "success" against specific, defined goals. This is most convincingly accomplished through the goal attainment model — which relies on judging the success of a program on the basis of the extent to which predetermined, and, ideally, quantified goals are achieved. In the goal attainment model, the program goals established prior to the implementation of the program serve as the yardstick against which success is judged.

As noted, Donabedian's structure-process-outcome model was originated for quality assurance evaluation. Etzioni's goal attainment and system models are most applicable to total organization or agency evaluation. The several typologies presented in the remainder of this section are modeled primarily for program evaluation.

James (1962) introduces five categories or criteria according to which programs may be evaluated. Suchman (1967) expands on his work. Together they are credited with seminal work in the field of program evaluation. The five categories of criteria defined are (a) effort, (b) performance, (c) adequacy of performance; (d) efficiency, and (e) process. The following paragraphs draw heavily on Suchman's definition of these criteria.

Evaluation of effort relies essentially on an "assessment of input or energy regardless of output." The assumption is made that an exertion of effort on a specific activity is a valid means of accomplishing the goal. Effort evaluations usually rely on counts of the activity(ies) being performed in the course of program implementation.

Performance is the end-result of effort; it is the effect produced as a result of the effort exerted. Evaluations reporting the number of obese patients losing weight after a diet program or the number of stroke victims able to regain full use of their limbs are examples of evaluations of performance. There are particular validity assumptions and problems with reliability involved in evaluations of performance. For example, assumptions are made about the causal relationship between the activity performed and the effect achieved.

Evaluation by the criterion of adequacy of performance examines the extent of effect achieved against the total amount of need. For example, if 95 percent of the obese patients in a given diet group lost over 20 pounds, an evaluation of performance would label the program very successful. However, if only a small proportion of obese people in the community were able to enroll in such a group, the adequacy of the program in terms of the community's need would be less than acceptable.

Efficiency refers to the cost in terms of resources required to attain the objectives. Efficiency is the ratio between effort and performance. Evaluating a program in terms of efficiency includes the question of whether the same results could have been attained with less cost had alternative methods been used.

Finally, process evaluation examines the mechanics of the program to determine how and why the program did or did not work. A most important aspect of program evaluation, process data have the potential to explain why results were, or were not, achieved. Here is the key to establishing the important causal link between program action and observed results.

Deniston and Rosenstock (1970) also offer five criteria for the evaluation of programs: (a) appropriateness, (b) adequacy, (c) effectiveness, (d) efficiency, and (e) side effects. The close parallel between the first four of these criteria and those of James is obvious. The added criterion of side effects involves those effects produced by the program's operation other than those related to the attainment of the objectives. These side effects may be desirable or undesirable, anticipated or unanticipated. Program evaluation requires that the side effects generated be identified and their implications considered in the net evaluation of the program.

Arnold and Blum offer categorizations of program evaluation based on the evaluative question asked or the use intended. Arnold (1971) specifies four levels: (a) evaluation for management control of program activities, (b) evaluation to determine program efficiency, (c) evaluation to determine the effect achieved, and (d) evaluation to determine the relevant goals for the future. The parallels of her categorizations to those of the others is apparent.

Blum (1974) identifies six levels of evaluation that also are comparable to those of Deniston and James.

1. Activity (Is the operation working?)
2. Meeting operational guidance standards or criteria.
3. Efficiency (Can the cost per unit of output be improved? Or alternatively, is the operation working at the cost agreed upon?)
4. Effectivity (How well is the operation producing the net outputs specifically desired?)
5. Outcome validity (How well has the intervention achieved the ultimate consequences or purposes for which the outputs were designed?)

6.   Overall desirability or system appropriateness (Does the desired result actually serve the overall best interest of the encompassing system?)

A BASIC GUIDE TO DEVELOPING AND IMPLEMENTING A PROGRAM EVALUATION

Many papers and texts are available that offer specific, detailed guidance for those interested in developing and carrying out evaluations of interventions or programs. In the literature are thoughtful discussions of theoretical issues, detailed technical and methodological directions, and reports detailing specific evaluations accomplished. In actual practice, though, the busy community health nurse has limited time to apply to extensive study of the evaluation literature. Often she or he passes up good opportunities for evaluations of interventions because of being overwhelmed by the potential complexities that surface as the evaluation effort is contemplated.

The purpose of the following paragraphs is to guide the community health nurse step by step through the thought and action processes that are essential to producing an evaluation. In effect what follows is a skeletal outline of the evaluation process — the basic steps required for an evaluation. As a skeletal outline it is not intended to reflect the state of the art of evaluative research. The community health nurse is encouraged to refer to the literature, which is generously cited, as he or she feels the need for a more extensive treatment of specific aspects of the evaluation process. The steps described in the following paragraphs might be used as a basic guide through the maze of program evaluation.

Most programs planned and executed by the community health nurse will have unique features — characteristics that set them apart from previous efforts. Indeed, it is because the community health nurse tries alternative interventions to realize his or her goals that evaluation is important. Just as each program has unique characteristics, so will the evaluations designed for each different program. And just as it is impossible to anticipate the particulars of specific interventions, it is impossible to anticipate the unique details of the companion evaluations that will evolve to assess the "success" of these alternative programs. However, there are certain general principles that can be applied and specific steps that each evaluation effort will incorporate. These steps are outlined here.

Step One: Give due consideration to the context within which the evaluation will occur, and assess the potential influence that the factors identified will have on the feasibility and success of the evaluation effort.

As any experienced community health nurse is aware, no program or intervention is designed or implemented in a vacuum. Before any nursing program or intervention is undertaken, the astute community health nurse first gives considerable thought to the existing or potential political, environmental, and economic circumstances that can be expected to thwart or support the planned intervention. Nor does the evaluation of the program or intervention occur in a vacuum: there are several important preliminary factors to consider. To ignore or fail to recognize these pre-evaluation issues seriously jeopardizes the successful accomplishment of the evaluation. Four such pre-evaluation considerations are identified below.

First, it is necessary for the community health nurse to objectively examine his or her motivation for undertaking the evaluation (Knutson 1969). Accurate recognition of motives is important because the major methodological choices to be made and implementation strategies to be used, employed later in the course of the evaluation effort, will be significantly influenced by the determined underlying purpose of the evaluation.

In most cases when a would-be evaluator is challenged with the question "Why are you undertaking this evaluation?" the response is something to the effect that "evaluation is good," "it's necessary to determine whether the intervention is achieving the desired effect," or "I want to know whether my effort made a difference." While these statements certainly reflect noble and legitimate reasons for undertaking an evaluation, they usually are an incomplete expression of motive. Often such mundane reasons as the requirements specified in the terms of a grant, a supervisor's mandate, or peer pressure (i.e., being the current vogue), are the real factors mobilizing the effort for an evaluation. These latter reasons, while perhaps not so high-minded or grandiose as the former, are nonetheless legitimate. The mistake lies not so much in having a mundane motivation as in failing to recognize and acknowledge it objectively for what it is.

Knutson (1969) cites a number of explicit and covert reasons for which evaluations are undertaken. He distinguishes between reasons that are organizationally oriented and those that are personally oriented. The former include

1.   To demonstrate to others that the program is worthwhile;
2.   To determine whether or not a program is moving in the right direction;
3.   To determine whether the needs for which the program is designed are being satisfied;
4.   To justify past or projected expenditures;
5.   To determine the costs of a program in terms of money or human flow;
6.   To obtain evidence that may be helpful in demonstrating to others what is already believed to be true regarding the effectiveness of a program;
7.   To gain support for program expansion;
8.   To compare different types of programs in terms of their relative effect;
9.   To compare different program methods or approaches in terms of effect;
10. To satisfy someone who has demanded evidence of success.

Personal reasons, according to Knutson, can be described as

1.   "the thing to do" if one wants to belong;

2.   a means of bringing favorable attention, better budgets, and better staff to one's unit;
3.   a means of gaining status and acceptance of peers and supervisors;
4.   a way of making one's job easier and more interesting;
5.   a step toward promotion;
6.   [a means to satisfy] a vague but urgent need to know if one is progressing.

Many aspects of the evaluation hinge on motivation. The choice of the program to be evaluated; the scope of the evaluation; the intensity, complexity, and level of critical analysis to be applied to the evaluation; and the time and resources to be committed are all influenced by a forthright answer to the query "Why is this evaluation to be undertaken?"

A second pre-evaluation concern is to take candid stock of the resources available. Only naïveté could explain the disregard of such factors as the availability of time, money, or needed additional personnel. Early questions for the evaluator are: Do I have one week, six weeks, or six months to devote to this evaluation? Will I be able to work full-time or only part-time on the evaluation? Is my budget best described as "shoestring," "generous," or "nonexistent"? Will I be able or do I want to allocate potential service funds to my study? Will I have access to outside experts, or computer services? What skills and expertise do I already have that will allow me to accomplish the evaluation? What skills do I need to acquire to accomplish this task? Again, frank answers assure a realistic atmosphere in which to proceed with the planning and implementation of the evaluation.

Third on the list of pre-evaluation considerations is the taking stock of potential obstacles to the development/implementation of the evaluation. The evaluator must re-examine his or her personal commitment to, interest in, and enthusiasm for carrying the evaluation through. At times all evaluation efforts are frustrating, meet seemingly insurmountable roadblocks, or simply lose their initial appeal. Only a sincere commitment to complete the evaluation will sustain the evaluator at these times.

Peer and superior support must also be assessed. Good questions to ask are: Do I have or can I expect complete support, reserved support, or non-support from my superiors? Do I have the support of my peers—or is my evaluation effort likely to be perceived as negativism or punitiveness? Is my work milieu generally one that is favorable, indifferent, or hostile to evaluation efforts? Again, realistic answers are important. An assumption of enthusiastic support from significant others that is later belied by apathy, indifference, or hostility at a critical point in the evaluation process could become the cause of evaluative failure. On the other hand, if the would-be evaluator has honestly assessed the degree of support or non-support he or she expects from peers or superiors, fewer surprises can be sprung.

In addition there is the political milieu in which the evaluation is to be attempted to consider. Relevant questions include: Are such politics operating as to preclude an objective hearing of my findings? Will only positive findings be accepted? Am I expected to report results that support a given position and to downplay or ignore less favorable findings? Who will be affected by positive findings? By negative findings? Have the motives of various opponents or proponents been realistically assessed? How will my present position or future role in the agency or organization be affected by positive or negative findings?

And fourth, the pre-evaluation period should be a time of beginning to do background reading. A literature review in the area of the projected evaluation will offer valuable insights into such matters as: Has such an evaluation been tried before? What techniques and tools were used? What were the problems encountered? How were they overcome, if at all? What were the findings? Did these earlier evaluators have suggestions for related future evaluations? Do these reports of evaluations provide any normative data that might be useful as I endeavor to develop specific objectives for my program or intervention?

Attempting to undertake any evaluation research project without giving due consideration to the work done before places the would-be evaluator in the proverbial situation of reinventing the wheel. On the other hand, over-reviewing the literature is not advised: at this stage it can result in stagnation, in never getting on with the task at hand, or in stifling of creative thinking. The best advice seems to be to review enough of the literature to be familiar with and comfortably conversant with some of the better work that has been done in the field, thus creating a sense of where specific advice, stimulation, or guidance might be forthcoming as the need arises.

The space expended on these four pre-evaluation matters reflects their importance. To insufficiently or unobjectively judge the motivation for undertaking the evaluation; the fiscal, time, and personnel resources available; the existing political milieu; and the relevant literature would seriously jeopardize an evaluator's chance for eventual success. Once a candid consideration of these factors has been made, the evaluator can move on to Step Two with confidence that the groundwork for the evaluation has been firmly laid.

Step Two: Prepare in writing a clear statement of the goals and objectives of the program or intervention in terms that are specific, quantifiable, and time referenced.

The importance of the skill required to accomplish successfully this second step of the general evaluation procedure often is misleadingly downplayed and underestimated. A common assumption is that the undertaking of the program or intervention indicates the prior establishment of a goal and specific objectives. Unfortunately, this assumption is often not based on fact. (The exception might be in those commendable instances in which the evaluation was anticipated and planned parallel with the program or intervention.) More often a program or intervention is instituted with only vague goals and unspecific, unquantified objectives. In these cases the evaluator is responsible for formulating specific, quantifiable, time-framed objectives before proceeding. The essential nature of this step is reinforced by Suchman (1967): "Given the basic importance of a clear statement of the program objectives to be evaluated, it is not difficult to understand why so many evaluation studies which fail to define these objectives prove unproductive. This is tantamount to undertaking a basic research project without first formulating one's hypothesis."

A brief digression is in order here to assist the aspiring community health nurse–evaluator as he or she confronts the substantial theoretical and applied literature on the function and formulation of goals and objectives. Perhaps in no other area of evaluation literature is there a more confusing proliferation of language. The evaluator will encounter such terms as goal, mission, objective, subobjective, intermediate objective, ultimate objective, ideal objective, practical objective, aim, steps, purpose, activities, long range goal, and short range goal. Recognizing the difficulty in communication resulting from the confusing overlap of terms, a committee of the American Public Health Association in 1970 published a useful glossary of evaluative terms that might serve as a starting point for the sorting out process. There is, for example, a level of consensus about the term goal, which refers to the "ultimate or idealized objective" or the statement reflecting the desired final state of affairs; it is often a philosophic value. Objectives are usually perceived of as on a continuum of generality — that is, orderable from the very general to the very specific. The chain of objectives for a program or intervention is often visualized as a hierarchy of intermediate steps to be accomplished in achieving the goal. James (1962) provides perhaps the most succinct delineation of the hierarchal nature of objectives:

These objectives are then considered as making up an ordered series, each of which is dependent for its existence upon an objective at the next higher level, and each in turn is implemented by means of lower level objectives. In this framework there is a descending order of objectives beginning at the ideal objective [James' term for goal] and ending at the lowest level at which the task is to be subdivided.

Suchman (1967) also provides a thoughtful commentary on the statement of evaluative objectives and their hierarchal ordering. Both the work of James and Suchman are highly recommended for further understanding of goal and objective terminology used in evaluation literature.

Finally, a summary introduction of the terms *value assumptions* and *validity assumptions* is in order. Value assumptions pertain to the general belief system by defining what is "good" within a given society. "Birth defect–free babies are to be desired" is a value assumption, for example. Validity assumptions are more specifically related to program objectives and are generally recognized as the "cement which holds (the) hierarchy of objectives together" (James 1962). Essentially, validity assumptions are those assumptions that are implicit in the hierarchal arrangement of objectives. One is made, for example, in the acceptance of statements such as "a baby is more likely be born free of birth defects if prenatal care is adequate." Prenatal care is here assumed to be linked to birth defect–free babies. Such an assumption remains valid only until it is disproved — by, for example, other factors being shown to account for birth defect–free infants.

James (1962) describes the relation of validity assumptions to the hierarchy of objectives:

An assumption of validity must be made whenever we move from a higher order objective to a lower one. Hence, every lower level objective must assume all of the assumptions we have made for all of the objectives above it on the scale. Any program which is based upon a set of false major assumptions cannot be rescued by its lower level objectives, although quite valid evaluations might still be made for each of them individually.

Value and validity assumptions offer a rich field for discussion. However, further consideration is beyond the scope of this chapter; the works of James and Suchman are recommended for a more detailed analysis.

Now we return to the issue of formulating good objectives for evaluations. Earlier the parallel was drawn between a hypothesis of basic research and a statement of objectives of evaluative research. Just as there exists an accepted convention for the formulation of the null hypothesis for a basic research question, so there exists an accepted form for the specification of objectives in evaluation research.

The importance of proper statement of the objectives cannot be overstated. In the final analysis, whether or not a given program or intervention is successful is determined by an assessment of the extent to which the stated objectives were achieved. To the extent that the objectives were stated in specific, quantifiable, and time-referenced terms, the conclusions will be readily forthcoming.

Compare the following two statements offered as alternative objectives for scheduled prenatal nutrition education seminars.

1.   To provide prenatal nutrition education to prospective mothers.
2.   By June 30, 19--, to increase from 60 to 90 the number of poverty-level expectant mothers residing within the two inner city census tracts attending four scheduled nutrition seminars and demonstrating by examination an assimilation of the course content.

Now, imagine it is your task to determine how successful the prenatal seminar effort was. Which statement would allow you to make an assessment of the degree of success achieved?

A close examination of the second objective reveals the elements that account for its usefulness (Sorenson and Elpers 1978). First, it is *time referenced* (by June 30, 19--). The *issue or variable* is clear (an increase in the number attending the seminars and assimilating the content). The *largest group* is specified (poverty-level expectant mothers in the two inner city census tracts). The *direction and amount of change* is indicated (increase the number of mothers from 60 to 90).

And, finally, the *resources to be used to effect the result* are exercised (four scheduled nutrition seminars).

This latter objective also implies some of the criteria to be used in assessing the achievement of the objectives (attendance and examination results). Evaluative measures are readily surmised, such as

1. number of poverty-level expectant mothers in the target area identified as of the starting date.
2. number of seminars held and number of prospective mothers attending.
3. number of expectant mothers completing the seminar sequence.
4. number of expectant mothers receiving a passing grade on examination.
5. number of mothers delivering healthy babies (i.e., Apgar Score = 8).

While it would have been difficult — probably impossible — to assess the success of the nutrition program based on the objective as first stated, the restated objective nearly begs for an evaluative judgment. The community health nurse–evaluator is encouraged to develop objectives incorporating as many of the discussed elements as possible. The better the objective is specified, the more naturally the remainder of the evaluation effort will fall into place (Suchman 1967).

The community health nurse–evaluator will probably encounter comparatively few difficulties in specifying the elements of time period, target group, issue or variable, and resources for his or her objectives. However, frequent difficulties arise in attempting to specify an acceptable, realistic level of desired change. Setting the degree of change targeted too low runs the risk of concluding success when, in fact, the extent of difference made by the program or intervention is insignificant. On the other hand, if the degree of change targeted is set too high, the evaluator risks concluding failure when actually a significant difference was made.

There is, unfortunately, no pat solution to this dilemma. Furthermore, in the field of community health, recognized optimal service levels are more often than not unsubstantiated. Several suggestions are offered here to assist the evaluator in specifying realistic levels for the change desired. One method is to find empirical data in a review of the relevant literature. A possible discovery is the level of a given condition as it has generally been found in several populations. Perhaps community, family, or individual client profiles with respect to the variable under investigation are available for comparison. The levels of the given condition in these several communities might be compared. Such information would, of course, be of special value if a comparable profile was available on the specific target group involved in the program or intervention. In this case the target for achievement could be set at the level found in the more "ideal" community, family, or individual.

Occasionally, standards or norms are available. In this fortunate case it will be comparatively easy to set a target for accomplishment of the objective. Lacking norms, arbitrary standards or rules might have to be called upon — though such a situation, of course, calls into play more subjectivity and personal judgment. Rather than abandoning an evaluation effort for the lack of accepted, generally recognized standards for success, it is usually better to create arbitrary but reasonable end-points and proceed. While these might prove less than accurate, data will still be amassed that might be used by colleagues in the future who are faced with a similar dilemma (Greenberg 1968).

Step Three: Identify the criteria to be used to assess the success of the program or intervention. Select the most appropriate method of study and techniques of data gathering for assessing the achievement of the objectives.

Earlier in this chapter five categories of criteria for program success were discussed: effort, performance, adequacy of performance, efficiency, and process (Edwards and Yarvis 1977). At the present stage of the evaluation the evaluator must decide which of these criteria will be applied to determine the program's degree of success.

To a great extent the wording of the objective begs the criteria to be applied. For example, the stated objective "to increase the number of poverty-level expectant mothers attending a nutrition seminar" requires an evaluation of effort; that is, a count of the number of such expectant mothers attending. Evaluation according to the assessment of effort expended is usually the easiest type of evaluation, often requiring merely good record keeping and counting. It should be noted that an assessment effort usually makes the assumption that the specific activity is a valid means to reach some higher goal (i.e., a validity assumption).

The following are hypothesized examples of other objectives for the nutrition program, the success or failure of which would be determined against the criteria of performance, adequacy of performance, efficiency, and process.

Performance:	To decrease the number of premature infants born to poverty-level mothers by improving the nutritional status of the mothers.
Adequacy of Performance:	To expand the nutritional seminar program to reach 85 percent of the poverty-level expectant mothers in the inner city.
Efficiency:	To decrease the cost of the nutrition seminars to expectant mothers from $18 per enrollee to $12 per enrollee.
Process:	To examine the content of two alternative teaching methods applied in the prenatal nutrition seminars to determine which one results in a higher success level as measured by test scores and infant health status.

As illustrated hypothetically here, a given program or intervention can, and usually does, have multiple objectives. The specific number and kind of objectives selected for a specific evaluation effort depends to a great extent on those factors identified candidly in the first step or pre-evaluation phase of the evaluation process.

Once the criteria according to which the success or failure of the program is to be judged are established, the evaluator moves on to the selection of the method of study and the specification of the techniques and tools for data collection. This step calls upon the evaluator's understanding of the general principles of research design and measurement, which cannot be detailed here. At this stage of the evaluation effort, the would-be evaluator is strongly urged to refer to one or more of the very fine research methods texts available.

The method or design is the basic plan of study — in effect, the blueprint for the overall development and execution of the evaluation. As Suchman (1967) points out, there is no single "correct" design. Different objectives require different methods or designs. There are, however, good and less good designs for a specific evaluation. In addition, a design well suited to one evaluation might be poor for another. Suchman goes on to point out that all research design represents a compromise dictated by many practical considerations. (Abdellah and Levine 1979; Campbell and Stanley 1966; Wandelt 1970; Treece and Treece 1973; Shortell and Richardson 1978) This point is particularly applicable to such a field as community health, in which experimental controls are so difficult to achieve.

Greenberg and Mattison (1955) offer a model representing the "ideal" experimental design from which all evaluation research study designs should be derived. Commenting on this model Suchman states (1967),

No matter what approach one uses or what concessions one is forced to make because of operational limitations, the basic logic of proof or verification will be traceable to this model. It is important to remember that there is not one but a set of experimental designs, and that there is no best way to design all evaluative studies.

The reader is referred to Chapter 7 and to the work of Campbell and Stanley (1966) for a thorough description and discussion of alternative experimental and quasi-experimental designs for research. Overton and Stinson's work (1977) might be profitably reviewed as well. These authors outline some of the central issues the evaluator should keep in mind as she or he attempts to apply experimental designs to program evaluation. The conditions for facilitating the use of experimental designs in evaluating health programs are worth reviewing.

The evaluator is forewarned that methodologic problems will surely crop up as the evaluation design moves from blueprint to execution stage. The literature is replete with descriptions of problems encountered in the course of devising and executing evaluations in the community health field (Klerman et al. 1973; Borgatta 1973; Greene 1977). A listing of just a few of the recurrent methodologic dilemmas encountered include obtaining equivalent control and experimental groups, sampling, matching, randomization, internal and external validity, isolation and control of the stimulus, experimental versus placebo effects, and the applicability of tests of statistical significance. As these dilemmas emerge, the evaluator must recognize the need to turn to research methods texts and, perhaps, to expert assistance.

Once the design of the study is mapped out, the techniques and tools for data collection must be selected. Technique here refers to the "process of making or obtaining individual observations of phenomena or entities. It is the process by which data are collected . . . . Tools refer to "the instruments used in the process of securing observations that are to comprise the data for the study (Wandelt 1970). The technique(s) selected will vary largely according to the design of the study; and the tool(s) selected will be those called for according to the technique(s) selected.

There are many and varied techniques available to the evaluator. Consider the following list of familiar and perhaps not so familiar technique(s) that might be incorporated into an evaluation (Wandelt 1970).

1. questionnaire
2. survey
3. participant observation
4. non-participant observation
5. record analysis
6. interviews
7. content analysis
8. nursing audit
9. process recording
10. diary keeping
11. work sampling
12. time sampling
13. activity or task analysis
14. Q-sort
15. critical incident

The evaluator is again referred to research methods texts and the periodical literature for an in-depth discussion of these techniques.

Tools for recording tasks must also be selected and developed. The tools required are dependent, of course, on the technique(s) selected. Again, the following list of tools suggests the wide variety:

1. rating scale
2. pre- and post-tests
3. video tape
4. encounter forms
5. interview forms
6. survey questionnaires

7.   observation checklist
8.   diary

Often the evaluator is led to the choice of technique or tool based on the literature review. At this stage it is likely the evaluator will want to return to a more comprehensive review of the literature to discover whether tools have already been devised that he or she might adopt or adapt. The evaluator is also encouraged to be aware of the need to pre-test tools. An advantage of adopting or adapting a previously used tool is that it is likely to have already been pre-tested; as such it will be subject to fewer bugs.

Step Four: Implement and administer the evaluation process.

Now the evaluator is ready to actually set the evaluation into motion. It is at this stage that the study techniques are applied. Data sources have been identified and the carefully selected and designed tools are applied in the field. This is the phase of data collection. Ideally, when the evaluation is planned in consonance with the intervention or program itself, data required for the evaluation are collected as the program is being implemented.

Data collection is done in different ways and by different people in different evaluations. Sometimes, where the budget permits, data collection might be hired from external sources. At other times the same person implementing the program or intervention will assume the duties of data collection. Whichever is the case, this phase must be monitored. Periodic checks must be made to see that data are being collected completely, uniformly, accurately, and at the specified time intervals.

If the earlier steps were carefully conceived, this phase should progress smoothly. However, the evaluator must continue to keep an administrative eye on the process. Once the gears are set in motion, problems can still emerge, which should be quickly recognized and remedied. Monitoring of the process also allows for feedback into the program even as it is being implemented. In those ideal situations when the evaluation mechanization is regarded as a part of the control component of a program, ongoing feedback into the program can be used to improve the program even as it is in progress (Zembach 1973).

Step Five: Analyze the data and interpret the results.

The evaluator has at last arrived at that step where a determination can be made whether the program or intervention is a success or a failure. That characterization is made after the data are consulted. The evaluation does not end with the collection of the data. The data must be computed, perhaps coded, tabulated, and manipulated. Tables and/or graphs might be prepared to display or present the data more meaningfully. Only after the data are examined in a purposeful manner can the assignment of success or failure be made.

Once the data is analyzed the findings are compared with the initially stated objectives. If the objectives were stated in quantitative terms, if appropriate techniques and tools were used, and if data collection was carefully executed and monitored, the determination of success or failure is relatively straightforward. To the extent that earlier steps in the evaluation process are weak, the interpretation of results becomes more difficult and subject to challenge.

The evaluator has a responsibility that goes beyond merely assigning the label of success or failure to the program or intervention. He or she should, for example, offer interpretations of specific findings that were, perhaps, unexpected or remarkable. The evaluator should also suggest what implications the findings might have for the specific program or intervention under investigation and for other programs. If specific methodologic problems were encountered, these should be noted. If the findings dictate that the program or intervention be interpreted as less than successful, possible explanations might be offered. While possible explanations might legitimately be brought forward, the evaluator is cautioned against mere rationalization or apologizing for lack of positive findings (Borgatta 1973). He or she should keep in mind that the evaluation might be a success even though the program or intervention is determined to be less than successful.

Step Six: Facilitate the dissemination of the findings and the implementation of recommendations.

Even after the results are in and the success or failure of the program or intervention determined, the evaluator has a further responsibility. The community health nurse–evaluator must attempt to bridge the persistent town-and-gown problem between the researcher and practitioner. Findings and specific application of these findings must be communicated to colleagues. The evaluation effort should be documented in writing and made available to both future researchers and practitioners.

It is at this time also that the evaluator must call upon change agent skills. If the program or intervention was shown to be effective or efficient, for example, this judgment must be brought to the attention of those in a position to act upon these findings. For example, if the pre-natal nutrition program for poverty-level expectant mothers was shown to result in healthier babies, it might be advisable for this program to be expanded to reach more prospective mothers. The community health nurse might bring his or her findings to the public health nursing district supervisor and even lobby for the expansion of the program.

If the community health nurse–evaluator is serious and determined to see that the findings from the evaluation study have an impact, several other strategies might be used. Results might be presented at staff meetings, talks might be made to other agencies or community groups, or letters might be written to government officials. Other strategies will suggest themselves as the community health nurse recognizes and seriously accepts the change agent responsibility of his or her role.

In the preceding paragraphs the evaluation process was segmented into seemingly discreet sequenced steps. It is important to point out here that, in fact, such strict time sequencing does not exist. In reality, aspects of several steps will often be under consideration simultaneously. The convention of labeling steps does, however, present a useful, workable outline to guide the community health nurse–evaluator through the evaluation process.

THE FUTURE OF EVALUATIVE RESEARCH WITHIN THE COMMUNITY HEALTH NURSE ROLE

All indications point to evaluation becoming an increasingly large portion of the community health nurse's role. Very few social programs today can escape scrutiny by those footing the ever-larger bills for these services. Community health nursing is no exception. As a profession, it senses the need to justify its costs and to establish its legitimacy in the eyes of the public. At one time, perhaps, the public was willing to accept on faith alone the need for newer, more sophisticated, and more costly public health programs. Today, increasingly insistent demands are being made for the value of services and programs to be demonstrated. Whereas once efficiency and effectiveness were assumed, today the taxpayer demands evidence. As the community health nurse seeks continued and increased support for new programs, he or she must accept the responsibility for evaluation.

It is misleading, though, to imply that the community health nurse undertakes evaluations of his or her services only under unremitting public pressures. Current literature is reporting more and more evaluations undertaken by community health nurses sincerely interested in finding out if they are making a difference, or if a specific program or intervention is successful in achieving its objectives. Community health nurses are recognizing evaluative research as a means by which they can have an impact beyond the specific program or intervention. Reporting findings from evaluative research studies is a means of communicating to colleagues better ways for accomplishing common goals.

As community health nurses seek advanced training and are more cognizant of their professional status, they sense a need for this self-evaluation. As they prove the value of their contributions, their sense of professional and self-pride increases. That is the real reward for accepting the increased responsibility for evaluation.

REFERENCES

Abdellah FG, and Levine E. Better patient care through nursing research. London: MacMillan, 1979.

Arnold MF. Evaluation: a parallel process to planning. In: Arnold MF, Blankenship LV, Hess JM, Administering health systems. Chicago: Aldine-Atherton, 1971.

Attkisson C, Hargreaves WA, Horowitz MJ, and Sorensen E, ed. Evaluation of human service programs. New York: Academic Press, 1978.

Block D. Evaluation of nursing care in terms of process and outcome: issues in research and quality assurance. Nurs Res 1975; 24:256–263.

Blum HL. Health and the systems approach. In: Blum HL, Planning for health. New York: Human Services Press, 1974.

Borgatta EF. Research problems in evaluation of health service demonstrations. In McKinley JB, ed., Research methods in health care. New York: Prodist, 1973.

Campbell DT, and Stanley JC. Experimental and quasi-experimental designs for research. Chicago: Rand-McNally, 1966.

Committee on Evaluation and Standards. Glossary of evaluative terms in public health. Am J Public Health 1970; 60:1546–1552.

Deniston OL, and Rosenstock IM. Evaluating health programs. Public Health Rep 1970; 85:835–840.

Donabedian A. Evaluating the quality of medical care. Milbank Mem Fund Quart 1966, 44:166–206.

Donabedian A. Some issues in evaluating the quality of nursing care. Am J Public Health 1969; 59:1833–1836.

Edwards DW, and Yarvis RM. Let's quit stalling and do program evaluation. Community Mental Health J 1977; 13:205–211.

Etzioni A. Two approaches to organizational analysis: a critique and suggestion. In: Schulberg HC, Sheldon A, Baker F, eds. Program evaluation in the health fields. New York: Behavioral Publications, 1969.

Greenberg BG. Evaluation of social programs. Rev Int Stat Inst 1968; 36:260–278.

Greenberg BG. Goal setting and evaluation: Some basic principles. Bull New York Acad Med 1968; 44:131–139.

Greenberg BG, and Mattison BF. The whys and wherefores of program evaluation. Can J Public Health 1955; 46:298.

Greene LW. Evaluation and measurement: some dilemmas for health education. Am J Public Health 1977; 67:155–161.

Highriter ME. The status of community health research. Nurs Res 1977; 26:183–192.

Hilleboe HE, and Schaefer, M. Evaluation in community health: relating results to goals. Bull New York Acad Med 1968; 44:140–158.

James GF. Evaluation on public health practice. Am J Public Health 1962; 52:1145–1154.

Keeler JD. The process of program evaluation. Nurs Outlook 1972; 20:316–319.

Klerman LV, Jekel JF, Currie JB, Gabrielson MD, and Sarrel PM. The evolution of an evaluation: methodological programs in programs for school age mothers. Am J Public Health 1973; 63:1040–1047.

Knutson AL. Evaluation for what? In: Schulberg HC, Sheldon A, Baker F, eds., Program evaluation in the health fields. New York: Behavioral Publications, 1969.

Overton P, and Stinson SM. Programme evaluation in health services: the use of experimental designs. J Adv Nurs 1977; 2:137–146.

Price J, and Vincent P. Program evaluation: what to ask before you start. Nurs Outlook 1976; 24:84–87.

Shortell SM, and Richardson WC. Health program evaluation. St. Louis: Mosby, 1978.

Sorenson JE, and Elpers JR. Development information systems for human services organizations. In Attkisson et al., eds., Evaluation of human service programs. New York: Academic Press, 1978.

Stanley DT. Excellence in the public service: how do you really know? Public Adm Rev 1964; 24:170–174.

Suchman EA. Evaluative research: principles and practice in public service and social action programs. New York: Russell Sage Foundation, 1967.

Treece EW, and Treece JW, Jr. Elements of research in nursing St. Louis: Mosby, 1973.

Wandelt M. Guide for the beginning researcher. New York: Appleton-Century-Crofts, 1970.

Woy J, Lund DL, and Attkisson CC. Quality assurance in human service program evaluation. Attkisson CC et al., eds., Evaluation of human service programs. New York: Academic Press, 1978.

Zembach R. Program evaluation and system control. Am J Public Health 1973; 63:607–609.

POLITICAL AND ECONOMIC CONSIDERATIONS FOR COMMUNITY HEALTH NURSING PRACTICE AND RESEARCH

One of the major tasks of the immediate future is to prepare nurses for cross-disciplinary leadership in health care. The greatest gains in achieving higher levels of wellness involve the 98 percent of the U.S. population who are not in institutions or domiciliary care facilities. Yet to date, only about 10 percent of employed nurses are working in community health settings where such opportunities for health care can be addressed.

The national move toward higher levels of wellness has begun in the lay community. This trend lends credence to the notion that the public is ready for the programs in self-help, home care, and community action that community health nurses are so capable of leading. In many areas, nurses have now opened private practices, begun home health agencies, and started local and state health department programs. Many more such efforts are needed before their impact on health will be felt nationally.

Chapter 9 deals with the building blocks necessary to develop the kind of power base that can make a difference within a community, region, or state. Through concerted actions taken by community health nurse leaders, both individually and in groups, the necessary political influence and economic support can be garnered to form health care structures based on the nursing model, as elucidated in Chapters 10 and 11. Chapter 12 points the way toward capitalizing on this strength for the betterment of the health of all people.

POWER AND CHANGE 9

Christine DeGregorio

Problems in the health care industry have been well documented in the literature. Depending upon one's perspective, these problems can be attributed to a number of causes, with just as many solutions: some solutions have been tried and others have not; some threaten the status quo, and others perpetuate it. The phenomenon of social power determines which policies are tested and for whose benefit. This chapter suggests changes in strategies that are appropriate and necessary for nurses to take if they are to gain social power and to assume a meaningful role in the development of health care.

Why is the role of nurses in addressing health care changes an important one? In the United States, nurses comprise over 50 percent of the health professionals involved in direct service. While delivering this care, community health nurses become familiar with consumer needs and frustrations in a variety of settings — homes, schools, places of work, and treatment facilities. Nurses can use the perspectives they gain to stimulate change in policy issues, or they can ignore them entirely. Many nurses are settling for the latter option, because they are not as visible in the planning and decision-making aspects of health care as they are in providing service.

Planning for change in the health system, as in other systems, involves competition among vested interests. The power held by different participants is not evenly distributed, so that some interests are served more promptly than others (Abramson et al. 1952). Because nurses are underrepresented in this highly political change process, the valuable resource they constitute is wasted, to the detriment of potential outcomes. But greater participation in planning is not enough. If nurses do assume responsibility in helping to shape health care, they will be only as effective as the skills they possess to intervene. Their ability to guide change will still be dependent upon their power in relation to that held by others in the health care power struggle. A corps of nurses who value health goals beyond their profession's self-interest and who understand their power resources in relation to those of others is needed. This combination of commitment to extraprofessional values and of political awareness will free more nurses to become risk-taking, responsible participants of a collaborative change process. The following pages address this combination.

Power is the ability to get others to act in a way that they might not act ordinarily. Its impact, or controlling capacity, is related to the scale on which

The author wishes to thank Helen McNerney for her assistance in supplying insights from her considerable and varied experience in nursing practice, administration, and education.

it is applied. Nurses are accustomed to intervening in situations that affect the will and behavior of individuals. For example, a nurse may convince an older person, who she believes is unsafe living alone, to move into a more protected environment; or a community health nurse may affect aggregates of people by providing health education in schools and workplaces. These examples show that control over the behavior of others is a by-product of service, and that this control is power nonetheless. Nurses are familiar with the uses and abuses of power in these circumstances.

A less familiar area, the one addressed here, is that of control at the policy-planning level, where nurses are not very visible. Yet, this level is where the gate-keeping decisions of health care are made.

Decisions at this scale establish parameters within which all other programming must fit. For example, criteria for Medicare coverage ensure minimum health benefits for persons 65 years old or over. Younger persons, unless handicapped, are not covered under Medicare, and no form of appeal, short of an amendment to existing law, can reverse this practice. The established criteria, then, allow service to some and not to others.

Another example where policies set by a few affect the services provided to many occurs when money is allocated to support various health priorities. Federal financing (and state financing, for that matter) historically offers greater support for service in disease-oriented institutions than to health promoting, home-oriented service. Once these parameters are set, subsequent operating budgets must conform accordingly.

Often allocations that might support research and development, planning, and coordination services are trimmed; and these restrictions affect programs negatively. For example, new approaches to service delivery may go untried; outmoded practices may be perpetuated because they are not evaluated; or poor management may cause fragmented or inappropriate service that wastes needed funds. All of these potential inadequacies manifest themselves at levels below that at which policies originate. Therefore, to make an impact on service at the individual and single-institution level, intervention at a higher administrative level may be necessary; and ironically, the participants most visible in setting policy at this scale are professionals, bureaucrats, elected officials, and others who are most distant from direct service. In other words, those closest to the clients, the direct service providers, are farthest from policy development.

If practicing nurses were engaged in higher-level decisions on behalf of their clients, the health system might be more responsive to consumer needs. To this end, nurses could apply power to affect the attitudes, and thereby the decisions, of key individuals in health care administration at many levels — community, state, and national.

An analogy may help to summarize some of the points of this section and to provide a transition to the next section. The phenomenon of power is quite similar to the characteristics of a drug. Each is complex. Like drugs, the effectiveness of power varies according to its makeup, how and with what frequency it is used, and upon whom it is employed. We often associate power with unjustified force or malicious behavior intended to cause harm. In actuality, power (like properly administered drugs) can be a lifesaving and protective force. Unlike drugs, however, power lacks a benign synonym, such as "medicine," to raise it above suspicion. Just as nurses need to know the principles of pharmacology to administer drugs and monitor for dangerous side effects, they need similarly to realize that power can indeed be dangerous. Also, nurses should know the principles behind power in order to employ it safely and to avoid abuse that might cause harm to others. To this end, the theoretical dimensions of power are presented first so that nurses can recognize power when it emerges and understand how power can be applied appropriately to the decision-making process. The examples that follow translate the theory into nursing practice.

TERMINOLOGY

A distinction needs to be made between social power and political power, since only the former is addressed here. Both forms of power are social in that interaction between individuals is a necessary part of them, and both create change in policy that affects social roles, rights, and the distribution of resources. Political power, however, is a narrow subset of social power, because it is circumscribed by party affiliation and franchise. It is a formal mechanism, so to speak, for organizing access to power over decisions in the public domain: nations, states, cities, and townships: People have the right to vote or not to vote. They may meet criteria for elective office or they may not. These are political contingencies that establish the parameters within which the play for power is made. If we put these special laws of order aside, social power uses a vast series of rules that are determined by cultural norms, folkways, and historical precedent. In a democratic society such as ours, there is much elasticity with regard to accumulating social power (Dahl 1960). Each of us must determine which issues are important and find ways to maintain control over their outcomes.

Other important distinctions in terminology need to be made among power, influence, and authority. The terms are related but not synonymous. As stated earlier, *power* is the ability to make others act as you wish them to, rather than as they would if left to themselves. *Influence* is power that has been actualized. If conformity occurs in response to the application of power, we may say that an individual, or group, has been influenced. The word *influence* can be used interchangeably with *dominance*, both evidence power after the fact. *Authority* differs in that it is a special type of power. It exists when capacities to influence others are inherent in a position, or rank, held by an individual or organization. It may eliminate some confusion to remember that authority is only one source of power, not power per se. In fact, depending upon the situation, authority (position) can either promote or impede control over others. If used wisely, however, authority can be a valuable resource to one's power supply.

Although influence is power actuated, power can exist in an inactive state called "potential power" (Dangzer 1964). Using potential power can influence behavior while risking no power loss. Obviously the use of power potential is the safest way to engage in power struggles, since, unchallenged, power results in wins, not losses. Depending upon the strength of power potential, however, the target for change may or may not be affected, and it may be necessary to activate power. In this latent state, power may be exerted as a threat of punishment or promise of reward, thereby subduing resistance and evoking conformance. The controlling signals may be given deliberately or not, as the following situations exemplify. In the first situation you will notice that an employee deliberately uses power in its latent state as a threat to affect the decisions of her seniors; while in the second, a supervising nurse effectively changes the behavior of another without intending to exert her latent power.

Consider an employee who threatens to resign her position to protest an agency ruling that she believes jeopardizes patient care. Although her motives may be noble, she loses all chance of subsequent influence if her resignation is accepted. The risks to her position and to her ability to affect future decisions are very high. Her power potential is the threat of resignation, which may or may not have enough force to change the policy in question. If the nurse's threat is successful in changing the policy, then the contest is won, and her position continues as a power potential. One should not be fooled, however, into thinking that the threat of withdrawing service will work as effectively a second time. The power wielded may have come from the surprise of confrontation and not from the fear of her departure. If applied again, her resignation may be welcomed in the hope that calmer decision making will follow in her absence.

In the second case, a nurse acquiesces to her superior's wishes every time a disagreement arises about patient management. She modifies her behavior because of assumptions she makes about her superior's status, experience, age, and the like; yet when collaborating with her peers, she exhibits a great deal of assertiveness and self-determination. Regardless of whether the supervising nurse encourages such passivity (she may indeed prefer a little professional challenge), her personal and professional attributes comprise a power potential that affects her underling's behavior.

These examples illustrate the complexity of power. Depending upon where in the decision-making hierarachy it is applied, the results will differ. The higher the position; the greater the impact. Also, whether the behavior or decisions of others are controlled through threats and promises or through actual force, there are varying degrees of control that can be maintained over a power supply. The skillful deployment of power involves knowing *when* and *how* to apply it, so that the desired outcomes are reached with a minimum of power loss.

THEORETICAL FRAMEWORK

Power is a complex phenomenon that exists in virtually all social relationships, except possibly those so brief that vested interests do not emerge. The exercise of power necessitates two or more contestants (individuals, collectives, or institutions) who are sufficiently motivated to compete with each other to achieve an objective that, if gained by one, is lost to the other (Alford 1975).

A situation that exemplifies this conflict is the issue of how to spend the public health dollar. In this conflict, multiple opposing interests seek control over a fixed amount of money. The participants in this struggle may or may not share the broader goal of better health for all; and they certainly have no consensus about what combination of services would meet society's needs best. Because of this division, a power conflict emerges. Proponents of health promotion strategies, for example, may argue the old adage, "An ounce of prevention is worth a pound of cure"; while disease-oriented special interest groups resist this approach, stressing that those most victimized by debilitating illness deserve greater attention. The result is a classic fight over limited resources, with multiple contestants who are motivated enough by their values to resist each other's domination in budget decisions. Each group of contestants has a clear health objective that requires considerable financial support but, because of the limited funds available, a gain in support by one side causes a loss for the other.

This example, illustrates the point made earlier, that in order for power to exist there must be two or more contestants, a shared objective (one focus over which there is division), and action and counteraction(s). Once these prerequisites exist, one can gain or lose power by manipulating three critical ingredients: motivation, capacity, and resistance. This notion is summarized in the equation:

$$\text{Power} = \frac{\text{Motivation} + \text{Capacity}}{\text{Resistance}}$$

where

power is the ability to get others to behave in a way they might not act ordinarily; motivation is the commitment one feels toward achieving an objective; capacity is the access to and skillful deployment of resources that subdue resistance; and resistance is the force that impedes one from attaining desirable objectives. Power can be increased by building motivation and capacity or by decreasing resistance.

A wise power contender has clear priorities and motivation for action, so that he or she can estimate the source, direction, and strength of any likely resistance and can anticipate the risks associated with various lines of action selected to overcome resistance.

The remainder of the chapter examines what each critical ingredient comprises and gives examples of how each factor contributes to a net gain or loss of power.

Motivation

Whether we choose to use it or not, we all hold some degree of power over others. Motivation is the stimulus that activates power when something we value is threatened. Without motivation, power lies dormant — both our own and that of the opposition.

The old adage "let sleeping dogs lie" contains a valuable lesson about power. If you have an opponent who could easily defeat you in a power dual, but who is weakened by preoccupation or inattention, nothing should be done to arouse interest in your objectives. Knowing that an opponent's disinterest can be the cause of your victory is a lesson in itself. Guard against dissipation of power that is attributable to your own distraction. This sort of watchfulness that safeguards what you value can only be achieved by having a clear sense of purpose. You need to consider answers to questions such as: What do I really value in life and in my career? Do any of these valued objectives have higher importance than others? Will certain strategies to achieve these ends create regrets that overpower the satisfaction of reaching them?

In practice, nurses often refrain from forcing prescribed health practices on certain clients, because they realize that the patient's own internal commitments have more lasting power than cases in which compliance results from the application of external pressure. For example, a nurse deliberately chooses not to pressure a patient, even though the impact of her uniform, expertise, and professional status might prompt immediate compliance. This passive strategy is deliberately taken to allow time for the client to want change for the right reason: to promote his or her own health and not the nurse's peace of mind. In another example, a nursing administrator may accept without argument the board of director's decision to reject a new service for the homebound, although it may very well be within her power to change their minds. The administrator purposely chooses not to contest the board's action, because higher value is placed on the services that might be cut to allow for the new. Both examples illustrate power brokers who know their objectives and motives for action. In each a stand is taken that does not jeopardize highly valued outcomes: a client's commitment to health in the first case and existing services valued by the community in the second. When motives are vague and goals are nonspecific, a power contender dilutes his or her own strength, making victory for opposing forces that much easier.

In cases when individuals, groups, or institutions combine forces to achieve valued outcomes, it is even more essential to bring priorities and motives sharply into focus. Commitment to collective goals and strategies is a key component in activating one's potential power. The organizational style of the group affects the degree to which consensus formation is permitted — which, in turn, affects readiness to act.

As conceived here, organization is narrowly defined as the framework within which information is shared, decisions are made, and action is taken. All participants may be involved equally, or they may share responsibility selectively.

When establishing an organizational structure, the decision of whether or not to exchange information freely and decentralize problem solving is important for maximizing power. If collective goals and strategies evolve from the free exchange of individual preferences, commitment is likely to be higher than if decisions are arbitrarily made by a few. A structure that allows for continuous revision to accommodate change in member composition, intragroup relations, and values and preferences will facilitate consensus formation and mobilization — collective motivation, commitment, and action. Further, an organizational framework that encourages a high amount of consensus requires less time on internal controlling tactics. Efficiency of power use is thereby maximized over the duration of a power struggle.

Motivation to use power, whether as an individual or as a group, is closely linked to having clear objectives and values. When these are not well defined, more is at stake than personal power loss. When an individual and the associations he or she joins have no clear mission, one can easily be exploited to fight for causes that are not really valued. Power can be transferred. A person can contribute his or her name, money, and other valuable assets to accomplish ends that are unclear. When a transfer of power occurs, that person can be held accountable for an outcome that results from a number of steps over which no judgment or control was exercised. Unfortunately, power is transferred more often than any of us would like to admit.

To avoid the inexcusable abuse of power that results from negligence, nurses must assess their personal and professional values and affiliate only with organized action or take only individual actions that contribute to accomplishing known desirable ends. Power should be invested like money. Only after weighing the merits and liabilities of a transaction should either money or power be transferred to others. In the case of power, however, bear in mind that the investment risks are greater than personal loss of control. Giving power to causes that one does not understand or value can only lead to an ultimate tip in the power equation. Uncontrolled action generally results in two kinds of power loss: (a) diluted strength that could have been saved for future objectives and (b) increased strength of resistance as potential opponents observe evidence of ineptitude. Both of these power losses are within one's control to stop, and the means to harness such power is to develop motivation. In summary, motivation can be raised by the following:

1. Developing a clear understanding of personal and professional objectives.
2. Establishing priorities for what is valued.
3. Remaining attentive to the actions of others that may affect the accomplishment of desired outcomes.
4. Developing a clear understanding of member values and commitments.
5. Forming a consensus about collective goals and strategies.

Since power does not emerge unless resistance is encountered when seeking a goal, and because resistance is so closely related to motivation, resistance is discussed next.

Resistance

As the equation on page 277 illustrates, the strength of power needed to accomplish an aim is equal to the resistance that must be overcome. Obviously, strength can be gained by simply minimizing resistance. As in the adage of the sleeping dog, one merely needs to withhold from engaging in strategies that arouse attention. Too often fledgling power contestants seek news coverage or other forms of publicity because of a misconception that it guarantees support. One does not necessarily lead to the other — as the following actual recent event exemplifies.

The establishment of a group home for profoundly retarded adults was pending before a local town council. A vocal neighborhood minority circulated a petition to veto the plan, which generated a great deal of publicity. This visibility mobilized a previously passive group of neighborhood residents, who surprised the sponsors of the petition by attending the public hearing and testifyied in defense of the home. In this case, publicity had a negative effect by increasing resistance to insurmountable proportions. Particularly unfortunate is that this type of destruction is self-generated.

Another kind of resistance that is self-induced is the alienation that springs from the way a confrontation is approached. The change process is greatly affected by the way power is applied. The most coercive approach pays no attention to the values and/or reasons that motivate resistance; instead, the things most needed for the opposition's survival, such as money, services, and information, are forcibly withheld until the opposition is broken. As an example, in a conflict between hospital administrators and unionized employees, the latter could threaten to withhold services until the benefits they seek are granted. As another example, a funding organization might cut allocations to an agency, expecting it to carry on independently, and instead, the agency administrator might threaten to cut programs unless the cutback is restored. If the services are valued by the funding organization or if it fears the potential negative press, the administrator's threat could influence the reallocation of funds.

A second use of power creates change by inducement, working on the forces that motivate the opposition. In this instance, symbolic rewards and information are applied usually over a period of time until the competitors' need to resist is lessened. Then one side may comply to the aims of the other, or both contenders may compromise to reach a third alternative that was not previously considered. When opposition is caused by fear or insecurity, status and praise can often convert resistance into support. When disbelief and misconceptions create opposition, they may be dispelled by education and trust-building experiences, such as in the situation of an administrator who relies on a staff member, held in high regard by her colleagues, to advocate the adoption of policy that would be rejected if presented by an authority figure.

Between the extremes of force and psychological inducement is a utilitarian approach to wielding power, in which resources like money, credit, and services are offered as payoffs to quiet resistance. When an employer offers a valuable employee higher wages to keep him from accepting a desirable position elsewhere, he is using this form of power.

Material rewards are used to evoke change in social behaviors as well. For example, free milk has been offered to low-income mothers so that they will improve their infants' nutrition during the early stage of development.

When the methods used to produce change leave no alternative but submission, the target of that change develops a great deal of resentment and resists being controlled regardless of the values sought. For this reason, one must give serious consideration to the risks associated with employing coercive tactics that allow no choice. Utilitarian approaches are more acceptable (that is, if you do that for me, I'll do this for you). Less alienation is generated so that the amount of resistance, also called counter-power, is proportionately lessened (Etzioni 1968). Normative inducements, though slow to take effect, produce negligible resistance because they persuade the opposition to value the same objectives the power contender seeks. Choosing a combination of strategies tends to be better than selecting one approach exclusively.

Power then, evokes change differently depending on how it is applied. Threats of punishment and promises of reward can be deployed forcefully or not. The range of methods discussed thus far — coercive, utilitarian, and normative — evoke resistance in descending amounts, respectively. An individual can minimize the resistance to his or her actions by applying power wisely.

To summarize, the change process is rarely, if ever, devoid of power struggles because almost always multiple interests compete for valued objectives. The amount of power needed to achieve one's aims is equal to the resistance that must be overcome. Resistance is associated with the degree to which contestants are motivated to compete for the changes they seek, and motivation can be manipulated to overcome the resistances that emerge. To this end, a wise use of power necessitates subduing resistance, which can be done in the following ways:

1. Maintenance of a low profile when attention to one's accomplishments will provoke resistance.
2. Diversification of power strategies that rely on the least alienating, yet effective, means to reach one's ends.

Of all the dimensions that interact to evoke power, *capacity* is the most complex to describe. Capacity is affected by the *resources* one has to confer on or withhold from others to elicit desired behaviors. Capacity is also affected by one's ability to make appropriate judgments given the constraints (opportunities) of *time* and *culture*. These two facets affect all the other dimensions that make up the power balance because they set the stage in which the action takes place.

Capacity

Having discussed the effects of motivation on power struggles, let us now examine the raw materials everyone has with which to subdue opposition when it does emerge. The discussion that follows concentrates first on power resources as they affect the ability to overcome resistance. Three points are presented here for consideration.

1. The fundamental elements that constitute the resource base so one can take inventory of his or her own supply (composition of resources).
2. The source and expandability of resources so that one knows how to build a power potential (acquisition of resources).
3. The mechanism of how resources impact on the pace and stability of change (application of resources).

Composition of Resources
In general, interest groups and organizations take on the attributes of people. They have collective instincts to strive for self-maintenance and social acceptance, just as people strive for physical sustenance, self-esteem, and love. Because the insecurity felt when these needs go unfulfilled is a great motivator for compliance, knowing the points of vulnerability at which the needs are most open to threat is necessary to neutralize opposition. In other words, know your opponent. It is also necessary to understand one's own capacity to threaten or satisfy the needs in question.

These "satisfiers" make up one's basic resource supply. They may be material and measurable things like money, services, or information, or they may be symbolic and intangible things like prestige, popularity, or position. Keep in mind that power can be depleted by misjudging one's capacity to threaten or satisfy the needs of competitors. This type of error in judgment can spring from many sources, but two of the most common are (a) being unaware of the extent of one's control so it is not deployed effectively and (b) misinterpreting what is most valued or feared by opponents. For these reasons knowing the range and effectiveness of the resources one possesses is critical.

When first taking inventory of these commodities, some aspects of the assessment process are particularly important to realize. First, all resources are time bound, because needs are transient. In other words, what works today may be outdated tomorrow. Recall the example of the nurse who threatened to resign as a tactic to change a policy that was thought to disrupt quality care. A threat of this magnitude alienates an employer and does not work repeatedly.

Second, resources are issue relevant. What is valued in the health arena may not be valued in another arena. Some examples of health-specific resources include professional licensing and special certification (*rights to practice*); access to third-party reimbursement, research and training grants, Medicare waivers (*supports to practice*); certificates of need, admitting privileges to hospitals (*acceptance*); and technical skills and knowledge (*expertise*). Without these resources physicians could not set up practice, hospitals could not expand services, nurses could not work as independent clinicians, scientific research would come to a halt — and the repercussions would go on and on. Examples of resources that are transferable to any situation include money; credit; control over jobs, services, and information; prestige; popularity; and so forth.

Next to money, which can buy most other power resources (social standing, position, visibility, information, services, expertise, etc.), knowledge is the most transferable commodity of the resource bank. This term does not refer to technical knowledge about a special skill that is readily gained in formal education. Rather, it refers to the knowledge of one's own motivations, resources, and weaknesses gained from prior exposure to crisis and change.

Experience accumulates from one conflict to another, and problem-solving skills accrue. This accumulation of knowledge affects the efficiency with which one employs resources and is therefore a critical factor for power potential. In other words, the capacity to make judgments about the timing and use of sanctions and rewards is itself a resource. In part sound judgments grow from the right mix of collecting data and the processing and dissemination of information (Etzioni 1968).

Data collection includes the sources for, accuracy of, and number of facts known about all the variables surrounding an objective. An example of data collection is the assessment of one's values, motivations, priorities, and tactics and those of the opposition, followed by the determination of the overriding context within which an action will take place. *Data processing* refers to the time and expertise each contestant has to devote to analyzing the information obtained. *Dissemination* pertains to facts and findings that are communicated to bolster support or thwart resistance and to the thoroughness and timeliness with which this occurs.

When the collection, processing, and dissemination of information are unevenly developed, an imbalance results that is destructive to problem-solving capacities. Collecting too much data can result in accumulating many bits of unrelated information that never congeal into a usable form. Information that nurses stockpile about consumer needs and frustrations is an example of this problem. The insights gained by nurses while providing direct service are rarely transmitted in a form that is useful to the planning/policy development process.

Too much processing without sufficient data collection can result in a view of the situation at hand that is not based in fact. Planning agencies often find themselves in this bind when they have an abundance of hardware and technicians for processing data but a shortage of time or professional staff to acquire new facts. Take for example, the decennial census. Until recently, planners and elected officials relied on information gathered early in the decade and outdated by the latter part of the decade because of the excessive cost of more frequent surveys. Now the U.S. government has agreed to take the national census at 5-year intervals. This technique should bring into better balance the aspects of data collecting and processing.

Further, the ability to acquire information is directly related to wealth. Richer governments, organizations, and their subdivisions have larger research and development budgets than do poorer ones. As a result, they have a greater capacity to research pending issues (collection), draw justifiable solutions (processing), and communicate findings (dissemination). Within the health care system, those who can afford to accumulate and analyze facts about controversial issues have a powerful advantage over those who have meager funds to support research and development.

What one does with available knowledge to maximize its impact in a power struggle, however, is not associated with money. Rather, the openness with which information is shared is an organizational issue. This facet of capacity was discussed earlier with respect to building motivation and commitment when individuals are engaged in collective action. The same principles apply to the knowledge resource. Information can be accumulated to benefit a few people or many; it can be distorted, withheld, or openly shared. The decision about disseminating information is a facet of capacity that affects one's ability to make the most of what one knows. Finally, bear in mind that power resources are complementary. Money can buy most of the other resources, and knowledge can contribute to such elements as prestige, trust, social position.

Acquisition of Resources

The evenness with which money, credit, prestige, and other power factors is allocated in society is a function of the social, political, and economic environments. The size of one's original resource base is, therefore, externally determined. Personal power depends heavily on the class an individual is born into, which influences such determining factors as access to education and aspirations to seek difficult challenges. Whatever the external controls, resources can be accumulated by working hard, taking risks, associating with the prestigious, and even marrying into money.

What is the first step in acquiring power? In the previous section, we saw that the services and symbols one has to withhold or confer in a power struggle are limited to the extent to which each is valued by the opposition; technical knowledge, prestige, etc. are powerful motivators of compliance only when they have special meaning for individuals or groups. Knowing this, it is probably best to stockpile a variety of influencing commodities, so that the resource base is responsive (flexible) and can be adapted to the range of circumstances (needs and fears) encountered. To expand power resources, an individual or group can (a) develop collaborations and trusting relationships with others who have the resources of money, services, knowledge, or social standing; (b) establish a positive image in the community or system; or (c) select opponents over whom one is dominant. Additionally, collectivities and organizations can develop coalitions or specially select members who will expand the resource base needed to overcome resistance.

Each of these means of building a power base has strengths and weaknesses. For example, when developing collaborative relationships, one has to anticipate which resources benefit others, then offer them as favors as a means of establishing some indebtedness. Instances of this process in nursing and other professional fields are commonplace. One nurse practitioner known by the author developed a specific expertise and reputation for helping clients. After this reputation was established, her professional colleagues (nurses, physicians, and teachers) began to rely on her for counsel in cases where they needed a resource. Her expertise, which she offered freely to help others, now gives her legitimacy, prestige, and access to critical information.

This sort of resource investing anticipates circumstances in which one might need favors returned. If the reverse is the case, and one is constantly indebted to others, the capacity to move freely in power relations is weakened.

The second means of expanding power resources, gaining visibility, is only desirable when the image built is a positive one and reinforces the objectives sought. Recall the example of the residents who tried to prevent a state government from purchasing a home for retarded adults in their neighborhood. The residents circulated a petition to rally protest and publicized the scheduled date for testimony. The original protestors were defeated because their use of publicity awakened powerful opposition to their aims. The purchase was resoundingly supported at the hearing, demonstrating that in this case the petition and the visibility it engendered raised community support for the purchase.

Third, power contestants can gain satisfaction, visibility, and support by providing evidence that they can accomplish their aims, even in the face of resistance. The point is to set yourself up for wins in the beginning, because success generates success. Choose the kinds of contests in which there is a good chance of success. In this manner, abilities to reach desired outcomes can be tested. Then, with some experience as a guide, one can tackle the remaining challenges.

For example, a strategy used in the community organization process is first to select an issue for which there is unquestionable support, such as demands made on slum landlords to raise housing standards so that they are in compliance with the law. This is an objective that crosses class, race, and age boundaries. Problem-ridden residents can easily mobilize the support of those either directly or indirectly affected by the violations; and both public law and social norms are compatible with the demand for changes. After cohesiveness has been developed within the neighborhood group, and leaders have been tested for their effectiveness, harder goals can be sought.

Nancy Milio, R.N., Ph.D., a community health nurse and activist, used this strategy to develop a progressive health center in Detroit (Milio 1975). First she assessed the values and resources of community residents. Next she mobilized mothers who shared a critical need for day care to form a child care center. With that success, trust and self-confidence were raised, so that the more serious problems of poverty, racism, and unemployment could be approached. When these critical life issues were under control, individuals were free to consider improving their health behaviors.

When collective action is used to mount a power offensive, individuals, organizations, and associations may gain resources in two ways: (a) by forming coalitions and (b) by selectively recruiting their members. With respect to the first method, developing coalitions occurs when two or more groups band together to maximize resources against powerful odds. Take, for example, home care agencies that work independently and, in fact, compete for clients and funding. When federal policies endanger their access to third-party payments (reimbursements) or when state policies create obstacles to maintaining well-qualified employees, such as the lowering of personnel licensing requirements, home care agencies have been known to form temporary alliances to fight their common enemy (or enemies). In so doing, their collective action raises power potential for dominating the obstacles that emerge. The capacity to change combatant relations into cooperative ones, when common interests are at stake, is a desirable skill that should be cultivated.

Professional groups like the American Nurses Association are made up of many individuals who share common schooling, expertise, and interest. Their resource base is made up of member fees and nonmonetary contributions such as service, information, contacts, and the like. When money is in short supply, a ready store of resources that are freely offered by members must be available. These resources might include, for example: an intimate understanding of opponents' strengths and weaknesses; prompt access to relevant information; social rapport that attracts the interest and commitments of others; time for various coordinating, lobbying, and service tasks; and experience in leadership, power tactics, and change.

Further, individuals have different types of assets that complement each other, and therefore, a deliberate selection of supporters can ensure variety and volume in one's resource base. For example, a group with the goal of improving school health services should probably include representatives from teaching staff, school administration, health personnel, parents, and, possibly, students. Through a mix of this nature, one obtains the following power assets: (a) expert knowledge (from teacher and health professional involvement), (b) experience with the social and power relationships currently underway (from administrators), and (c) consumer self-interest for follow-through support (from parents and students).

Any of these three member types may also possess charisma, community connections, and other power-maximizing advantages. If the organization restricts membership so that all available assets are not tapped, one's power potential will be hampered from the outset. (But even when the membership is sizable and varied, no reliable power base exists if demands on individual commitments are unclear.) Of course developing a consensus about group goals and strategies before securing agreements about what members have to offer is always necessary because their commitment to give of themselves will vary with the cause.

In summary, the evenness with which resources are initially distributed in society is determined by social, economic, and political forces over which one has little control. The power base can be expanded by taking deliberate action, however, once clear objectives emerge and are focused upon. Five strategies are useful:

1.   Develop relationships with resource-rich associates.

2. Control one's own visibility, maintaining a low profile when it subdues resistance and heightening public awareness when it guarantees support.
3. Accumulate success by starting with challenges that are easily met.
4. Cultivate the facility to form coalitions with others, when mutual threats arise.
5. Select members wisely so resource deficits are minimized.

Remember that the depletion of power resources is affected by the amount of resistance one confronts and the rate and efficiency with which resources are expended.

Application of Resources
The impact of the resources used on the pace and stability of change is important. As stated earlier, coercive measures keep opponents from seeking refuge from change and make no attempt to manipulate the values, reason, and judgment that otherwise might prompt resistance. They are, therefore, relatively fast acting. For instance, New York State law rules that a child must have specific immunizations before entering school. By refusing admission in this way, the law coerces parents to have their child immunized. In another example, health promotion campaigns use legal restrictions and financial disincentives as coercive measures to achieve health objectives where other methods have failed. Legal restrictions such as limiting alcohol consumption among minors and reducing the highway speed limit are two examples where compliance to laws helps control unsafe behaviors, and thereby promotes health.

In contrast, health promotion strategies that require lasting changes in lifestyle necessitate noncoercive methods. Often called normative strategies, these appeal to opponents' reason for resistance, their strongly held values, and norms. These methods are often slow to evoke compliance because it takes time to change attitudes. Patterns of food, tobacco, and alcohol consumption are behaviors deeply rooted in consumers' concepts of self. Changing practices of this nature usually means giving up something pleasurable. The coercive approach of posting No Smoking signs in restaurants may influence behavior over dinner, but it takes noncoercive measures like education, peer example, and even encounters with victims who have suffered ill effects like lung disease before lasting change is effected. This change strategy needs time to appeal to underlying motivations, values, and judgments that produce opposition.

Since the way resources are applied greatly affects the length of time that achievements last, a power contender should select strategies (coercive or noncoercive) that are compatible with the results sought. In other words, match strategies to objectives. Once again, this necessitates knowing precisely what one wants to achieve. A vague goal, such as "nurses should be powerful," is grossly inadequate because what you set out to achieve is difficult to measure. Powerful to do what? Restating the goal so that it is measurable helps determine what has to happen in order for one to feel successful. Saying, "Nurses need to participate in developing policies where they work," brings the objective a bit more into focus. All nurses who sit on policy committees can be counted and all policies that affect nursing practice can be listed. Then, one can set out to increase the quantity and quality of nursing performance in decisions that matter.

To summarize this point, a specific definition of success must be developed before one can decide how to apply his or her power. These judgments directly affect success in achieving results. An example may help to clarify this point. A decision to enact a law requires a shorter time than does the implementation of, and adherence to, the law. If the aim of an organization is simply to get a law enacted, coercive tactics may be very effective. If, on the other hand, an organization's objective is to change attitudes and behaviors to conform to a new policy, tactics that reeducate and are normative will be more effective than force.

Further, sometimes fast-acting coercive tactics are necessary; rescuing a suicidal client, for example, may necessitate protective force. But time-consuming approaches to change must inevitably be used when objectives call for compliance over time, such as ensuring that the pay scales of nurses are on a par with other workers on the same level. Wage parity assumes a belief system that values people equally. Usually compliance to change methods comes from a combination of strategies, some coercive (food and drug legislation) and some normative (nutrition classes). Guiding change in health care (policies and behavior) is similar to the case of stopping smoking; change must appeal to underlying motivations, values, and judgments.

In summary, this dimension of capacity builds on the earlier points about motivation and clarity of purpose. Skillful judgments are needed to select the right mix of resources so that desirable changes are attained and sustained.

A key element to measuring power is the range of actions from which one may select to pursue the desired objective. Range forces one to look beyond personal and organizational characteristics of competing interests and their power resources to the social processes at work that restrict or expand possible actions. The combination of single acts that make up the action and counter-action of a power conflict is derived from many individual judgments about which confronting behaviors are acceptable in the given circumstances. Each judgment is affected by the social context surrounding an action, as well as the amount of time available for completing the action. The factors indicate the effects of the social context and the time horizon on the contestants' power potential, which are the last items for discussion in this chapter.

Social Context

The power of individuals and collectives to guide change in their own best interests is affected enormously by social and political institutions and by tradition. Frances Fox Piven, well known for her work in welfare rights, summed up this phenomenon effectively when she stated:

What some call superstructure, and what others call culture, includes an elaborate system of beliefs and ritual behaviors which defines for people what is right and what is wrong and why; what is possible and what is impossible; and the behavioral imperatives that follow from these beliefs. Because this superstructure of beliefs and rituals is evolved in the context of unequal power, it is inevitable that beliefs and rituals reinforce inequality by rendering the powerful divine and the challengers evil (Piven and Cloward 1977,1).

Applying this quote to the discussion about power, the social context impacts power potential both positively and negatively. On the positive side, having shared values and norms about how to behave (what constitutes appropriate behavior) sets up "rules" so that opponents in a power conflict anticipate the resistant behaviors of the opposition. When these rules are abandoned, as in the case of international terrorism, one's ability to make good tactical judgments about counteraction is drastically reduced. The chaos that accompanies the violation of norms presents a risk to the potential power of all parties, because it reduces everyone's ability to predict behaviors.

Abiding by norms that perpetuate inequality, however, has a negative impact on power outcomes. Take the examples of traditional parent/child, creditor/debtor, and supervisor/employee relationships in which roles of dominance and submission are acted out respectively in a predetermined fashion. In cases of this sort, individuals react automatically based upon a common understanding of what they perceive their opponents to expect, so that the designated submissive parties are expected to lose (Warren 1968).

Both the positive and negative effects of norms are of particular importance to nurses because their professional and sexual roles are changing and beliefs about how they "should" behave are less commonly shared. Although the overwhelming majority of nurses are women, no common values and perspectives should be taken for granted. Today's role change opens new opportunity and challenge, but it also causes amibivalence and conflict. Nurses engaging in collective power actions need to evaluate thoroughly their internal values about acceptable and unacceptable behaviors. (This evaluation is part of consensus formation discussed in the preceding section.) They also need to consider how opponents will respond to departures from tradition and select methods (actions) that offer the least risks and the most gains to their power potential.

When nurses challenge the status quo by assuming expanded roles, they disturb two traditions — sexual and professional — which are both undergoing changes in society. When assuming nontraditional behaviors, they remove the limitations that tradition has destructively enforced. At the same time, however, they risk antagonizing counterattacks from threatened proponents of the status quo who may be within, as well as outside, professional and sexual boundaries.

To reiterate this point, changing traditions and deeply rooted norms provide as much of a burden as they provide opportunity; competitors in a power match must select actions in their scheme to guide change according to their best power advantage. Sometimes traditional ways are more advantageous than new behaviors, and sometimes the opposite is true. A reanalysis of resistance is needed for every new opponent and every new objective. Careful reflection about the values of self and others will help in the selection of actions on their own merit and in the avoidance of knee-jerk responses to uphold or defy custom whether old or new.

Poor judgments that alienate factions within a support group can result in another form of self-inflicted power loss, and, since challengers of tradition have built-in disadvantages, they cannot afford this type of depletion. The skillful employment and conservation of power is critical to achieving success. Because of the imbalance of power created by the social context, the odds are always against success. Said another way, powerful (traditional) interests can afford an occasional mistake in judgment; weaker (innovative) ones cannot.

Time Horizon

Throughout this chapter, power has been described as a social phenomenon that is inextricably connected to change. Power is a "latent force" that is activated to obtain an outcome that would not have occurred by chance. The power process is a contest of wills between two or more parties (individuals, groups, etc.) who are sufficiently motivated to take risks and confront resistance in order to gain their objectives. The time frame in which this contest occurs is the final point for consideration. The critical impact of time on the process and outcome of power disputes is examined along two dimensions: the effects of available time on (a) motivations and (b) resource mobilization.

We know from previous sections that the motivation to resist dominance by another is a precondition for the phenomenon of power to emerge. The complexities behind what stimulates or retards motivation in individuals and groups is well beyond the scope of this chapter; however, we can briefly establish that motivation is related to personal, social, and psychological factors. The amount of dissatisfaction one feels (a personal factor), for example, can motivate change; the amount of motivation aroused depends to some degree on the optimism (a psychological factor) one has that taking action will relieve the dissatisfaction.

Perceived crises, that is, significant problems needing quick resolution, can prompt or subdue motivation. They can also influence commitment in a power contest. If one sees that the perception of crisis will stimulate motivation or subdue resistance among supporters, it might be wise to describe problems in crisis proportion in order to persuade quick action. Problems in health care have existed for decades, yet only when recent national goals focused on the "crisis" in health care, did we witness a mushrooming bureaucracy to plan for, and coordinate, change.

In contrast, when a short time horizon overwhelms people, thereby threatening to dilute motivation, "actual time" and "perceived time" can be manipulated to offer hope. For example, one may assume a grant deadline is inflexible and make a decision to withhold proposal development for a later submission date. There might be, however, enormous leeway if foundation personnel become interested in helping.

Time that is actually rigidly set can also be stretched through sound planning. People often set objectives that are too grandiose and all-encompassing for a given time period; but, if these are subdivided, more realistic, attainable goals emerge. The achievement of a set of goals raises hope and commitment for the next phase by offering positive reinforcement.

Any successful change process requires that specific tasks be articulated and responsibility for them be designated in advance. What has been said about time and motivation can also be applied to time and resource acquisition. For example, in a crisis when time is limited, resources may flow from unanticipated sources, such as when a family is affected by a serious problem. It is common for help to come from neighbors, relatives, and friends who were previously uninvolved. The same mobilization of resources can occur with power resources. Power potential may be vastly expanded because of the need for brief but intensive action.

The dynamics of motivation in a brief time horizon can also be restricting to the participation of individuals and their resources if they fear that failure is imminent and that their efforts will be futile. As with motivation, power contenders may overcome the fear of failure and stimulate resource acquisition by expanding the time frame or by seeming to stretch a rigid one. The aim is to convince people that action is indeed feasible.

Put more simply, *perceived time* may not be the same as *real time*. People sometimes misjudge the time required to perform a task — usually underestimating what can be accomplished within a certain amount of time. An individual or group must manipulate circumstances, including the time horizon, to maximize the power potential.

Clear objectives and established criteria for what a group considers successful are fundamental in order to motivate and mobilize for change. Unclear expectations about the aims sought and about how to measure success deprives a challenging interest group of the "lifts" that clarity of purpose and procedures can bring. These lifts are stimulants for motivation of members and the resources they have to offer and, as such, translate into power.

CONCLUSION

It is appropriate and necessary for nurses to engage in guiding the future of American health care. However, if they intervene without the requisite skills for managing conflict and change, their attempts to control processes they do not understand will be ineffective. This chapter introduces the complexities of social power to prepare nurses for the responsibilities of planning change with others. Theoretical considerations are presented along with practical examples of how to contribute productively to the change process. The key factors enhancing and depleting effects on power for attaining desired goals are motivation, resistance, and capacity as well as the social context and the time horizon. As described, these factors affect power as weather conditions affect the sailing of a boat. That is, the skipper must have a specific destination always in mind; but wind shifts, currents (tides), and natural land formations may require a certain amount of tacking back and forth. In planning for change, one needs to know the destination (goal) chosen, but deliberate, incremental sidesteps may be required to reach it. Just as the skipper tests for wind conditions, a nurse must test for resistance. As the skipper manipulates the angles of a sail and weight distribution of the boat, one must manipulate motivation, power resources, judgments, and time to achieve one's goals.

REFERENCES

Abramson E, Cutler HA, Kautz RW, and Mendelson M. Social power and commitment: a theoretical statement. Am Sociol Rev 1958; 23:15.

Alford RR. Health care politics. Chicago: University of Chicago Press, 1975.

Dahl R. The analysis of influence. In: Adrion C, et. al. Social science and community action. East Lansing: Michigan State University, 1960.

Dangzer H. Community power structure. Am Social Rev 1964; 29:707.

Etzioni A. The active society. New York: Free Press, 1968.

Milio N. Care of health in communities: access for outcasts. New York: Macmillan, 1975.

Piven FF, and Cloward RA. Poor peoples' movements. New York: Pantheon, 1977.

Warren DI. Power, visibility and conformity in formal organizations. Am Sociol Rev 1968; 33:951.

LEGISLATION AND POLICY

10

Barbara E. Hanley

INTRODUCTION

Politics: The Route to Professional Status

Political participation provides the key for nursing's achievement of professional status. Over the past century, nursing's advancement toward this goal has been characterized primarily by activities to improve the quality of patient care. While concerns such as professional ethics, quality assurance, and continuing education are indeed of value, professional autonomy — the hallmark of a profession through which comes the power of self-regulation — will be acquired by nursing practice only through participation in the political process. The health care system is shaped by political decisions and subsequent policies. Recognition of nursing and its unique contributions to the system will take place only if nurses ensure its inclusion.

Community health nursing contains a rich tradition of community leadership in social movements on clients' behalf, and yet nurses frequently do not identify their activities as political. The current national climate of fiscal constraint and conservatism will challenge the political ingenuity of nurses to effect innovations in both clinical practice and agency policy and function. For community health nurses, this means survival and development of programs as well as preservation of jobs.

The purposes of this chapter are twofold: (a) to provide a sound conceptual framework for political involvement and ideas for implementation and (b) to provide a review of the legal basis for practice and the roles of state and federal legislation and regulation.

Politics as Role for Community Health Nursing

Incorporation of political involvement as an integral element of the community health nursing role can be viewed as the challenge of the eighties. The decade of the seventies was a time of consciousness raising when nursing became aware of its potential power and began to educate its members. It also heralded the start of an era in which baccalaureate education would be required for entry into professional nursing practice. In nursing as in other professional

fields there is a positive relationship between education and political participation. Academic education provides both the necessary reasoning and communication skills as well as the opportunity for political participation (Hanley
1983).

The effectiveness of academic settings as political training grounds depends
upon faculty and their ability to both serve as role models of the politically
involved nurse and provide opportunities for students to participate in political
activities. The role that university-affiliated faculty and students took in the
recent lobbying for funding of nursing education and research bears witness
to the potential of the university as a successful mobilizing center for political
activity. Certainly the successful results of lobbying by faculty and students
alike increase the likelihood of further political activity to eventually attain other
goals, such as direct third-party reimbursement, enactment of legislation for
development of community nursing centers, and changes in Medicare reimbursement criteria to include nurse-initiated interventions for home care. Thus,
the university should provide the base for initiating the prospective nurse into
the need for political involvement and the conceptual framework for political
activity.

CONCEPTUAL FRAMEWORK

This section presents a conceptual framework for community health nursing
involvement in politics. The key concepts in the framework are nursing expertise, political/legal boundaries of practice, policy decision-making process,
and action strategy (Fig. 10.1). Before discussing these terms, however, we
turn to the definition of politics as used in this chapter.

Definition of Politics

It would hardly be an exaggeration to say that our lives are surrounded and
shaped by political decisions. Current nursing literature exudes references to
"the politics of nursing." The media are replete with references to the "politics
of power," the "politics of health care delivery," "foreign politics," "state politics," etc., etc. Definitions of politics are as numerous as there are readers of
this chapter. Distinctions are therefore essential to enable us to build a framework for political involvement.

Most broadly, Deutsch (1965) describes politics as dealing ". . . with the
organized effort of society to change the probability of outcomes. In this sense,
politics is always the study of *Power* . . . particularly the study of the power
of any society over its own fate." A political system may be defined as any
persistent pattern of human relationships that involves power, rule or authority. Political systems therefore include not only formal government, but
the pattern of human relationships which influence its decision making." A

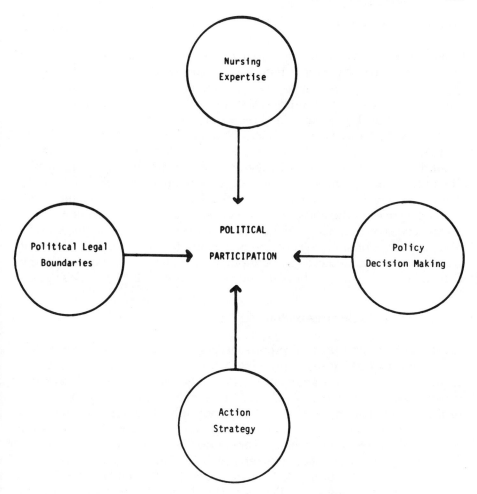

Figure 10.1.   Conceptual components of political involvement

more workable definition of politics might then be "[a] process by which decisions about governmental outcomes are made" (Milbrath 1976). A definition of politics on a secondary level might comprise the actions of individuals, interest groups, and classes on their own behalf and in relation to each other through the wielding of power and/or authority.

Both levels are relevant to community health nurses. The first level may affect legislative or regulatory decisions on the scope of practice, licensure requirements, or funding levels available for community health agencies and programs within which a community health nurse may wish to work. The second level of politics could encompass decisions within a particular employment setting on how workloads will be assigned and what the appropriate lines of authority will be.

Professional Expertise

Consciousness of one's nursing expertise is an essential quality for community health nurses participation at both the primary or secondary political levels. Awareness of one's competence is essential to professional autonomy. It is also the core from which community health nurses must approach all political systems: institutional, legislative, and regulatory on federal and state levels.

Far too often nurses fail to recognize that their basic competence for practice coupled with solid clinical experience and various modes of continuing education has yielded professional expertise. Nurses are the experts in nursing. The unfortunate devaluation of nursing accompanying the label of "women's work" has led to some nurses' low self-image and resultant failure to take leadership roles in the decisions determining when, where, and how nursing care will be given. Nursing experts must provide the direction for the evolution of their profession and practice. Accountability to the consumer implies vital collaboration, communication, and input from interested and involved parties. Others may offer support but only nurse experts can speak for nursing.

Political/Legal Boundaries of Practice

Involvement in any political process necessitates awareness of the political/ legal context. This means knowledge of the laws, regulations, and policies within which decisions are made. Community health nurses in practice are constrained by a number of political/legal considerations. An understanding of the bounds placed by these factors is not only an essential component of conceptualizing the role of a nursing care provider, but is also an important prerequisite to political activity. A community health nurse planning a career and concurrent practice should therefore consider factors such as these: federal regulations (e.g., Medicare); federal legislation (e.g., Rural Health Clinic, National Health Planning, and Resource Development Acts); state legislation (e.g., dealing with nurse practice acts, continuing education, expanded practice, third-party reimbursement, public health and local health ordinances). Regulations accompanying laws also carry the weight of law and should be taken into account. At the institutional level, practice parameters include institutional policy and job descriptions.

An overview of these areas can provide a political assessment tool to determine the extent of freedom for innovation in a particular practice setting. It also provides a base of information from which activities to bring about desired change can be planned.

Policy Decision Making

Within each political system lie both formal and informal decision-making mechanisms. Thus, institutional administration, state and federal legislative and regulatory bodies, and health-planning agencies all possess written and unwritten codes or processes for decision making. It is important to differentiate formal organization as a "planned structure representing . . . patterned relationships among participants in the organization" from the informal "relationships which occur spontaneously out of the activities and interactions of members of the organization" (Longest 1975). Longest (1975), in his work on this area, states that "the key to institutional policies is an understanding of the basics of informal organization and how it affects the formal authority relationships inherent in the [hospital's] formal organizational pattern."

Thus, the small group networks and their resultant dynamics provide the arena and the groundwork for key decisions. The importance of knowledge about informal networks in each sphere must not be underestimated. Corridor conversation among groups within the executive, mid-management, and staff levels — including cross-communication — may result in decision prior to the planned meeting. The open committee, board, or staff meeting or legislative hearing may provide the trappings of the process, it may be after the fact. Nurse members must therefore be aware of and involved in both levels of the system.

Action Strategy

All of the concepts outlined to this point would be meaningless without an action strategy. A community health nurse must have a plan of action — identifying the issues where there is motivation for action, political assessment of the situation, and selection of a goal, the development of a support base, and a course of action to most effectively use resources to accomplish that goal. An action strategy should incorporate all of the concepts presented thus far. Professional expertise and a knowledge of political/legal constraints enable the community health nurse to understand the situation and the factors causing it. An understanding of the decision-making process facilitates the choice of action. The development of a support base provides the resources to carry out these activities.

The following portion of this chapter provides some guidelines on developing a course of action to most effectively use resources to accomplish a goal.

ACTION STRATEGY FOR POLITICAL INVOLVEMENT

An action strategy for political involvement is made up of four phases:

1. Motivation for action on issues
2. Political assessment
3. Developing a support base
4. Action

Keep in mind that each of these phases can be modified to fit into the institutional, local, state, or national political settings.

Motivation for Action on Issues

How important an issue is to an individual is a key motivational factor in whether or not he or she will become politically involved. The community health nurse's role, full of such salient concerns, provides an excellent situation for political activity. Virtually any experience in community health nursing increases the awareness of the influence of health policy, whether local, state, or federal, on practice. For example, the current climate of economic conservatism has caused reductions in programs. The implication of this event for community health nurses has been twofold: first, a loss in patient services; second, a loss in employment opportunities due to elimination of positions. Hence, the community health nurse's perception of health policy as directly affecting both the client advocate role and individual economic well-being serves as a motivational factor for political participation. For the community health nurse, salient issues abound.

1. Keep issue narrowly focused and defined.
2. Include nonessential element as a "negotiating" option.
3. Remember that change will be best achieved in small steps.

Political Assessment

This phase involves critical assessment of all actors involved — that is, administrators, legislators, committee chair and members, and staff who serve in supportive roles to the actors. Given the goal is to provide information to and thereby gain the support of the policy maker, learning as much as possible about the policy maker will help create an effective case. Factors to consider are

1. What is the nature of the policy maker's power and influence? (e.g., ranking or nonranking minority? Does he or she chair the group? Who among the members is interested in the issue?)
2. What is the best approach route? (e.g., who is a close contact of the chair? Is it better to approach a staff person for help in gaining access? Would a letter or making an appointment be effective?).
3. What is the individual or group's history of support for health or nursing issues? Find out by checking existing policy, voting records, and deliberations on related issues that may provide clues.
4. More generally, are party politics involved? If so, which group dominates? What is the affiliation of supporters of each side of the issue involved? Is

the atmosphere open, conducive to change, supportive of the nursing position?

5.   What are the positions of other professional and health related groups (such as the AMA, American Hospital Association, of insurance companies, etc.? (are they supportive, neutral, opposed?)

Developing a Support Base

Integral to achieving goals in any political system is the development of a support base. In any endeavor for change, one person alone accomplishes little. Social action theory identifies organization as an essential step for political mobilization, with consciousness that an inequitable situation exists serving as a key intervening variable catalyzing the process (Klein 1980).

Support from Nurse Colleagues

Consciousness refers to an awareness that an inequitable situation exists and that political activity provides a viable means for change. Mary Kelly Mullane (1976) in Politics Begins at Work discusses the notion of a "critical mass," a small number of committed individuals who actively participate in a political endeavor to achieve goals. The size of the critical mass varies according to the setting — from one to two in a small, executive-level committee to a half dozen in an agency or institution to a dozen coordinating a nationwide mobilization effort aimed at attaining congressional support for major legislation. Support bases are built, not discovered. The development of the support base is a key endeavor for the nurse change agent. A logical first step is to identify nurse co-workers or local colleagues supportive of your goals — in other words, to work toward a critical mass.

Professional Organizations

Policy change on any level beyond a specific institution requires the support of formal organizations. With their extensive legislative and policy-making networks, specialty nursing organizations and, more specifically, the professional nursing organization are of critical importance here. Membership in and coordination of effort with the appropriate level of the American Nurses Association (district, state, or national) take on major significance. Similarly, activity through the Public Health Nursing Section of the American Public Health Association may provide nationwide nursing support. These organizational endeavors, as well as individual nurse interactions with legislators, serve to educate the policy makers on the role of the nurse in health care, to underline the specific health problems in each respective district, and to provide the nursing perspective on solutions to these problems. Communication of this nature increases the likelihood of support for nursing when key legislative and policy decisions are being made or when opportunities for relevant committee positions arise.

Non-Nurse Support

Nursing needs to do more to develop what Freidson (1970) terms a "strategic elite," a cadre of influential supporters outside of nursing who will in time of need exert influences in behalf of nursing. Relationships with local legislators, health planners, local businessmen, news writers and editors, and other community and state decision makers should be fostered. Similarly, clients and health consumer groups, when informed of the issues, can lend needed weight to a cause. Closely related to the development of a strategic elite is the building of a coalition. *Coalition building* for a support base can be very effective, yet often difficult because of the breadth of issues facing groups. It is therefore best to concentrate on a single issue, focusing the appeal upon the nature of the group approached. Thus because of their health problems a senior citizens' group may respond to the importance of nursing services in a satellite clinic, while an influential local business would be concerned about cost effectiveness and keeping workers on the job.

Media

Media coverage of nursing issues and events is a vital aspect of support. Letters to the editor provide an excellent forum for airing of health policy concerns and a means of presenting nurses' concerns to the public at large. Getting a local newspaper editor's support can be a major factor in obtaining the interest of legislators and policy makers, particularly in controversial situations.

A second means of going public with a policy concern is to issue press releases to all newspapers that serve a targeted audience. News editors can fit these in when space allows. They should always be provided with a name and phone number on the chance that additional information will be sought.

Feature writers are always looking for interesting material. New nurse roles, health service programs, and policy concerns fit this category, and the coverage helps develop a positive, accurate public image of nursing. Other media tools include appearances on TV and radio talk shows. Publicizing nursing roles, goals, concerns, and accomplishments will serve to inform the public and hopefully increase the likelihood of their support of nurse policy recommendations. All too often nurse roles in health movements such as home care, hospices, and health education either remain invisible or are prompted by other health providers.

In summary, a broad base of support is essential to build enough momentum for change. Four general principles serve as guidelines for developing broad support.

1. Organize nurse colleagues.
2. Work in conjunction with the professional organization and nurse specialty groups.
3. Build coalitions among consumer and other supportive groups.
4. Go public through newspapers, radio, TV

Action

Once policy goals have been established, necessary tasks should be outlined and delegated to subgroups. For example, if the goal is to persuade a state legislator, tasks might include

1. Planning letter-writing party.
2. Identifying and initiating media contacts (e.g., letters to the editor, press releases).
3. Developing a telephone tree for activating the group on short notice.
4. Planning a public information night, inviting the legislator.
5. Requesting endorsement letters from coalition members.

The group leader(s) will coordinate the endeavor and facilitate communication of information.

TYPES OF POLITICAL PARTICIPATION

Political activity can be viewed on a continuum of degrees of personal commitment (see Fig. 10.2). Successful experiences at the lower end, along with the perceived importance of the issues and of one's participation, encourage movement toward the upper end of the continuum. Once a problem and the decision-making structure involved have been identified, the community health nurse is ready to assess methods of communicating with — and participating in — the power structure.

Policy-making Politics

The first level of activity, policy-making politics, is embodied in the community health nurse as an outsider to the decision-making body who provides information. The simplest method of providing information is by writing letters to an appropriate authority. The more complex activity of directly meeting with and providing information to policy makers and their staff in an effort to gain their support is known as lobbying. For instance, the community health nurse may wish to explain to local health-planning officials the nursing view on a proposed cutback in nursing home beds, or brief a local representative of a state legislature on the need for a baccalaureate education as a minimum entry level requirement for an R.N. Further along the continuum, the community health nurse may choose to make a formal presentation of testimony before the appropriate decision-making body that is based upon a well-formulated rationale and molded by a sense of the power base and constituency for whom she or he speaks. At the local level, this body could be a Health Systems Agency board; at the state or national level, it could be the appropriate legislative body.

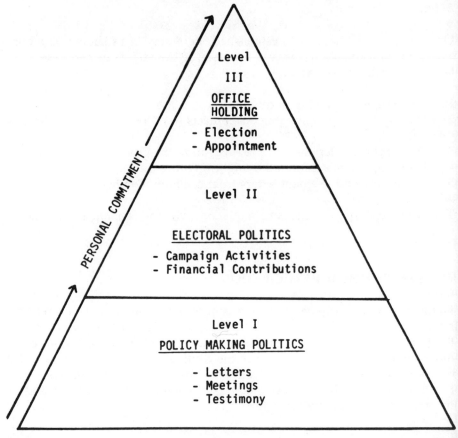

Figure 10.2.   Levels of political activity (applicable to institutional, local, state, or national spheres)

In short, the principles behind communicating with legislators can be summarized as follows.

1. Serve as an information resource to the policy maker.
2. Learn to negotiate, compromise.
3. Aim for incremental change; consider presentations to garner support.

Electoral Politics

A second level of activity available to the community health nurse is to become involved in electoral politics: influencing the election of members to decision-making bodies. The leap from policy making to electoral politics, its natural complement, is a short one. The types of activity included in this level are campaign oriented, such as volunteering time to send out mailings, hosting fund-raising events (e.g., cocktail parties, teas), or door-to-door canvassing for votes or financial contributions. Only recently has organized nursing moved into electoral politics, with the 1974 establishment of Nurses' Coalition for Action in Politics (N-CAP), the political action arm of the American Nurses Association, and the subsequent establishment of state-level counterparts.

Political action committees with their separate accounting mechanisms allow organized nursing to endorse as well as make financial contributions to supporters of nursing and health care. Decisions for endorsement are made on the basis of voting records and feedback from nurses on the quality of support provided by legislators and their staffs. Political action is therefore a means to ensure the election and re-election of legislators supportive of nursing's causes.

The Nurse Policy Maker

The ultimate level of political involvement for the community health nurse is membership in a decision-making body. The range of possibilities exist, extending from membership on a commission, committee, or board; to key staff positions in regulatory bodies (e.g., city, state, or federal health departments or legislative bodies); finally to running for local elected office (e.g., a school board, health officer, city council, or state or national office. Increasing though still small numbers of nurses are being elected to state legislatures and national commissions. Their potential effectiveness in roles as nurse–policy makers is perhaps best exemplified in the accomplishment of Marilyn Goldwater, R.N., Delegate, Maryland House of Delegates. Her sponsorship and support helped to eventually enact landmark legislation that provides for insurance reimbursement of nurse midwives and nurse practitioners in the state of Maryland. Several R.N.'s have served as congressional staff members. Nurse membership in Health Service Agencies (HSA) boards is growing. Indeed, with nurses' increasing perception of the importance and viability of the nurse–policy maker role, this trend marks the beginning of a future wave.

In summary, community health nurse practice for the future necessarily incorporates political participation on three levels: policy making, politics, and electoral politics and office holding. A nurse's discovery of an effective action level begins with these steps:

1. Conducting a community political assessment (see page 298).
2. Keeping abreast of health and professional policy issues via professional publications, memberships.
3. Joining a local political club; participating to the extent possible.
4. Initiating action on issues of concern (by following the action strategy discussed here or developing an individual plan).

5.   Noting references in the attached bibliography for more specific information on political participation.

LEGAL BASIS FOR PRACTICE

The second section of this chapter considers some legal and regulatory issues and their ramifications for nursing practice — both existing and potential. In their excellent work *Legal Accountability in the Nursing Process*, Murchison, Nichols, and Hanson (1978) encourage integration of legal concepts into the nurses' framework for practice. These authors view law as a dynamic force to support decision making and thereby strengthen autonomous practice. In development of such a framework, both statutory law and the common law of tort have a role.

Statutory law refers to the laws enacted by legislative bodies such as Congress or the state legislature. An important distinction in statutory law is that between consolidated and nonconsolidated law. The former term refers to the organized bodies of state or federal laws regulating health, education, labor, taxation, etc. Laws not falling within these specific bodies are termed nonconsolidated. Consolidated law is frequently implemented by a commissioner and a respective regulatory body. Regulations drafted by these bodies carry the weight of law. Nurse input to development of both legislation and regulations is of paramount importance, since sections may influence nursing.

The Nurse Practice Act is contained in that section of state consolidated law dealing with practice acts for the licensed professions. A view of the Nurse Practice Act in relation to the other practice acts is instructive. Nurses may gain access to the practice acts through contact with state legislators, the public library, or the state capital legislative library.

Implementation of statutory law is usually authorized to a commissioner and regulatory body such as the state department of health and the United States Department of Health and Human Services. Regulations drafted by these bodies carry the weight of law. Thus, nurse input to the legislative process cannot stop upon enactment of desired legislation; the implementation of new and existing legislation through the regulatory process remains a less publicized yet crucial avenue for system change.

The Department of Health and Human Services and most state agencies have a mechanism to publicize proposed regulations or changes in existing ones and allow a formal period for public response or testimony. Copies of proposed regulation changes are available to interested parties on request. Depending on the magnitude of the proposed change, there is variation in mechanisms for public response. For major change, public hearings are often held in which interested individuals or groups may present testimony. However, such opportunities are often late in the process and may be of limited value because the respective agency and governmental officials or staff may have already conducted extensive investigation into the issue. Similarly, regulatory bodies may make "emergency rulings," thereby skirting the usual public notification and response period. Such was the case in 1976 when the New York State Commissioner of Health signed the regulation which enabled physicians' assistants to prescribe any medications with the exception of controlled substances, despite the opposition of legislators, legislative staff and organized nursing. Input from nursing experts relating to current health and practice issues is essential for the development of quality health policy.

Nurse membership on state health policy committees or task forces offers several advantages. It provides the opportunity to participate in agency policy discussions and to develop allies within agencies and related state organizations who may be supportive of nursing's position. Further, such membership facilitates learning the informal network behind agency decision making. Communicating one's interest in membership with either local legislators or those on key committees may be useful in obtaining such membership. All ANA constituent nurses' associations and many specialty nursing organizations have legislative and other programs already involved in health policy negotiations. Coordination of health policy activity with the professional nursing organization has high priority because of the need to coordinate activities, share information and present a united nursing position on issues.

The *common law of tort*, or decisional law, is that body of law established by courts when they rule on cases brought before them. Statutory law, particularly in the form of the state nurse practice acts' definitions of nursing practice, outlines what nurses may do. Common law, created by court cases of neglect or malpractice, analyzes what the nurse did do, and through the doctrine of precedent, establishes law to govern future conduct. Legal authority for practice thus finds its source in both statutory and tort or common law (Murchison et al. 1978).

Tort law deals with deviant behavior that leads to injury or property damage to another individual, whether intentional or unintentional. Its intent is to restore equality between the involved parties through a financial compensation. Professional malpractice or negligence cases therefore are included here. Murchison et al. (1978, 42) use the terms interchangeably, defining them as "the failure of a professional person to act in accordance with the prevalent professional standards or failure to foresee possibilities and consequences that a professional person, having the necessary skill and training to act professionally, should foresee."

A key principle of tort law is that every person is responsible for the torts he or she commits. For nurses, therefore, the presence of physicians' orders or protocols will not remove legal liability. Although there has been an increase in litigation against nurses, there has also been an increase in the number of nurses held *solely* responsible; in high technology roles — e.g., nurse anesthetists, nurse practitioners, emergency room nurses, and critical care nurses — indicating that nurses have undertaken more risk as well as responsibility. (Sheeran 1979).

The concept of legal liability or responsibility must be integrated throughout the nursing process:

Assessment of the client's status involves establishment of the nurse client relationship and recognition of the nurse's basic legal responsibility for his well being, in interaction with the client, his family, other care providers and institutional policy;

Nursing clinical judgment will include recognition of only those actions within the scope of his or her ability and legal constraints;

The decision to act or not to act is based on one's legal duty as identified through consideration of professional standards and institutional policies;

The nursing action undertaken must be consistent with that of professional nursing colleagues;

Evaluation of the client's response to the nursing action must include legal consideration for the quality of care given to the client, with a long term goal of improving client care (Murchison et al, 1978).

Accurate and thorough documentation of one's rationale through each phase of the process is essential for both protection of the nurse in the case of litigation and, more positively, as an evaluation tool for quality nursing care with precedent setting value for the future (Gelb and Palley, 1979).

Unprofessional conduct includes both personal and professional dereliction of an ethical, moral or legal nature. Examples include negligence in nursing practice, the knowing or unknowing misrepresentation of clinical competence (although a client may not have been injured), or of performing acts beyond the scope of practice as defined in the nurse practice act. Examples of the laws' positive influence are the current cases establishing precedent in "compatable worth" wage disputes as well as in cases of alleged "practice of medicine" by nurse practitioners. For the latter, strong definitions of nursing practice serve as an umbrella for the growth of nursing practice.

Judgment in malpractice cases is based on the "prevalent professional standard of care" in the given region. Keeping abreast of standards of care, as developed by the professional organization and attending continuing education programs, will therefore serve to decrease the likelihood of litigation. The most basic precaution, however, is the maintenance of positive nurse-client interactions. Litigation tends to occur in situations of poor provider-client communication.

To reiterate the points made within this section:

1. Be familiar with applicable laws and regulations; incorporate them into a plan of action.
2. Maintain clinical competence through continuing education.
3. Maintain positive nurse-client relationships.
4. Be aware of clients' rights; obtain their informed consent.
5. Carry professional malpractice insurance.
6. Follow proposed changes in legislation regulations and participate in the process.

Table 10.1   From Idea to Law

Legislative Process	Action Input
I. Introduction of bill	Bring ideas for legislation for sponsorship to legislator (Possible as individual, better as organization)
II. Bill assigned to appropriate committee/ subcommittee for action Committee role is research, public input in the form of hearings	Key stage for letters, visits, testimony from nurses, their organizational support and coalitions
III. Bill reported from subcommittee/ committee to full house for floor debate, vote	Letters, mailgrams, visits, especially to uncommitted legislators to win their support
If passed by both houses, bill moves to governor/president for action (Congress and some state legislatures have a conference committee with representatives from both houses to iron out any differences in language of the bill form passed.)	Work with staff of conference committee (between houses) if one is called to resolve differences
IV. Executive action Governor or president signs the bill into law or vetoes it. Veto can be overridden by ⅔ vote in both houses.	Extensive input to the executive from governmental agencies and interest groups supporting or opposing the bill

Law: Direct Versus Indirect Influence on Practice

Law influences nursing both directly and indirectly. State nurse practice acts are the best example of direct effect legislation. Each state defines the practice of nursing, legal title, and requirements for licensure within its jurisdiction. The authority for interpretation of and enforcement of the nurse practice act is delegated to the state Board of Nursing. Regulations for practice as defined by the board thus carry the weight of law and form a vital part of a nurse's legal framework.

Examples of legislation that indirectly affect nursing are found in the fields of education, health, insurance, and labor. Policy developed in these areas, while possibly not directly addressed to nursing, may have crucial ramifications for nursing's practice and future evolution. This principle is best exemplified by insurance legislation, which determines eligibility for direct insurance reimbursement for health services. Although it does not directly state whether or not a nurse can develop a private practice, by controlling access to monies of third-party payors, it effectively sets limits on the practice undertaken by nurses. Another cogent example is the legal basis on which pharmacists fill prescriptions. If pharmacists are only allowed by law to fill the prescriptions of authorized physicians, a prohibition against primary care nurses writing prescriptions becomes redundant. The legal/regulatory realm is therefore a dynamic arena in which decisions in the broad areas of education, health, and insurance will either directly or indirectly shape the health care industry — and the practice of community health nursing.

State-Level Laws and Regulations

States provide both statutes and regulations that define the scope of nursing practice in each state. This section covers some of the most prominent forms of state-level activity and illustrates the applicability of the conceptual framework previously presented.

Nurse Practice Acts

Nurse practice acts are the best example of direct effect legislation. The purpose of nurse practice acts is twofold: (a) they protect the public welfare by ensuring that nurse health care providers have attained a minimum level of competency to practice, and (b) they protect the profession by restricting the title and practice of the profession to those who have met specified criteria.

Review of the history of the evolution of nurse practice acts reveals three distinct phases of nurse licensure. The first phase from 1900 to 1938 was characterized by permissive licensure whereby the title "graduate or trained" nurse was reserved for those licensed as such; others could practice nursing for hire but could not use that title. The mandatory licensure phase for those practicing nursing for hire began in 1938 and continued until 1971. The third phase, currently in effect, has been characterized by revisions in nurse practice acts to extend definitions of nursing practice to reflect expanding roles of nurses. As of spring 1978, nearly every state had made some attempt to deal with this major issue.

To understand the problems faced in this third phase, one must view the nurse practice acts in the context of all health practice acts. The first nurse practice legislation was enacted in 1903 and within 20 years all states had some form of permissive licensure. However, medical practice legislation had been enacted in all states by 1895. As the first to legally define its practice, medicine preempted all acts it deemed appropriate. Medicine therefore assumed exclusive control of the gate-keeper functions of diagnosis, prescription, and treatment (Murchison et al. 1978). All other health occupations have been forced to define their practice so as not to interfere or overlap with the practice of medicine.

Viewed in this context, the nature of nursing's problems becomes clear. Despite nursing's demonstrated competence to cost effectively provide essential health care services, which may include some gate-keeper functions, legislative and regulatory prohibitions serve as an obstruction. The crux of the expanded role issue is whether a nurse, by performing functions involving diagnosis and treatment, is practicing within the scope of nursing or encroaching upon medicine's domain. The ANA, in fact, suggested the original disclaimer for nurse practice acts against nurses performing any diagnostic or prescription acts. This action has been interpreted by Bullough (1976) as a kind of anticipatory self-discrimination — a response often seen in ghetto populations and here found in the nursing profession. At the time that the disclaimer was suggested in 1955, there was no real pressure from the medical profession for the role of nursing to be thus defined.

In a study of state boards' attempts to resolve this issue, the Trandel-Kovenchuks (1978) have identified three approaches. The *nonamendment approach* essentially favors a more liberal interpretation of the statute or a slight modification; the *authorization approach* recognizes nursing's expanded role through specific changes in the state's statute; and the *administration approach* allows nurses to perform expanded functions as authorized by the professional licensing boards through various mechanisms.

However, in their 1978 review of state nurse practice acts, the Trandel-Kovenchuks disturbingly identified clear trends toward defining nursing practice in terms of physician involvement and supervision of expanded nursing practice. Indications for this trend include (a) the determination and promulgations of rules and regulations by joint medical and nursing boards, (b) the requirement for use of protocols, and (c) the necessity of a written agreement between the physician(s) and the nurse regarding the details of the supervision of the nurse that is submitted to the Board of Nursing (p. 41). This trend, although related to the underlying issues of reimbursement for additive versus substitutive care raises the question of whether or not nurses are moving closer to their goal of professional autonomy.

Nurses involved in these state legislative and regulatory issues are cautioned to

1. Use general language — the more specific, the less room for future evolution, which is occurring in all health provider roles.
2. Avoid use of the term *supervision*; substitute with terms such as *collaboration*.
3. Avoid descriptive titles; use "professional nurse" as consistently as possible.

As the knowledge explosion continues, more and more of what is incorporated into "expanded practice" will be incorporated into generic nursing preparation. Hastily drafted restrictive legislation and regulations portend an even more restrictive future. In summary, nurses interested in expanding their role through legislation should

1.   Participate in the policy process, utilizing the framework from the first section of this chapter.
2.   Be reticent to introduce or support enactment of legislation that has potential for future restriction.
3.   Resist being forced into hasty policy making by medical influence, which is often strong in regulatory agencies.

Nursing Education
Sharing the limelight with expanding nursing practice as a major legislative concern of the decade is the issue of basic educational preparation for entry into practice. At this time the issue continues to be debated on its merits across the country. States such as New York have spearheaded the movement, while and others (e.g., Pennsylvania, Ohio, and Wisconsin) have developed models for implementation. Unfortunately, the resultant foment has served to divide the nursing community, thus dissipating its scarce resources of energy and money.

Integral to the subject matter of this chapter, yet frequently overlooked, are two key points:

1.   The initial socialization of nursing students to a sense of power and ability to change the system must take place within an academic environment.
2.   Although nurses and nurse administrators recognize the difference in the capacity of nurses based on educational preparation and experience, the public will continue to view the products of 2-, 3-, and 4-year programs similarly because nurse practice acts make no distinctions.

Therefore, until the issue is resolved with a baccalaureate seen as entry level preparation for the practice of professional nursing and practice acts are appropriately amended, initial socialization of nurses will continue to be inappropriate and scarce funds from both federal and state sources will continue to be dissipated in support of a nonsystem.

Less controversial now, though still of concern (as it is frequently misunderstood in itself or confused with entry to practice) is mandatory continuing education. Essentially, mandatory continuing education is a key concept in the current trend toward accountability to consumers. Health care providers will thereby increasingly validate to consumers their competency, in a health care system in which a knowledge turnover occurs every five years, by participation in an approved continuing education mechanism to re-register their licenses.

Nursing's endeavors to develop systems initially of voluntary and then mandatory continuing education have been. Each state has some voluntary system of continuing education in process, while legislative endeavors are underway in many states to make them mandatory. Further, the ANA has developed a nationwide program (Continuing Education Approval + Recognition Program) with the acronym CEARP to ensure a uniform system wherein continuing education units (CEUs) are transferable and records interchangeable across the country. Within this system, contact hours, which are 50 minutes of class time, are the unit of measurement; and ten contact hours equal one CEU. Although some states allow the recognition of CEU for varying forms of educational activities, not all of these may be transferable. Overall, however, a uniform system is well underway.

Insurance Reimbursement

Access to third party reimbursement is a major indicator of professional autonomy level as it determines practice options. As nursing specialization increased rapidly in the early seventies, state nurse associations initiated legislative activity to obtain insurance reimbursement.

Although ANA had advocated inclusion of nurses among reimbursable providers since 1948, the first success was in 1973 when nurses in the state of Washington became eligible for disability insurance payment. Then in 1979 New Mexico and Utah obtained reimbursement for nurse midwives and Maryland and Oregon enacted legislation covering both nurse midwives and practitioners. Recent ANA data reveals that as of June 1983, a total of thirteen states have nurse reimbursement legislation: nine cover nurse midwives including Alaska, Maryland, Montana, New Jersey, New Mexico, New York, Pennsylvania, West Virginia and Utah; and four cover nurse practitioners — Maryland, Montana, Mississippi and Oregon (McCarty 1983). Only California covers psychiatric nurse specialists while West Virginia covers primary health care nursing services which are defined as "non-salaried registered nurses in private practice, nurse midwives and midwives" (McCarty 1983, p. 1). Since 1981 in Washington state, R.N.'s are reimbursed if, when acting within the scope of their licenses they provide a service covered by the contract when performed by a physician (McCarty 1983).

The reimbursement of nurse services is therefore limited to their substitutability for physicians services. Given the atmosphere of fiscal austerity, further advances will be made based only on the cost-effectiveness of nurse services in direct competition with higher priced physician services. Fagin (1982) noted that increased visibility of nursing reimbursement at the state level was impeded by state law, regulations and nurse practice act interpretation. She then emphasized the precedent-setting value of including nurse services as a competitive force for lower cost, high quality health care in proposals for federal legislation and regulation.

State Regulatory Bodies

State regulations, as noted earlier, carry the weight of law. Knowledge of which bodies make which regulations is, therefore, of great importance. The regulation of most agencies will have indirect effect upon nursing.

Charged with implementation of the relevant nurse practice act, the role of the state board for nursing has direct impact on nursing practice. The state board functions as a state administrative body usually appointed by the governor. Within the framework of protection of the public welfare, its responsibilities include the licensing of nursing practitioners and the overseeing of nursing education programs via the processes of accreditation and registration. Both processes are based on minimum standards of safety and competency — in distinction from voluntary professional programs for certification of practitioners and accreditation of programs, which are based on excellence. More specifically, the state board functions include minimum program standards, registering programs, conducting licensing, reviewing infractions of the nurse practice act, and revoking or suspending licenses (Stahl 1974). It should be noted that it is within the jurisdiction of the board of revoke or suspend licenses, but actual prosecution of cases is undertaken by other agencies.

Membership on the state board is predominantly registered nurses, with state variation ranging from all registered nurses to a combination of registered nurses, licensed practical nurses, and other health professionals. A number of trends characterize membership on state boards, one being the expansion of the number of non-nursing health professionals on boards, a second the inclusion of consumers. While both of these developments undoubtedly promote a fuller understanding of nursing and give nursing members access to other perspectives on issues, they must be evaluated in light of the nature of board functions. So long as boards continue to control educational standards, acceptance of applicants for license, and disciplinary measures over existing nursing personnel, it is essential that nursing maintain controlling membership on its boards. Otherwise nursing would be relinquishing control over its profession, a step not to be taken lightly. This same point applies to a third suggested development concerning state boards: the abolition of individual boards for professional groups and their replacement by amalgam boards to govern all health professionals. Membership on these proposed boards would consist of consumers or state employees.

In most states, there is a mechanism by which proposed changes in regulations are formally announced. Copies of such changes are available to interested parties. Depending on the magnitude of the proposed change, mechanisms vary for public response. For major change, public hearings are often — though not necessarily — held in which involved parties may offer testimony. At least there is a theoretically reasonable time period in which the public may respond. However, because state regulatory agencies may sometimes have their own agendas inconsistent with nursing's interest, it behooves nurses to offer their services as committee or task force members. Such participation is essential to ensuring nurse involvement in the development of regulatory policy. It is also a key way in which to develop allies within the agencies who can be invaluable to nurses in learning the informal network of agency-planning decision making.

Federal-Level Laws and Regulations

While definition and regulation of nursing practice and licensure are within the purview of the state, federal legislation also influences nursing in the following ways: first, it sets a critical precedent for the development of state legislation. Second, it shapes federal health programs. Several of the chapters in this book comment upon the increasing involvement of the federal government in health care financing and delivery over the past two decades. Such governmental expansion has repercussions on the practice of all health providers. This is particularly true since the federal government has become a prime financer of health care delivery. By determining which providers can be reimbursed, government regulations effectively limit or expand the practice of professionals — particularly nurses. It is therefore critical that the federal government recognize the full scope of practice of the community health nurse as a legitimate health care role reimbursable under federal programs.

This section presents several examples of federal legislation with direct and indirect effects on nursing.

Nurse Training Acts

Perhaps the type of federal legislation having the most direct effect upon nursing practice has been the funding of nursing education. Federal subsidy of nursing education, although originating in the 1940s, became critical to nursing with the enactment of the Nurse Training Act of 1964. With the passage of subsequent bills, subsidies to nursing expanded to include monies for activities such as research. The nurse training acts have played an important role historically in the development of community health nurse programs. Since 1956, the nurse training acts have provided a source of funds for Master's programs, research, and financing study of community health nursing in the senior year. Thus, the expansion of study in the field of community health is strongly linked to funding levels of nurse training acts.

Federal funding for nursing education peaked in 1972–73 and has since then declined. Given community health nursing's dependence upon government funds, this is of great significance. The most dramatic attempt at a federal change in policy toward funding occurred in 1978, when President Jimmy Carter not only vetoed a bill for continued funding, but attempted to rescind all the then current support for nursing programs with the exception of those for advanced training. The attempt was unsuccussful because of the immediate political mobilization of nurses. The episode taught nurses the critical political lesson of being legislatively aware and involved in order to protect essential programs; and the outcome manifested their potential political effectiveness.

Rural Health Clinic Services Act of 1977

The Rural Health Clinic Services Act (RHCSA) was passed on December 13, 1977 with the explicit purpose of providing medical services in areas with an insufficient number of physicians. The RHCSA amends sections of the Medicare and Medicaid laws to allow for expanded reimbursement of nurse practitioner as well as physician assistant services. Historically, Medicare has covered medical and other health services apart from the hospital and skilled nursing facility services in the second section of its provisions. That section provided a strict definition of reimbursable "medical and other health services," which included

1. physician's services.
2. services incident to a physician's services that are without charge or included in the physician's bill.
3. outpatient hospital services incident to a physician's bill.
4. diagnostic outpatient hospital services.
5. outpatient physical therapy services.

Nurse practitioner services were thereby excluded from reimbursement, unless incident to physician services and included in the bill. Under the RHCSA, nurse practitioner and physician assistant services are reimburseable under specified conditions. These include that the services must be provided under the medical supervision of a physician, must be legally permitted to be performed by a nurse practitioner by the state in which the clinic is located, and must be in accordance with any medical orders of a physician. In addition, the reimbursable services must include services that would be covered if they had been provided by a physician. Finally, the rural health center, not the nurse practitioner, is reimbursed for the services. The nurse practitioner must be employed by or compensated by the clinic to be reimbursed.

Limitation of reimbursable nurse practitioner services under the rural health act has important implications. First, as the law adresses only medically oriented nursing acts, recognition of the nurse practitioner role is limited to that of a physician extender. Recognition of the unique importance of nursing functions through reimbursement remains beyond reach. Second, the needs of the community as client remain beyond its scope. This failure to provide for community diagnosis in isolated rural areas is serious because they frequently lack resources essential to health care delivery. Absence of a thorough assessment of a community's health needs and resources makes development of a functional plan to provide essential and comprehensive health services extremely difficult.

The failure of the RHCSA to reflect a comprehensive health care philosophy demonstrates the more basic failure of the United States to develop a national health care policy. Thus, although the National Health Planning and Resource Development Act of 1974 (PL93-641) provided national impetus and a framework for efficient use of present health resources and collaborative planning toward the evolution of a comprehensive, yet cost effective health care system, this philosophy is conspicuously absent in the rural health clinic act.

Despite these limitations, the rural health clinics act remains the first federal step recognizing payment for the practice of nursing in expanded roles. Further, its reimbursement restrictions may not be as formidable as they appear. The "supervision" requirement can be met by a physician's periodic review of the nurse practitioner's records. Although the physician does not have to be on-site, there must a physician on-call for consultation and emergencies.

National Health Planning and Resources Development Act of 1974

Encompassing a more broadly defined view of the health care system, this act (Public Law 93–641) recognizes preventative as well as illness care. It has provided a national impetus and framework for efficient use of present health resources and collaborative planning toward the evolution of a meaningful and cost effective health care system. Espousing a regional concept for provision of health services, it is philosophically closer to the community health view of community as client. Neither the Comprehensive Health Planning Law nor regional medical programs of the 1960s had a regional focus.

The work unit and key avenue for local and regional health care decisions under P.L. 93–641 is the Health Systems Agency (HSA). Law requires the HSA boards to comprise 60 percent consumers and 40 percent care providers. Two important implications follow: first, the consumer predominance establishes a natural base from which nurses can launch a social action movement; second, nurse membership as providers on the board increases the likelihood of public awareness of nursing roles and their inclusion as vital components of cost-effective quality health care delivery. To date, however, evidence demonstrates a general lack of nurse involvement. Health, Education and Welfare data from May 1979 show that nursing is dramatically under-represented proportionately in the mandated 40 percent health provider membership. In an effort to identify the existence of institutional impediments to nurse participation in HSAs, an exploratory study was done on the six HSAs of North Carolina. Findings indicated the variation in nurse participation levels was evenly distributed: low (2), medium (2), and high (2). Receptivity of the agency staff to nurse participation, however, was uniformly high. While these findings are preliminary and a larger study must be conducted to test for significance, there is a strong suggestion of discrepancy between nurse participation and receptivity of such involvement (Landsberger and Hutter 1980). Also, presumably, when nurses accept this role and become involved in HSAs, they will be accepted.

Although state planning activities have suffered severe cutbacks in recent years, they remain a functional arena for community health nurse input.

Diagnostic Related Groups

The prospective reimbursement system for diagnostic related groups (DRGs) in hospitals through Medicare marks the beginning of another new era in health care. Within the next few years, the system is expected to extend to nursing homes and ultimately to home health care. While visiting nurse services have effectively costed out home care services, Mundinger (1983) in her recent study identified a discrepancy between the types of home care services needed by clients and those ordered by physicians on hospital discharge. The resulting dilemma is that the services rendered differ from those ordered, while the necessary nursing services are not reimbursible. This situation reflects the need for further research documenting the cost effectiveness of nursing services actually provided so that these services will be continued when home care nursing budgets undergo increasing scrutiny required in prospective reimbursement systems.

Community Nursing Centers
Federal legislation has been introduced to develop community nursing centers (CNCs) through existing visiting nurse associations and health department structures, as well as newly established practice units. The purpose of the CNCs is to provide nursing services in an independent ambulatory setting to keep clients from institutionalization in hospitals or nursing homes. Although if successful the CNCs would prevent costly institutionalization, budget office opponents to the bill cite the increase of costs because of the new clients eligible to use this service who are neither hospitalized nor using services now. This proposed program as defined holds a unique opportunity for community health nurses to demonstrate a nursing-based cost effective alternative to the traditional medical system. Further, this program is consistent with a prospective payment system. Enactment, however, will require a concerted lobby effort utilizing principles outlined in Table 10.1.

SUMMARY

Excellent works exist on the legislative and regulatory processes; and courses are being developed on nurse roles in these areas. Readers are referred to these for additional information. Getting involved, however, through direct or indirect roles in local or state health planning agencies, private corporations, and legislative or regulatory bodies as staff, legislators, or lawyers, remains the most important step toward political power.

Responsibility for development of a profession rests with those who practice it. Accurate representation of issues that need legislative action can only come from within the profession itself. Community health nursing is in a strong position to take charge of its destiny by joining the political arena in behalf of itself and the public. Understanding the means for doing so is the obligation of each nurse leader as well as the discipline as a whole. The framework and review of legal basis for practice, state and federal legislation, and regulation presented here provides the background for knowledgeable entry into the political arena.

REFERENCES

Bullough B. The law and the expanding nursing role. Am J Public Health 1976; 63(3):

Deutch KW. On political action and political theory. Am Pol Sci Rev 1965; 65:1.

Fagin CM. Nursing as an alternative to high cost care. AJN 1982; 1:56.

Freidson E. The profession of medicine. New York: Dodd, Mead, 1970.

Hanley BE. Nurse political participation: an in depth view and comparison with women teachers and engineers. Doctoral dissertation, University of Michigan 1983. University Microfilms.

Klein E. A social learning perspective on political mobilization: why the women's liberation movement happened when it did. Doctoral dissertation, The University of Michigan, 1980.

Landsberger BH, Hutter R. Some institutional factors promoting and impeding nurses' participation in HSAs: a study in one state. In: Nauger BL and Huggins K (eds). Abstracts in nursing research in the South. Vol. 1. Atlanta, GA: SREB, 1978.

Longest B. Institutional politics. J Nurs Adm 1975.

McCarty P. Nurses eligible for direct payment in thirteen states. The American Nurse 1983; 6:15.

Mullane MK. Politics begins at work. RN 1976; 39:7.

Milbrath LW. Political participation: how and why do people get involved in politics? Chicago: Rand-McNally, 1976.

Mundinger MO. Home care controversy. Aspen Systems, 1983.

Murchison I, Nichols T, Hanson R. Legal accountability in the nursing process. St. Louis: Mosby, 1978.

New York State Nurses Association. Third party reimbursement for non-institutional nursing service introduced. NYSNA Legislative Bulletin, April 10, 1980, p. 1.

Sheran P. Malpractice in nursing. The Michigan Nurse 1979; 10:8.

Stahl A. State boards of nursing: legal aspects. Nurs Clin NA 1974; 9:3.

Trandel-Kovenchuk D. Trandel-Korenchuk K. How states recognize advanced nursing practice. Nurs Outlook 1978; 26:11.

ECONOMY AND COST METHODS

11

Judith S. Warner

The community health nurse practices nursing in the broadest of possible senses. Clients of the community health nurse include the individual, the group or family, and the community. Practice settings range from home to health center to school or place of work. Patient care includes not only sick care but also prevention of illness and promotion and maintenance of the highest possible level of health and well-being. The community health nurse must function as an advocate for the patient to government agencies, individual health care providers, institutions, and community service organizations.

Employment settings within which the community health nurse can function include the home health agency, community service agency, health maintenance organization, school system, hospital, government health department, planning agency, or university. In each of these settings the role can vary from clinician to administrator to supervisor. But while the primary focus for the community health nurse is always, like that of other nurses, the health care of the client, the skills needed to accomplish this objective extend far beyond the traditional complement of nursing skills. One discipline in which the community health nurse should be well versed is that of economics and the general concepts of cost analysis and measurement.

Why Economics?

Every health care professional in the United States today must be concerned about rising health care costs. Governmental and nongovernmental actions occurring at local, state, and national levels to combat rising costs have already or will eventually impact upon all health care professionals.

Health care expenditures in this country have risen dramatically in recent years. In the 10-year period 1966–1976, total health care expenditures increased 235 percent ($42.1 billion to $141.0 billion) (Gibson and Fisher 1978). While it is true that expenditures for other goods and services have also been rising, the proportionate share of our nation's resources devoted to health care has been increasing. In 1966, 6.5 percent of this nation's output of goods and services, as measured by gross national product (GNP), were health related. By 1976, health-related activities accounted for 8.6 percent of GNP.

In itself, this trend toward relatively higher health care expenditures in the United States is not problematic if that is how Americans choose to spend their income. However, while the relative share of health care expenditures has been rising, so has the proportion of those expenditures financed by public funds. In 1966, only 25.7 percent of such expenditures were financed publicly; in 1976, public expenditures for health care accounted for 42.7 percent of total expenditures. The situation has thus developed where more money is being spent on health care services, but the proportion of money spent directly by private individuals has declined. The reason, of course, is the growth of public programs such as Medicare and Medicaid that finance health care for the aged, disabled, and poor. The significant point here is that Americans are faced with a situation where more of every dollar they earn is being spent on health care but a government which seems distant, unaware of, and unresponsive to their needs as *they* see them is determining how and how much of this money is to be spent.

This situation has prompted critical response from the public on the appropriateness of the government's spending for health care programs. Much of their questioning is directed toward legislators who are faced simultaneously with growing appropriation requests for financing and providing health care services and demands for cutbacks in public spending. Legislators have attempted to restrain rising costs through stricter budget review procedures and regulatory actions such as the National Health Planning and Resources Development Act of 1975 (42 U.S.C. 300).

These actions have many implications for both consumers and providers of health care services. There is considerable debate on all sides about what impact these restraint measures will ultimately have upon the quality, availability, and cost of health care services. The public's concern over rising health care costs, and more specifically, over rising public expenditures, is becoming a more vocal, hence political issue. Health care providers can expect to be affected to the extent that regulatory actions directly limit their practice. Further, this is of particular interest to community health nurses in that they are often employed in public agencies or agencies dependent upon public funds for operation.

Community health nurses in school systems, public health departments, and public planning agencies are usually directly and completely dependent upon government appropriations for funding of their positions. Those in voluntary health agencies may also find their positions dependent to varying degrees upon public monies. Studies in the Rochester, New York, area have shown that over 45 percent of voluntary health agency revenues come from local, state, or federal government sources (McMeekim 1976).

As administrators in such agencies community health nurses must be able to justify the staff's positions. As clinicians they should be able to demonstrate the effectiveness of their services. These justifications must often be addressed to financial analysts or policy makers who are not attuned to the nursing process, particularly the scope of community health nursing. Therefore, it is in the interest of community health nurses to be able to *explain* and *justify* professional concerns in the vernacular of the decision maker. The ability to accomplish this depends upon an understanding of economics and knowledge of the tools and techniques of this discipline to determine and evaluate the costs of a program or service, and to demonstrate its value.

This ability is valuable not only in publicly supported programs but is also an invaluable tool for community health nurses in other employment settings. In private health clinics, home health agencies, or other such settings community health nurses may similarly be faced with having to justify their services relative to alternative allocations of resources by their employers.

Another reason why community health nurses should be concerned with economics and cost analysis relates to their role as patient advocates. In this capacity community health nurses attempt to mobilize the patient's resources for self-help and to coordinate any other available services. The community health nurse is accountable to the patient for facilitating the best health care possible. This responsibility includes evaluating what community services are available to the patient, whether they are being used effectively, and what new services are justifiable. Any such program or service assessment should include a cost analysis and statement of the overall economic impact of a proposal for new services. The community health nurse should be capable of analyzing not only community health nurse–initiated proposals for change but also the proposals of other health care providers, planning agencies, and regulatory bodies that wish to alter the mix and number of services in the community health nurse's practice area.

The objective of this chapter is twofold: (a) to familiarize community health nurses with the basic principles of economics and (b) to arm them with a working knowledge of cost-benefit and cost-effectiveness analyses. The former are very general in nature and applicable in many settings. The latter are usually, to the surprise of most people, simple to perform; and although broader, more complicated applications are possible, the community health nurse will be able to handle the basics with little trouble.

PRINCIPLES OF ECONOMICS

We are all familiar with the concept of scarcity. It is a fact that all working individuals face each payday as they decide how to spend their earnings for food, clothing, housing, and everything else they wish to purchase. There is never enough money for everything, so priorities must be set. Relative values must be assigned to a new television set, a vacation, or a car insurance payment.

Community health nurse program administrators are equally familiar with the phenomenon of scarcity. Instead of formulating a household budget, they must decide among alternative program services. They must set priorities and decide on the relative value of more home health visits versus expanded physical therapy schedules and other alternatives.

On an even broader scale, society at large must deal with the reality of scarcity. During time of war, we often hear the "guns versus butter" argument. A country cannot produce sufficient military equipment for war and also continue to produce a high level of goods for private consumption. The problem is one of having limited *resources* available for producing goods and services.

The purpose of economic theory is to deal with this problem of scarcity. Economics recognizes that society has limited resources and that decisions must be made on what it will produce with them. Economic theory analyzes how these decisions are made under different cultural or political assumptions. For example, one would not expect decisions on the quantity of health services to be produced in a year to be made in the same way in the Soviet Union or Great Britain as in the United States.

By understanding the decision-making process in terms of the allocation of resources for production one is able to analyze the probable outcomes of a particular decision: Who will benefit and who will suffer as a result? For example, if the budget for a school health program is cut in half, what will be the immediate effects in terms of employment, student health, and attendance? What will be the long-term effects upon the labor market as school nurses compete for other positions? How will the community's health status be affected if children are less strictly monitored for immunizations? While economics certainly cannot predict the future, it can forecast what can be expected to happen given differing assumptions.

In order to understand how an economist views the production of health services, it is necessary to introduce and define the basic terminology of economics.

Factors of Production

Economists classify the resources that can contribute to the production of a good or service into three types: land, labor and capital. These are called factors of production. *Land* and *labor* need no further definition. *Capital* represents the machinery and physical plants that are necessary for production. In the health care field, hospital facilities, x-ray equipment, and ambulances are all examples of capital equipment. In addition, it is recognized that expertise is necessary to organize the factors of production to produce a service and this is called *entrepreneurship*. A person is viewed as an entrepreneur when he or she establishes a business rather than, for example, choosing to work for another person.

In order to attract each factor of production into service it is, of course, necessary to pay for it. The monetary returns on each factor of production are called respectively *rent* (land), *wages* (labor), and *interest* (capital); the return to the entrepreneur is called *profit* (Wonnacott and Wonnacott 1979; Samuelson 1980; Waud 1980). Without these returns, the factors of production would not be available to produce goods and services. Consider this example: Nurse practitioners represent a type of labor. In return for offering this labor to produce a service, nurse practitioners receive a salary from their employers.

It is possible for a person to perform two functions. Nurse practitioners in private practice would be such an illustration. These persons would represent both labor and entrepreneurial talent. They should expect an income from their practice that would reimburse them both for their labor and their entrepreneurial functions. Otherwise, there would be no financial incentive for these practitioners to remain in private practice.

Industries are often characterized by the relative amount of the factors of production used by them. Agriculture is seen as land intensive. Health care is usually characterized as labor intensive. This is particularly true in the production of nursing services. For example, a recent operating budget for a county health department in New York State (1980) reported 80.4 percent of the nursing program's expenditures in salaries, overtime, and benefits.

Product and Factor Markets

Most simply, in the United States, the decision on what combinations of factors of production should be used to produce what goods and services takes place in a free market system. Two types of markets exist: product markets and factor markets. Product markets are those in which entrepreneurs offer goods and services to consumers and it is decided how much of these will be produced. For example, how many nursing services will be produced in the United States? Factor markets are those in which factors are offered to produce these goods and services and it is decided how much of each factor will be used. For example, how many nurses will be employed to produce the nursing services in this country? The two markets are closely related. The number of nurses employed depends on the amount of nursing services demanded by consumers. At the same time, the amount of nursing services available in the product market is constrained by the number of nurses available in the factor market.

Within this context, the community health nurse offers labor in the factor market and receives a wage. Within a product market the community health nurses employer (or the nurse if functioning as an entrepreneur in private practice) offers nursing services and is reimbursed for these services (either directly through fees, or indirectly through tax revenues budgeted for nursing services).

Market Structure

In order to analyze the basic principles at work in factor and product markets, economists typically construct a model wherein the assumption is made that buyers and sellers in the product and factor markets are unorganized. This model represents pure competition. It represents a world with no labor unions and no monopolists. It represents fiction.

The model of pure competition makes further assumptions. It assumes that each buyer and seller in a market is aware of price, that no discrimination among buyers or sellers exists, and that resources are perfectly mobile between different factor markets. These assumptions imply, for example, that consumers of health services are fully aware of price when they purchase a service such as hospital care; that consumers are free to purchase hospital services wherever they choose; and that factors of production in the health care field (e.g., physicians, dentists, and nurses) can easily move into other areas of employment. These assumptions are in striking contrast to the real world. Once the basic forces at work in a factor or product market are understood, the assumptions of pure competition can be lifted and the impact of monopoly, discrimination, immobility of resources, and other realities of the health care field can be analyzed.

Laws of Supply and Demand

The forces that affect decisions in the product and factor markets are *supply* and *demand*. Economists think of these as continuums along which varying quantities of a commodity are demanded and supplied at different prices. If one looked at the factor market for community health nurse services one could imagine two continuums:

1. Demand — this would represent how much community health nurse time employers would be willing to pay for at varying wage levels. One expects that at a relatively low wage employers would hire more nurses than at a higher wage. At a relatively high wage, an employer would tend to find other types of workers to substitute for community health nurses. A plotting of the demand by all employers for community health nurses could be shown on a graph as pictured in Figure 11.1(a)
2. Supply — this would represent how much time community health nurses would be willing to work at different wages. One expects that community health nurses would usually offer more time at higher wages than at lower ones. Higher wages could both draw more nurses into the labor market and increase the amount of hours each community health nurse would be willing to work. In Figure 11.1(b) a graph similar to that for demand shows the variations in supply of all community health nurse services at different wages.

It is possible to visualize similar demand and supply schedules for nursing services as a product. The demand by consumers for nursing services might be expected to be higher at lower prices and the supply of nursing services to consumers might be expected to rise as price increased. Figure 11.1(c) and 11.1(d) depict these schedules.

Much can be said about the slope of the curves in Figure 11.1. Economists refer to the *elasticity* of a curve, referring to the *responsiveness* of quantity sup-

Factor Markets

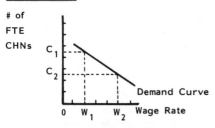

11-1a Demand for CHNs by Employers. At wage OW_1 an employer would demand OC_1, FTE CHNs. At the higher wage of OW_2, an Employer would only demand OC_2 FTEs. The employer would substitute less expensive personnel For CHNs at the higher rate.

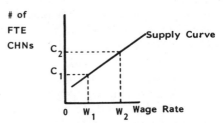

11-1b Supply of CHNs at Varying Wage Rates. At wage OW_1, CHNs would offer OC_1 of FTE CHN time to employers. If the wage rate increased to OW_2, more CHNs would be willing to work and those already working might increase hours they were willing to work. This would result in CHNs being willing to supply OC_2 of FTE CHN time.

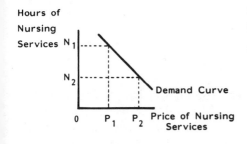

11-1c Demand for Nursing Services by Consumers. At a price of OP_1 consumers would demand ON_1 hours of nursing services. At the higher price of OP_2, they would only demand ON_2 hours of services.

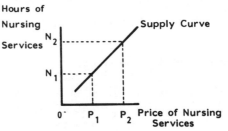

11-1d Supply of Nursing Services by Employers. At a price of OP_1, employers would be willing to supply ON_1 hours of nursing services to consumers. At a price of OP_2, they would be willing to supply ON_2 hours.

Figure 11.1. Demand and supply in factor and product market (FTE = full time equivalent.)

plied or demanded to a change in price. Several forces are at work in determining this elasticity. Most important of these is the *availability of substitutes*. For example, demand for health care services, particularly sick care services, is relatively inelastic because there is a limit to the effectiveness of substituting home or other alternative health remedies for professional care. Interestingly enough, however, one can see how the introduction of physicians' assistants and nurse practitioners who are capable of performing some physicians' services could increase the elasticity of demand for physicians' services.

The concept of elasticity is important in helping us forecast changes in supply and demand reflecting changes in price, both in factor and product markets. For instance, if there is a wage increase of a given magnitude and we know from other experience the approximate degree of responsiveness of the labor supply on the one hand, or employers' demand for such labor on the other, then we should be able to predict the impact that the wage change will actually have. The greater the response to the change, the more elastic the curve. Conversely, if the quantity demanded or supplied does not change appreciably, the curve is said to be inelastic.

Inelastic curves are presently more typical in the health care field, particularly in terms of demand for services. When people fall ill they wish to be seen by physicians regardless of the price. While their demand curve is not totally inelastic (i.e., the same at all prices) it is relatively so; faced with a doubling of medical costs and, say, beef prices, they are much more likely to become vegetarians than to risk their health. As noted above, however, the increasing availability of substitute health services is beginning to affect this traditional situation — with immediate implications for community health nurses.

Production Decisions

The major reason for being concerned with the laws of supply and demand and models such as pure competition is to understand how decisions are made to produce certain goods and services and not others. In pure competition, the decision maker on what or how much is produced is price. In any factor market or product market, supply and demand for a commodity interact until, at an equilibrium price, supply equals demand. If price is above an equilibrium point, there will be an excess of goods offered for sale; the market has produced more than consumers are willing to buy at that price and it will drop as the sellers compete with one another to sell their goods. As price drops, consumers will buy more but some sellers will begin withdrawing their products or services from the market because they are not getting a sufficient return on them. If the price drops even further and goes below the equilibrium level, there will be an excess demand for the goods or services, consumers will want to buy more than is available, and in competing with each other they will begin to bid up the price. This in turn will induce sellers to offer more for sale. These processes are depicted in Figure 11.2.

This very straightforward set of interactions shows price to be the determinant of what should be produced. The great economist Adam Smith referred to the market mechanism as the "invisible hand" determining production.

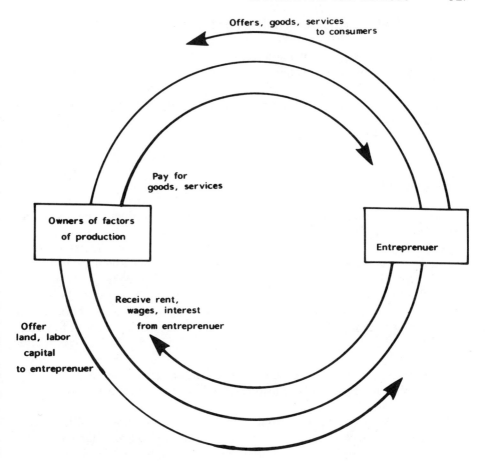

Figure 11.2.   Interrelationship between factor and product markets

Within this frame of reference, a student of economics can understand how producers of goods and services decide how much to supply. The major criterion is profit. Firms will not produce goods and offer them for sale unless they can earn a profit.

This begins to point up some of the problems that economists face in studying the forces determining the production of health care services. For instance, the very concept of profitability sounds strange in an industry where nonprofit firms are common and there is strong philosophical conviction that profit should *not* be a determining factor. Also, the relatively inelastic demand for health care is strikingly different from that for cars or television sets or even beef, where possession is not literally essential to well-being. Thus it is evident that the production of health care services in the United States is a very special case.

UNIQUE CHARACTERISTICS OF THE HEALTH CARE INDUSTRY

A number of economists have studied the health care industry. Herbert Klarman (1965), Victor Fuchs (1966), and Burton Weisbrod (1961) were among the forerunners in identifying those characteristics of the health care economy that make it unique. This section describes some of these unique features and serves as an introduction, for interested readers, to the more detailed discussions of these characteristics in the works of the above authors.

External Effects

Economists describe an *external effect* as the impact of another person's actions upon you. In the pure competition model price is left to decide how much of a particular kind of good is produced and who produces it. This is generally considered a satisfactory situation as one consumer's well-being is ordinarily not directly affected by how his other neighbor spends income. However, this is not the case for certain types of health services, particularly in the area of public health. It most definitely does affect a consumer if a neighbor fails to obtain proper immunizations or treatment of contagious diseases. It threatens the consumer's own well-being. The health care industry is thus categorized as one in which external effects are common and, as a result, these effects must be taken into consideration in the decision-making process determining how much of different kinds of health service must be produced and who will consume them.

Further, the existence of external effects creates a situation in which society decides that the open marketplace is not an appropriate mechanism for deciding upon the production and consumption of public health services. The decision whether or not to produce these services is taken out of the marketplace and put into the hands of the government representing the populace at large. Public health departments use monies appropriated through taxation to produce these services and offer them to the public. If a price is ever charged for a service such as a vaccination, it is generally only nominal and not intended to generate revenue to cover the full cost of the program. Even these minimal charges are often waived if the purchaser is unable to pay.

The alternative would be a private firm's offering public health services such as vaccinations to the public. It would purchase vaccine, employ public health nurses, and sell its "product" (i.e., immunization) in the marketplace at a price representing the balance of demand and supply. Anyone unwilling to purchase immunization at the market price would go unvaccinated and the public would suffer the potential cost of these carriers of polio, tuberculosis, etc. in its midst.

Due to the existence of external effects and the resulting justification for public health programs, community health nurses are often employed in government programs in which the benefits to the whole society leave room for little debate over the appropriateness of the government's intervention or subsidization. This, however, does not excuse community health nurses from accountability to the public for their performance or their particular programs. First, the community health nurses' duties in a public health department have varying degrees of external effects. Therefore, justification of tasks that benefit any individual client more than society at large are subject to challenge. Funding for these activities may be the first to be deleted in a budget review process. Second, even with traditional public health programs, budgets are not open ended. Pressure for restraint in government spending can, and increasingly does, affect even these programs. The result is a need to justify each program. In the example of a private firm involved in providing a vaccination program, the justification took place in the market. Services were provided to the point where demand equaled supply. Justification was automatic; the returns from producing the commodity covered the cost of producing the services, including a profit for the entrepreneur. Justification of appropriations for a public health program is not automatic for there is no marketplace. The mechanisms that have been developed to evaluate expenditure levels include cost-benefit and cost-effectiveness analysis, which will be discussed below.

The justification of public health programs in terms of external effects is generally accepted. The justification of government involvement in other kinds of health services on the basis of external effects is not as widely accepted. The argument for such intervention in personal health services recognizes an external effect related to psychic well-being. The consumer "feels better" if his neighbor receives the personal health services that the consumer thinks the neighbor should receive. This is typically stated as health care being a right: all people should have access to it regardless of ability to pay.

This argument opens a pandora's box. One obvious problem is defining the appropriate amount of personal health care. How much is a person entitled to, regardless of ability to pay? As the standard of living has risen in the United States, the definition of even the minimal amount of health care has expanded, and the cost of financing this care for those who cannot afford to pay requires an increasing governmental involvement in the health care system.

Another obvious problem is that the decision on how much to produce for whom is somewhat further removed from the marketplace. While suppliers of services may still be in the private sector, demand for their services is not comparable to the elastic demand curve for goods for which consumers must pay directly out of their pockets. Medicare and Medicaid have provided a seemingly open-ended source of funding for certain types of services. To suppliers, this has meant that all consumers can demand the same amount of services, at any price; because they are not paying for them directly. This eliminates the constraint upon production of health services that decreased demand at higher prices exerts in the private marketplace. It has led to a similar situation in the production of public health services, and here too some other mechanism for deciding upon amount of production must be found to replace the automatic mechanism of demand and supply in the marketplace. This search has led to such developments as new reimbursement techniques for hospital care and capital investment review procedures.

Consumer Information

One of the assumptions made in the ideal, purely competitive economic model is that perfect information is available to the consumer. This means that the consumer is fully aware of all the potential places where a service can be purchased, the relative quality of those services, and the prices at which they are sold by various producers.

This assumption quickly falls apart in the health care field: the consumer does not have perfect knowledge of available health services nor of their prices. Consider, for example, physicians' services. Physicians' fee schedules have not generally been available in the past because it has been considered unethical by the medical profession to advertise fees. In other types of markets advertising is a major source of product information for the consumer.

Equally or more difficult to obtain is information on the relative quality of various health services — and it may also be extremely costly to the consumer. Learning that a given store has sold you an imperfect dishwasher may be expensive and irksome, but usually remediable; quite different is the cost of discovering that an inadequately trained dentist has extracted a healthy tooth.

This entire problem of gathering and getting information on the quality of health care services is immense, and is an area in which the consumer may not be capable of meaningful judgments. Deducing poor workmanship in a dishwasher that will not work is fairly easy and straightforward; whether or not a patient dies, however, is not an indication of a physician's competency. Consequently the complexity and costliness of this problem have generally resulted in the consumer ceding responsibility for it either directly to the health care professional or to the government. Health care providers often decide for their patients what services they require and where they should obtain them. This is most often illustrated by the case of a physician advising a patient of the need for surgery and appropriate facilities for having it performed. It is seen also in the community health nurse's role as a patient advocate. Having assimilated all of the information on community services that are available to the client, the community health nurse then advises the client which should be considered. While the emphasis is on the patient's taking responsibility for the decision, the collection and assessment of information can be performed by the community health nurse.

Government involvement in this process of identifying competent suppliers of health care has traditionally been through its licensing functions. From an economic standpoint licensing, by restricting entry into a field, restricts supply and, as in the examples given previously, this interference with the normal economic forces creates an artificial situation. Economists continually debate the real nature of this situation and its effect upon health care delivery. Most studies have concentrated on the licensing of physicians, on which subject there are two schools of thought. One theory is that physicians and other professionals benefit from it because their supply has been sufficiently restricted to assure them excess profits. The second school of thought refutes the existence of excess profits for physicians through empirical evidence. It does not necessarily disagree that licensing can lead to excess profits, it simply holds that this has not occurred in the case of physicians (Lindsay and Leffler 1976).

What does this mean for the community health nurse? Licensing, no doubt, does restrict the entry into the field of professionals, or even institutions, when standards such as educational training or facility requirements have not been met. Licensure cannot be expected to ensure that all licensed professionals are equally competent, but it does provide some minimal safeguards. The community health nurse, as a patient advocate, still has a responsibility to gather information on the varying levels of quality of practitioners and services that a patient may use.

Perhaps more importantly though, the entire theory of licensing has a message for the community health nurse. There are strong theoretical grounds to support the contention that the licensing process can be subjugated by the licensees for their economic interest. When this occurs, licensing continues to protect the consumer against inadequately trained professionals, but it also acts against the consumer's interest by restricting supply and causing the prices of services to stabilize at a higher level than if freedom of entry and competition prevailed. It is important for the community health nurse to safeguard against this process in community health nursing. Restrictive entry measures in the name of quality control must be analyzed to assure that the supply of community health nurses or, at broader levels, nurse practitioners or registered nurses, is not so limited as to create a shortage. Entry controls should be counterbalanced with assurances of adequate openings in satisfactory programs to meet demand for services.

One last note on consumer information has to do with those incompetent professionals who still enter the system despite licensing safeguards. Identification of these practitioners cannot just be left to the marketplace; the price to be paid would be beyond monetary value. To avoid this unsatisfactory situation, professional boards exist to review questionable practices. Most professions have historically had an internal (self-policing) mechanism for review, but government involvement in this process has recently come about through the professional standards and review organizations established in a section of the Social Security amendments of 1972 (42 U.S.C. 1320(c)).

Uncertainty of Demand

Another unique characteristic of the health services industry is the uncertainty of demand by consumers for one of its products — illness care. Illness is unpredictable. Sickness is a potential threat, physically and financially, to us all, but an individual cannot predict with certainty the timing or extent of an illness. Statistically, however, predictions can be made for the entire populace, or large segments of it, and the economic response to this situation has been the pooling of resources through insurance to minimize the risks to any one person.

The impact of insurance upon the demand for health services is interesting. It was originally stated that demand varies according to how much a consumer (or aggregate of consumers) is willing to purchase at different prices. The higher the price the less a consumer is expected to be willing to purchase. Insurance coverage lowers the *effective price* of covered services to the consumer. The consumer can therefore be expected to demand more of the covered services than if he or she was paying the entire cost out-of-pocket. It is true that ultimately the cost is passed on to the consumer through premiums, but at the decision-making point the consumer acts on the basis of the lower effective price.

The existence of insurance not only lowers the effective price of a covered service relative to its true price; it also lowers the price of the covered service relative to uncovered services. This makes the uncovered services appear relatively more expensive than they actually are. This distortion illogically and inappropriately increases demand for covered services relative to uncovered services, leading to a maldistribution of health care resources that is not based upon true cost differentials.

This latter point is particularly critical to community health nurses in their roles as clinicians. In any case where the community health nurse provides a service that is not reimbursable under health insurance but that *would be* if provided by another type of clinician (e.g., physician or physician's assistant), the consumer pays an effectively higher price for the community health nurse's service. This restricts the ability of the nurse to "compete" with other health professionals in providing care. Growth in the utilization of community health nursing services may consequently be limited because of the distortion in relative prices to consumers. This emphasizes the importance of obtaining reimbursement approval for nurse clinician services under private and public health insurance programs. An indication of progress in this direction was the passage of the Rural Health Clinic Services Act of 1977 under which patients seeking services at rural clinics staffed by nurse practitioners without on-the-premise physician supervision can be reimbursed under Medicare. (42 U.S.C. 405.2401). However, this is an area in which community health nurses still have much to achieve.

Existence of Nonprofit Firms

Another characteristic of the health care field that deserves special attention is the existence of many nonprofit firms. One of the basic assumptions of economists is that all firms will base their production decisions upon expectation of earning profits on their output. It is this profit motive that encourages efficiency in businesses.

A number of studies have been made on how service levels are decided in the absence of a profit incentive (Jacobs 1974). Various theories exist. Hospital administrations are seen as attempting to maximize quantity of services in some models; in others, quality of services is maximized. Another alternative views the hospital as designed to serve the interests of those connected with it, i.e., physicians on staff, and that decisions within the hospital are made to serve special interest groups.

This situation is relevant to community health nurses primarily because of its impacts upon the environment within which they must practice. It may be of particular interst to community health nurses employed in hospitals in helping them understand some of the underlying rationale for policy decisions in those institutions.

Summary

The economist is concerned with the efficient production and optimal distribution of goods and services in a world of scarce resources. Analysis of production and distribution begins with a simple framework of pure competition and then proceeds to more complex market structures such as the world of health care. The economist's observations provide a unique and interesting perspective for community health nurses, enabling them to understand the factors that influence demand for and supply of services in the health care field — including their own. An understanding of these factors is essential to community health nurses as employees; as entrepreneurs, and as patient advocates, and the ability to explain and use this knowledge is vital to the growth and control of their profession.

METHODS OF COST EVALUATION

Economic theory has shown us that, in a world of scarce resources, their every use must be justified. In the purely competitive model we saw that this justification process takes place automatically in the marketplace. However, for many reasons, amount of health services to be provided in this country does not take place in a purely competitive market structure. Therefore, cost-evaluative procedures have been developed for assessing the appropriateness of output decisions.

Two evaluation procedures that have been developed are *cost-benefit* (C-B) and *cost effectiveness* (C-E) analysis. The remainder of this chapter discusses these two procedures. The terms C-B and C-E will not be interpreted in as strict a sense as they have been elsewhere. For example, as originally conceived, C-B was proposed to analyze questions from the perspective of the entire society. However, the same technique can be used for making evaluations from an employer's or an employee's standpoint. Similarly, C-B and C-E are most often applied to program evaluation; however, the techniques have other uses such as assisting an individual community health nurse in a decision on whether or not to invest in additional training.

Basically, the term C-B will be used to refer to methodologies in which *both the costs and the benefits* of a given action, program, or project are expressed in monetary terms and then compared. C-E will refer to analyses when *only the costs* of an action, program, or project are quantified monetarily. These costs are considered in conjunction with process or outcome variables.

Both C-B and C-E have certain data requirements in common when applied to program evaluation as well as each having unique requirements. The format in which data are available may influence the decision to use C-B, C-E, or neither. In an ideal situation, before budget reporting systems are set up, some thought is given to what evaluations will be required for the project or program. The community health nurse may be in a position to influence the format in which data are collected in an agency. For example, as an administrator, the community health nurse may be able to influence the form in which a budget is presented or information collected, suggesting methodologies that will facilitate later C-B or C-E analyses.

Often, though, the community health nurse will have to cope with analytical modes in which data are presented in an awkward format. This will most often be the case when nurses have to evaluate a program over which they have no direct control. In other cases evaluation questions are only raised after a reporting system has been initiated. The emphasis must then be on how the system or its output can be modified to fit the data requirements of C-B and C-E.

The ideal format for cost data collection for C-B or C-E is *program budgeting.* References for this approach appear at the end of this chapter (Levey and Loomba 1973; Hanlon 1974). In program budgeting, cost centers are identified for the various programs of an agency or department. For example, Hanlon illustrates the cost centers of a public health department as potentially including food protection, epidemiology, maternal health care, vital records, laboratories, public health nursing, and air pollution control. All costs for a program or activity are reported within a cost center. This would include personnel salaries and fringe benefits, equipment, supplies, travel, etc.

All costs can be categorized as *fixed* or *variable.* This differentiation should be kept cleanly in mind as it is most important for cost analyses. If the costs associated with a given activity fluctuate as the level of activity varies, then the cost is considered a variable cost. If costs do not change with activity levels, they are considered fixed. For example, as the number of home nursing visits increases in a public health nursing department, travel costs increase but rent or utility rates for department space do not. Travel would be considered a variable cost but rents and utilities would be fixed costs.

The importance of understanding fixed and variable costs is in deciding which costs should be included in an evaluation process. Generally, only the variable costs are considered in C-B or C-E. The classification into fixed and variable costs will depend upon the situation. For example, in evaluating the cost of more home health visits we have just seen that travel expenses are variable and rent is fixed. If, instead, we were evaluating adding an additional well-child care clinic site, rent would be a variable cost since adding a new clinic site would increase the rent paid by the public health department. Therefore it would be a relevant cost in the decision-making process.

The *relevance* of the cost is the important point. If cost records are maintained in great detail, it permits the isolation of the relevant costs. It is always possible to combine detailed costs for decisions that are broader in nature but not vice versa. For example, to evaluate a home health community nursing department, a community health nurse might need standard cost items such as salaries, benefits, employee reimbursement, and rent for the entire department's operations. However, if departmental records were not broken down for various programs within the department, the community health nurse could not respond to questions on the relative cost-effectiveness of different departmental services such as physical therapy field work versus hospital liaison activities. The greater the detail in a reporting system, the more flexibility it retains.

COST-BENEFIT ANALYSIS

As stated above cost-benefit analysis is a means of evaluating the uses of scarce resources when a purely competitive market does not exist. We have seen that it is often not in society's best interest to have production decisions in the health care field made in a private market, competitive or not.

In C-B analysis all of the costs of an action are compared to all of the benefits, and both costs and benefits are expressed in monetary terms. Traditionally the analysis was intended to be performed from the entire society's viewpoint. However, some economists have utilized the conceptual approach of C-B analysis for decisions where the costs and benefits to an individual are considered (Kushner 1974).

This section examines the tool of C-B analysis. C-B can be performed with varying degrees of sophistication depending upon the time, funds, and data available. The National Institute on Drug Abuse (NIDA) has provided an excellent example of a detailed cost-benefit analysis (Rufener et al. 1977a, 1977b). The objective of the NIDA study was to evaluate the cost versus benefits of its treatment programs over time. The discussions in this section will utilize the NIDA study to illustrate both the level of detail at which cost-benefit can be applied to a problem and how data can be abstracted from secondary material for simpler applications.

Definitions of Costs and Benefits

The first step in any cost-benefit analysis is to define the relevant costs and benefits to be measured in the study. There are four categories to be considered: direct and indirect costs, direct and indirect benefits.

The *direct costs* in C-B analysis represent the actual operating costs or cash outlays for the program or action being evaluated. It is important to consider whether or not one wishes to look at program costs in a given year or over a period of years. For example, in the NIDA study the costs of various drug treatment modalities were compared with the benefits of these modalities (elimination of drug abusers). The NIDA study estimated the direct costs per addict of each treatment modality over time. This involved a system of estimating operating costs per addict in each modality in one year and then estimating the number of years of treatment for each addict and their respective relapse rates.

In contrast, if one were evaluating programs in the United States in 1981 that facilitate the early detection of cancer, the direct costs would include the operating expenses in 1981 alone of programs to educate the public on cancer, plus screening tests. These costs would be based on budgetary information collected from cost centers relating to cancer in a myriad of health facilities across the country. In this case, a community health nurse would explore secondary sources of data such as the American Cancer Society. If the evaluation were limited to the nurse's area, as would more likely be the case, local agencies might be surveyed for actual program costs.

It is also possible that there may be some *indirect costs* associated with a program or action. If a person loses time from work to participate in an educational or screening program, there is an implicit cost to society. This implicit cost is the lost work time of the person and is measured by the earnings foregone by the program participant. These forgone earnings would be considered indirect costs of the program involved.

Indirect costs do not always exist. For instance, if a person attends a public education program on cancer detection in his or her free time, no work loss occurs: there is no indirect cost. Even if there are some indirect costs associated with a program, they may be very difficult to measure and thus are often excluded from C-B. The NIDA study did attempt to measure the indirect costs of the various treatment modalities. This was done by estimating the average yearly earnings of a drug abuser, the likelihood of the abuser being employed, and the amount of time the abuser would lose from work over the duration of the treatment program.

Benefits in the C-B analysis are also measured in terms of costs. The benefits of a program are the costs that are eliminated. Therefore, it is necessary to measure the direct and indirect economic costs of the disease or condition one is trying to alleviate in order to perform a cost-benefit analysis.

The direct costs of a disease would be the actual costs of treating the disease. The direct costs of cancer would include physician's costs, hospitalization costs, chemotherapy, radiation treatment, nursing home costs, family counseling, and any related expenses. In the case of drug abuse the direct costs, as estimated by NIDA, include not only the medical costs of treating drug addicts but also the other expenses to society caused by drug addicts, such as law enforcement and judicial system and correctional institution costs.

The process of estimating the direct cost of a disease such as cancer or a condition such as drug abuse is difficult. It is not something an individual community health nurse would undertake. However, much secondary data that can be useful in an analysis are available either from government sources or specialty societies such as the American Cancer Society.

Once an estimate of direct costs of a disease, etc. is available, it is necessary to decide how much of these costs might be eliminated through the program being evaluated. The amount of these reduced direct costs would be the *direct benefits* of the program. It may be extremely difficult to attribute reduced costs to a program, particularly if it is an educational program for the general public. Consider the problems of estimating the amount of cancer eliminated through cancer education. It is somewhat simpler in the case of treatment programs for diagnosed groups of patients. For example, in the NIDA study if the drug treatment programs rehabilitated every participant the direct benefit of the program would have been all of the costs of the drug abuse that would have been incurred by those abusers had they not been treated. Since a relapse rate was expected, the estimate of direct benefits was adjusted to account for this factor.

In order to estimate the *indirect benefits* of a program, it is necessary to know the indirect costs of a program or disease being treated. The indirect costs are again measured in terms of earnings lost to society. However, in this case the earnings are lost because of the disease or problem being addressed and not because of the program. For example, the indirect cost of cancer would be the productivity losses of persons with cancer. In the case of a cancer patient who receives treatment and returns to work full-time, the indirect cost in terms of productivity cost to society would be the time out of work and would be measured by the earnings lost while out of work. For patients who can only return to work part-time, the loss in productivity would be the total projected time lost over expected lifetimes as measured by loss of earnings. For cancer patients who die, the productivity loss would be the loss of earnings over what would have been their expected lifetime without cancer.

The indirect costs of drug abuse as measured in the NIDA study were earnings lost through unemployment caused by drug addiction, as well as earnings lost due to emergency room treatment, in-patient hospitalization, mental hospitalization, drug-related deaths, absenteeism, and incarceration. Any of these indirect costs that would be eliminated through a program would be considered indirect benefits of the program. All of the problems inherent in estimating direct benefits from direct costs also apply in this case.

Present Value and Discounting

If all of the direct and indirect costs and benefits of a program occurred in one year, or if the researcher were only interested in the impact of a program in one year, it would be relatively simple to compare costs and benefits. However, the benefits of a program such as cancer screening generally occur over a span of years. In such cases, it is necessary to discount the value of benefits enjoyed in the future to their present value.

Present value means the value to us now of a sum of money that will be earned in the future. We say that future earnings must be *discounted*. For example, $100 that will be earned next year is worth less than that to us now. What it is worth now depends upon the current interest rate. If the interest rate is 10%, the $100 is worth $90.90 to us at present since if we put $90.90 in the bank for one year it would yield $100.

Through discounting future earnings, we are trying to avoid overestimating costs. If a person died in 1981 who would have been expected to work two more years at $25,000 a year, the loss to society in 1981 is less than the $50,000 he would have earned. If one considered the indirect benefit of the program to save this man's life to be $50,000, one would be overestimating the benefits. The formula for discounting earnings is

$$PV = \frac{S}{(1 + r)^t}$$

where PV = present value of dollar to be received in the future
     S = amount of dollars to be received in the future
     r = discount rate
     t = number of years until money is received.

Methods of Comparison

There are several alternative means of analyzing the costs versus the benefits of a given decision. The most straightforward comparison is simply to calculate *net differences* between the costs and benefits in any given instance. For example, the costs of a cancer prevention program would be subtracted from its estimated benefits. If a community health nurse were comparing developing a cancer prevention program with other uses of funds, an array of net differences for each alternative use of the funds would be constructed. From an economic perspective, the best alternative would be the project with the highest numerical gain — where benefits exceed costs by the greatest amount. The advantage of the net difference method is that it keeps in perspective the actual dollar amounts involved.

Another method of expressing benefits versus costs is as a *rate of return* on an investment. If $50,000 were available in a budget for a new program and several alternative uses existed for the funds, one might estimate the expected benefits of each alternative. Assume alternative X's benefits were estimated at $40,000, alternative Y's equaled $60,000, and alternative Z's equaled $100,000. The rate of return in each case would equal the benefits divided by the costs. For alternative X, the rate of return would be 80 percent; for alternative Y, 120 percent; for alternative Z, 200 percent. In evaluating these options the community health nurse would generally find any rate above 100 percent acceptable and would rank those projects with the higher returns the better investments. It is important in this process to remember what rates of return represent in cost-benefit analysis. In financial markets, a return of even 10 percent on an investment may be acceptable because one invests money that one expects, with a given probability, to get back at the end of the investment period. This is not typically the case with projects in which the community health nurse may be involved. Fifty thousand dollars spent on a drug education program is never directly, entirely reclaimable. Therefore, one would hope to reap benefits at least equal to costs. To accomplish this, one must have a rate of return of at least 100 percent.

A third means of comparing costs and benefits is the *ratio method*. Continuing the example above of $50,000 available for a project and alternatives X, Y, Z having projected benefits of $40,000, $60,000, and $100,000 respectively, we can illustrate this technique. In each case, the ratio of benefits to costs is calculated.

Alternative X: Benefits : Costs
$40,000 : $50,000
0.8 : 1

Alternative Y: Benefits : Costs
$60,000 : $50,000
1.2 : 1

Alternative Z: Benefits : Costs
$100,000 : $50,000
2 : 1

Any ratio above 1:1 is acceptable in economic terms with the greatest ratio being preferred. This approach alleviates the problem of confusing acceptable rates of returns in financial market investments with acceptable returns in project evaluation.

Both the ratio and rate of return methods are criticized for abstracting from absolute values. They offer convenient summary methods for project presentations, but the dollar amounts involved should always be included. For example, one may be discussing different programs that all may be initiated in a given year. The ratios of benefits to costs of each program may be 2:1.

However, one program may entail costs of $500,000 with $1,000,000 in benefits, while a second program may only involve costs of $50,000 and benefits of $100,000. Obviously, the two programs cannot be evaluated as identical simply because they have similar cost-benefit ratios.

Alternative Perspectives

All of the examples to this point have concentrated on evaluating programs from society's point of view. The objective has been to see if the benefits to society exceed the costs. This is the traditional perspective for cost-benefit analysis. However, cost-benefit theory can also be used to analyze decisions from other perspectives such as those of the employer or the employee.

One such use that illustrates these different perspectives is evaluation of nurse practitioners in an area. From society's viewpoint, the costs of utilizing nurse practitioners includes the cost of their education, and even the loss in income that society experiences while registered nurses are enrolled in a nurse practitioner program. This last item reflects the fact that if practitioners were not enrolled in training programs, they would be holding productive jobs in society. Therefore, society loses the contribution of their output while they are in training. The benefits to society of having the nurse practitioners trained are their future contributions to productive output as measured by their earnings and the economic costs that are not incurred due to the preventive aspects of their practice. These benefits would depend upon the type of practice. For a community health nurse, the benefits might include lower morbidity rates due to better preventive health programs, savings in terms of reduced numbers of drug addicts, or reduced nursing home costs due to home care programs. As in any conventional cost-benefit analysis all of these measures would be translated into monetary terms.

Cost-benefit theory can also be used to evaluate the use of nurse practitioners from the perspective of an employer. The costs to the employer of utilizing a nurse practitioner would include all attendant expenses that the employer would not otherwise have. This includes items such as the nurse practitioner's salary, fringe benefits, additional office space, supplies, and telephone expense. The benefits from the employer's perspective would be additional income and/or free time that the employer has with the nurse practitioner in his or her employ. To maintain a nurse practitioner in a practice, an employer would minimally expect a benefit-to-cost ratio of greater than 1:1 or a rate of return of greater than 100%. In other words, benefits should exceed costs.

Cost-benefit analysis could also be used by an employer as a framework within which to make a decision on whether or not to invest in training an RN in expanded care skills. In this instance the costs to the employer would include items such as tuition costs and higher operating expenses both while the RN was enrolled in a program and after his or her return to the practice. Any projected costs over time would be discounted to their present value. The nature of these increased operating expenses would depend upon the individual situation. If the employer was hiring a temporary RN to assume duties while the original RN was in training and at the same time continuing to pay the original RN's salary, the temporary RN's salary would be considered a relevant cost. If upon completion of the program the original RN returns to the practice at a higher salary and assumes original duties plus additional tasks, the increase in salary would also be a relevant cost. All of the relevant costs would be compared to the benefits of having the RN with expanded care skills in the practice. These benefits would be the same as in the previous illustration: additional income and/or free time to the employer. The analysis of benefits versus costs would also parallel the previous illustration.

Cost-benefit theory can also be used by nurse practitioners by and for themselves to evaluate decisions on training. A community health nurse may be facing the question of investing in additional education. The costs to the nurse would be the direct expenditures incurred in the training, such as tuition, books and transportation, that would not otherwise occur. An indirect cost would be income lost while in training. This would represent the salary after taxes that the community health nurse would make if not in school; less any scholarships received. Utilizing the C-B framework, the community health nurse would compare these costs to the benefits received from training. These benefits would be measured by the expected increase in future earnings after the training. These future earnings would, of course, be discounted.

Several points are important in these applications. First, in deciding upon relevant costs and benefits, it is only those that are solely attributable to the person or project being evaluated which are included. Second, it cannot be stressed enough that this is a purely financial analysis. In the case of community health nurses evaluating whether or not to invest in further training, a good rate of financial return on the investment may be considered as relatively unimportant. However, it is still a consideration that they should be aware of, particularly if there is a considerable investment in time and money involved.

A further aspect of C-B analysis deriving from its being purely financial in nature is that only those factors that can be expressed in monetary values can be included as costs and benefits. In the case of the community health nurses deciding upon investing in additional training, the benefits were stated solely in terms of increased earning power. There can be many other benefits to them impossible to express in dollar amounts. How does one put a dollar value on the satisfaction they experience in being able to care for patients as advanced practitioners with advanced skills and methods? This same problem is inherent in measuring the indirect economic cost of a disease. The costs used in this section have measured losses to society in terms of productivity. This is appropriate within the general reference base of economics; where everything is analyzed in terms of its productive value. It is less than satisfactory from other perspectives (e.g., ethical and religious); no one can place a value on human life. Economists recognize this problem and are working upon alternative valuation procedures.

This point helps to clarify the role of cost-benefit analysis to the community health nurse. It is only one perspective. It provides one means of evaluating questions. Based upon society's current concerns with health care costs as outlined in the beginning of this chapter, it is an important perspective. However, it does not provide all the answers. As a final aid in understanding C-B analysis, the following problem summarizes a case example of C-B analysis utilizing secondary data sources such as NIDA.

PROBLEM

Community health nurses wish to evaluate the costs versus the benefits of a drug education program in their school system in 1980.

Step 1. Estimate Program Costs
  a. Direct program costs would be obtained from the operating budget of the program.

  Direct Costs = $250,000

  b. The community health nurses decide if there are any indirect costs associated with the drug education program and if they could be estimated. In a simple analysis, the presence of these costs could simply be noted and estimation ignored.

  Indirect Costs = $0

Step 2. Estimate Program Benefits

Since NIDA data are available on the costs to society of a drug abuser, a suggested approach would be to develop an outcome measure of the number of abusers eliminated under the program and multiply this by the appropriate cost figures.

  a. *Develop outcome measures*
  The community health nurses must estimate the number of drug abusers they hope to eliminate through the program. One approach might be to estimate how many of those exposed to their program may be turned away from drug abuse. Local expertise may be available to develop this estimate. Otherwise national data on prevalence could be combined with assumed effectiveness rates. Assume 2500 young adults are exposed to the program, 30 of whom are potential long-term abusers and 3 of whom will not become long-term abusers as a result of the program.

  Number of Drug Abusers Eliminated = 3

  b. *Estimate the economic cost of drug abuser to society over lifetime*
  The community health nurses must estimate the direct and indirect costs

of drug addicts. The best approach is to look for secondary data that can be used. In this case, NIDA data can be abstracted from their study for inclusion.

Direct Cost Per Abuser Per Year   = $10,000
Indirect Cost Per Abuser Per Year = 12,572
Total Cost Per Abuser Per Year   = $23,172

c. Calculate cost per year for all potential abusers in region who may be reoriented under program
These will be the direct and indirect benefits of the program.

Total cost per abuser × number of abusers = total cost per year
$23,172   ×   3   = $69,516

d. Estimate number of expected years of abuse of each estimated abuser. NIDA data show an average of 20 years of drug abuse per addict.
e. Calculate the present value of $69,516 a year for 20 years.
In order to do this, one would discount the $69,516 in cost of each year to the present. Using the formula for discounting mentioned in the section on present value and discounting, the present value would be $399,483.

Step 3.   Compare the Costs and Benefits of the Program

Costs = $250,000.00
Benefits = $399,483.35

a. Net Difference approach

Benefits − Costs = Net Difference
$399,483.35 − $250,000.00 = $149,483.35

b. Rate of Return approach

(Benefits ÷ Costs) × 100 = Rate of Return
($399,483 ÷ $250,000) × 100 = 159.8%

c. Ratio approach

Benefits:Costs
$399,483:250,000
1.6:1

Step 4.   Analysis

The benefits outweigh the costs of the project. Additional points that could be considered in evaluating the funding of the program are

a. The project would cost $250,000. What would be the benefit-to-cost ratios of other projects for which the $250,000 could be used?

b. The $399,483 in eliminated costs to society are incurred over the lifetime of the addicts. However, how much of this cost would actually have been borne by the community which is funding the project and how much would actually have been borne by later generations? Should only a portion of the costs be considered in estimating benefits? If an alternative project has the same net difference and rate of return as this project, yet all benefits accrue to the home community, might it not be preferable?

COST-EFFECTIVENESS ANALYSIS

Cost-effectiveness analysis can be a more flexible tool than C-B because the requirements for its use are not as difficult to meet. In C-B, both the costs and benefits of an action must be expressed in monetary terms. In C-E, only the costs of an action or program must be in financial terms. These costs are expressed instead on a per-unit basis in which the unit of measurement may either be a process measure such as number of visits or an outcome measure such as lessened morbidity.

Basic Approach

C-E analysis is process of evaluating alternative means to an objective. It consists of four basic steps.

1.   Definition of the objective.
2.   Measurement of costs and effects of alternative means of reaching the objective.
3.   Expression of costs on a per-unit basis.
4.   Comparison of results.

Statement of Objective
The initial step in conducting a C-E analysis is to define the objective or objectives of a program. They should be stated in measurable terms so that success or failure can be determined. It is important to define the *level* of success that will be considered an acceptable outcome of a program. For example, the objective of a program may be to decrease the number of pregnancies among unmarried teenage girls in a given geographic area. Prior to any program, the pregnancy rate of the target group may have been 100 per 1000 teenage girls. A reduction in the rate of pregnancy to 50 per 1000 teenage girls may be defined as a target for the program.

The objective does not necessarily have to be defined in terms of costs. In the above example, costs were not directly involved in the process of determining success or failure of a program. However, they can still be incorporated into the evaluation process.

Measurement of Costs and Effects
The second step in C-E is to *measure* the costs and effects of alternative means of reaching the objective. The costs are measured in the same way as in cost-benefit analysis and can be both direct and indirect. The direct costs are the operating expenses of the program. Salaries, training costs, supplies, rents that would not otherwise be expended, etc. are included. The indirect costs are any earnings forgone as a result of participation of the program under study. For a more detailed explanation of direct and indirect costs, refer to the discussion of them under C-B analysis, above.

Costs in C-E analysis are combined with some measure of the *effectiveness* of the program under study in meeting its objective. It is at this point that C-B and C-E differ. It is not necessary in C-E to devise estimates of the economic cost of the problem. For this reason, C-E is much easier to implement than C-B. For community health nurses attempting cost analyses independently C-E is preferable to C-B unless information such as the NIDA data discussed under C-B analysis is readily available.

Both process and outcome variables can be used in conjunction with costs in C-E analysis. The choice is dependent upon what is being evaluated and what data are available. The use of a process measure enables community health nurses to make statements about the effectiveness of one approach versus another as a delivery mechanism, while the use of outcome measures generally allows them to evaluate the impact of programs upon the health status of patients. For example, in the classic case of evaluating the cost-effectiveness of kidney dialysis versus transplants, the number of years of life gained under either alternative was used as the unit of measure (Committee on Chronic Kidney Disease 1967). More often, however, measuring outcomes is difficult and problematic; and as a result community health nurses may have no option but the use of process measures, such as number of visits or number of patients.

Process measures may be preferable to outcome measures when outcome is assumed constant under all circumstances. A study published by Sidney Garfield et al. (1976) illustrates this situation. An innovative Ambulatory Medical Care Delivery System was evaluated against a traditional system. The assumption was made that the outcome of medical care delivered under the two systems was constant; that is, patients received adequate treatment under either system. Given this condition a process measure, e.g., the number of patients, was utilized as the unit of measure for comparison of costs.

Expression of Costs on a Per-Unit Basis
The third step in C-E is to *express costs* in terms of the process or outcome measure selected. In this step, the costs of each alternative are presented in terms of the number of dollars expended per unit of outcome or process measure. In the example of programs to decrease unmarried teen pregnancies, the result of step three would be a list of alternatives expressed in average costs per decreased pregnancy which would be the result of dividing the costs of

alternative means of reducing pregnancies (e.g., alternative A, $5,000; alternative B, $7,500; alternative C, $8,000; and alternative D, $15,000) by the reduction in number of pregnancies under each alternative (A, 10 per year; B, 50 per year; C, 75 per year; and D, 90 per year). In this example the results work out to be $500 per pregnancy, $150 per pregnancy, $106 per pregnancy, and $166 per pregnancy, respectively.

Comparison of Results
The fourth step is to *compare* the results. The criterion for selecting the optimal result is generally to choose the least costly means of attaining the target level of the objective. In the case of alternative means of reducing the number of pregnancies, the least costly alternative within the target range of success is alternative C. This is not the most effective alternative in terms of number of pregnancies eliminated, but it was within the target level. The ultimate decision on which alternative to select would have to take into consideration whether or not the greater effectiveness of alternative D is worth the higher cost.

Role of Alternative

One of the most important prerequisites for cost-effectiveness analysis is that there must be relevant alternative programs or actions by which to measure. A description of one program in isolation is meaningless; *comparison* is the core of the concept. It is possible to make some comparisons to national averages. If, for instance, one were comparing the cost of physician visits in a rural group setting, it might be interesting to see how costs compare to the national average or the average cost per visit in nonmetropolitan areas. However, this tells the evaluator little about the value of continuing to fund a particular clinic. It would be of greater practical importance to know the cost per visit if a nurse practitioner was utilized or the cost per visit if the clinic was located elsewhere.

COST-EFFECTIVENESS VERSUS COST-BENEFIT ANALYSIS

It is impossible to conclude any discussion of C-E and C-B without a general comment on their relative value. Cost-effectiveness is most definitely the simpler of the two analyses to perform. As stated earlier, it is not necessary in cost-effectiveness to develop a dollar value for the benefits of a program. Therefore, it is recommended for community health nurses who wish to do cost analyses entirely on their own. However, it should be recognized that the use of process and outcome measures, even in conjunction with program costs, rather than benefits expressed in dollar values limits the applicability of cost-effectiveness.

With C-B it is possible to evaluate alternative uses of public funds with all costs and benefits expressed in the same terms — dollars. In C-E analysis, on the other hand, the cost of drug treatment programs may be expressed in terms of cost per rehabilitated abuser and the cost of a kidney dialysis project may be expressed in terms of cost per years of life gained. How can one compare cost per rehabilitated abuser with the cost for a year of life and come to a conclusion over the better use of funds? Obviously, one must have the common basis for comparison that is inherent in C-B (dollars), but not in C-E. Though C-B is cumbersome to utilize it is more universal in application. For the evaluation of any program involving a sizable expenditure it would be advisable for the community health nurse to explore the extent to which existing C-B data could be used in an analysis or to see if funds are available for the collection of such data by outside consultants in order to permit the making of proposals and decisions on an indisputable, factual basis. Community health nursing, like many other forms of health care, is largely motivated by altruism, but it exists in a world activated primarily by economics. Until community health nurses can understand, use, and explain these economics they will be limiting the extent to which they practice their own ideals.

REFERENCES

Committee on Chronic Kidney Disease. Report. Washington, DC: U.S. Government Printing Office, 1967.

Fuchs V. The contribution of health services to the American economy. Milbank Mem Fund Quart 1966; 44:65.

Garfield SR, Collen MF, Feldman R, Soghikian K, and Duncan J. Evaluation of an ambulatory medical care delivery system. N Engl J Med 1976; 294:426.

Gibson RM, and Fisher CR. National health expenditures, fiscal year 1977. Soc Sec Bull 1978; 41:3.

Hanlon, JJ. Public health administration and practice. 6th ed. St. Louis: Mosby, 1974.

Jacobs P. A survey of economic models of hospitals. Inquiry 1974; 11:83.

Klarman H. The economics of health. New York: Columbia University Press, 1965.

Kushner J. A benefit-cost analysis of nurse practitioner training. Can J Public Health 1974; 67:405.

Levey S, and Loomba NP. Health care administration: a managerial perspective. Philadelphia: Lippincott, 1973.

Lindsay C, and Leffler K. The market for medical care. In: Lindsay CM, ed. New directions in public health care. San Francisco: Institute of Contemporary Studies, 1976.

McMeekim S. Monroe County health care funds flow analysis—1974. Rochester, NY: University of Rochester School of Medicine, 1976.

Office of Management and Budget. Budget preparation report 112. Rochester, NY: County of Monroe, 1980.

Rufener BL, Rachal JV, and Cruze AM. Management effectiveness measures for NIDA drug abuse treatment programs. Volume I: Cost benefit analysis. Washington, DC: U.S. Government Printing Office, 1977a.

Rufener BL, Rachal JV, and Cruze AM. Management effectiveness measures for NIDA drug abuse treatment programs. Volume II: Costs to society of drug abuse. Washington, DC: U.S. Government Printing Office, 1977b.

Samuelson PA. Economics. 11th ed. New York: McGraw-Hill, 1980.

Weisbrod BA. Economics of public health. Philadelphia: University of Pennsylvania Press, 1961.

Waud R. Economics. New York: Harper & Row, 1980.

Wonnacott P, and Wonnacott R. Economics. New York: McGraw-Hill, 1979.

CHARGE FOR THE FUTURE

12

Judith A. Sullivan

In the mid-80s, community health nursing marks its one-hundredth anniversary in the United States. During its first 15 years the domain of practice was established and the concepts identified that were considered basic to this practice. Concepts such as simultaneous concern for the group, family, and individual, involvement of clients in self-care, attention to prevention, identification of major health issues, and the seeking out of those at risk remain the foundation of this practice today.

The circumstances surrounding this practice have varied markedly over the past century, rendering it at times prominent in developing policy as well as in implementing programs in health care, but at other times dormant in presenting new solutions to current problems. Examination of these different time periods can reveal the critical elements for a vital practice with voice in the policy-setting arena. This is the charge for the future.

Three factors stand out as co-requisites for professional vitality: the presence of a public mandate, the establishment of a base of power and influence, and a sound economic grounding. A public mandate develops from demand for a service coupled with perceived competency of the provider. In establishing its credibility and public support, each professional group must speak for itself. To the extent there is a match between demand and the components of service offered, there is likely to be public support — both direct and indirect.

As novel as it may have sounded in the 70s, the marketing of services has become a reality in the 80s. Not only are there competing providers of services, but the total pool of resources is smaller. Although these factors may seem threatening, precisely because of the community-oriented context of practice, community health nursing can argue for its high level of cost-effectiveness in raising the baseline of health in a community by seeking out those most likely to benefit from scarce resources.

In the presence of increased competition for a share of the health care dollar, therefore, community health nursing can increase the odds for success by marketing a service that carefully links the provision of care to the majority (demand) with a community-wide survey of need. Any legislator or insurance executive could perceive services developed in this way as the best return for an investment. Demand for a service that only a few need, however, can wither without a continuous effort to faster public awareness of those needs and the

349

methods available to meet them. Marketing methods are useful for building and maintaining a knowledgeable public constituency.

Establishing a base of power and influence is a step beyond gaining general public awareness. The people in a position to translate the public mandate into political and financial support for community health nursing are likely to be located in elected governmental offices, the philanthropic voluntary sector, and the health-oriented business community. To maintain leadership in these fields, these individuals need to find responsible and effective means to promote their own political, ethical, and/or financial survival. For them, a public mandate together with objective evidence provided by the profession of quality and cost efficiency of service presents a compelling combination. Their support of this kind of service in effect maintains the public trust in the supporter, whether politician, benefactor, or business executive.

The common factor in the first two requisites of a vital practice is communication about practice in a form prepared for and adequately directed to the intended recipient. Highly technical reports are useless for a public presentation, and primarily subjective appeals would not gain the favor of those in positions of power and influence. While within the discipline, selected individuals (political liaisons, those selected for prestigious boards and institutes) may be given special responsibility for communication, all community health nurses must become articulate in each of the languages necessary for professional survival: the public language, the political/factual language, as well as the intra-professional language for the advancement of practice theory. Nurses' ability to present broad-based communication not only multiplies the effect but also establishes every clinician's stake in public support.

The third requisite of professional vitality is the maintenance of a sound economic base. In a world of dollar currency and progressive inflation, the survival of work aimed at the public good depends on the strength of the financial base from which its suppliers are reimbursed. Attainment of this base is achieved through persuading those in power positions to influence the direction and amount of resources allocated to health care. Providing information to decision makers on the value of practice is not, however, enough to procure adequate salary levels.

The prices of services are established in two ways: by the cost of a salary to an employer in the factor market, and by the cost of a unit of service in the product market. In either case, the value attached to service should be negotiated by nurses themselves in response to public demand — and not by other professionals, who may pay the nurses at a lower rate than demand implies or who may not fully understand nursing practice.

Accountability within the profession demands adherence to ethical standards and the acceptance of responsibility for basing practice upon the accumulation of supportive research findings. By setting standards and conducting its own research, a practice discipline lays the groundwork for maintaining internal surveillance and winning public trust. In both areas, community health nursing long ago established its credibility.

The public demands personal services at reasonable cost, combined with a commitment to adequate health services for the poor and isolated. Community health nursing has the capability of providing and continually improving upon the personal services offered to the majority of the population, whether in schools, workplaces, homes, or clinics. In addition, community health nursing can continue to survey the ever-changing health needs of a community and adjust programs to accommodate these needs. Because of the generalist approach within community health nursing, the target of service may be any age, sex, or race; services may be defined for individuals, families, or groups; and the nurse may provide services alone, with other nurses, or in interdisciplinary groups. From such a flexible base of practice, community health nursing is in a position to respond to both public need as well as demands of private citizens. Further, with creative management, synthesis between these two can occur, resulting in programs with a high level of client involvement, outreach components to locate those in greatest need who may not seek out the program, and a measurable upgrading of health status within the community.

Health care in the United States has become a complex of poorly coordinated multiple systems — not pre-planned by level of care or by type of provider. By exerting leadership in the areas of need that community health nursing was designed to address, redirection of the care of clients can be accomplished. The greatest support for this change will come from the clients themselves, although public policy and economics will play a decisive role. The charge for the future is clear. The challenge is to fulfill the promise of leadership by community health nursing within its second century.

INDEX

Note: Illustrations, tables, graphs and figures are denoted by the page number followed by f.

Greek mythology, community health nursing
    roles, 3–5

Hall, Lydia, 139f
Health *See also* Interaction Model of Client
        Health Behavior
    definition, 59, 61, 62, 133
    human responses to, 133–134
    theoretic formulations, 135–144f
Health care industry
    costs and expenditures, 319–321, 351
    economic characteristics
        external effects, 328–330
        uncertainty of demand, 331–332
Health care policies *See also* Change, process
        of
    nurses role, 273–274, 292
    power, coercive vs. noncoercive measures,
        287–288
Health diaries, 233
Health outcome
    client singularity and, 159–160
    determined by interaction model, 148f, 157
    identification by nurse, 158–159
Health planning agencies, local, 130–131
Health promotion, 56
Health risks *See* Risk factors, health
Health screening research
    infants and young children, 179–181
    school age children and youth, 181–184
Helicy, 49
Henderson, Virginia
    nature of nursing, 52–53
    views of individual, nursing,
            society/environment and health,
            140f
Henry Street Settlement
    establishment, 8–9
    staff roles, 11–12
Hierarchial and simultaneous regressions,
        230–232f
Highriter, Marion, 176–177, 246–247f
Hilbert, Hortense, 175–176
History of community health nursing
    earliest documentation, 3–6
    1800–1900, 6–9
    1900–1910, 9–16
    1910–1920, 16–24
    1920–1930, 25–30
    1930–1940, 30–34
    1940–1970, 34–38
    1970–present, 38–41
Holistic concept, 135, 145, 157
Home Health care *See also* Individual client,
        care of

factors leading to proliferation, 130–131
    nursing research, 192–195
Hospital
    care, compared with home care, 193
    costs, 130
    establishment of community health nursing
            training programs, 7
Human response to health, 133–134
Hygeia, 3, 4
Hypothesis *See also* Research, public health
    definition, 47, 210
    revisited, following completion of project,
            223

Illness, client perception of, 150
IMCHB *See* Interaction Model of Client
        Behavior
Incidence
    defined, 77–78
    differences, use in establishing risk, 83
Individual client *See also* Interaction Model of
        Client Health Behavior
    early theorists' view of, 136–144f
    perception of health, 164
    power to evoke health care changes, 289–
            290
    relationship with nurse, 61–63f, 161
    care of
        client health care responsibilities, 131
        decisional control, 146
        expansion toward, 129, 130
        nature of community health nursing
                role, 132–133, 169–170
Industrial nursing, 15
Industrial Revolution, 9
Infants *See* Children; Maternal-childhood
        nursing
Influence, defined, 275
Information, health, approach to delivery,
        154–155
Inherited/biological risk factors, 84
Instruction, health care, 180
Insurance *See also* Medicaid; Medicare
    impact on demand for health services, 332
    third-party reimbursement, 311
Interaction Model of Client Health Behavior
        (IMCHB)
    application to community health nursing
            research, 165–169
    goals and objectives, 158–159
    major elements, 146–148f
        affective response, 151–152
        affective support, 152–154
        background variables, 148–149
        client singularity, 147–148

Date Due